Non-random Reflections on Health Services Research:

On the 25th anniversary of Archie Cochrane's
Effectiveness and Efficiency

Non-random Reflections on Health Services Research:

On the 25th anniversary of Archie Cochrane's *Effectiveness and Efficiency*

Edited by

Alan Maynard

formerly Director of the Centre for Health Economics
University of York
and Secretary of the Nuffield Provincial Hospitals Trust

and

Iain Chalmers

Director, UK Cochrane Centre
NHS R&D Programme
Oxford, UK

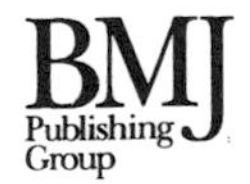

First published in 1997
by the BMJ Publishing Group, BMA House, Tavistock Square, London WC1H 9JR

British Library Cataloguing in Publication Data

A catalogue record for this book is available from the British Library

ISBN 0-7279-1151-1

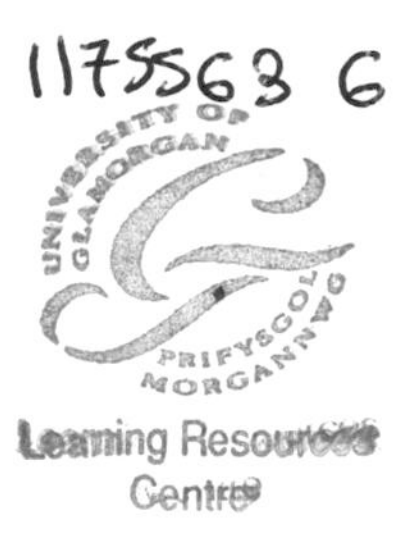

Typeset, printed and bound in Great Britain by
Latimer Trend & Company Ltd, Plymouth

Contents

Contributors vii

Foreword xiii

Acknowledgements xv

Introductory reminiscences 1

Archie Cochrane's legacy: an American perspective 3
KERR L WHITE

A reminiscence of Archie Cochrane 7
RICHARD DOLL

Archie Cochrane: an appreciation 11
DICK COHEN

Archie and the Nuffield Provincial Hospitals Trust 14
GORDON MCLACHLAN

"What have Communism and Catholicism against randomised controlled trials?" 18
ANDRÉ ROUGEMONT, ETIENNE GUBÉRAN

Some reactions to *Effectiveness and Efficiency* 21
HUGH F THOMAS

Part 1: Epidemiology 29

1 Response rates in south Wales 1950–96: changing requirements for mass participation in human research 31
JULIAN TUDOR HART, assisted by George Davey Smith

2 Cochrane and the benefits of wine 58
RICHARD DOLL

3 The epidemiology of asthma 75
MICHAEL BURR

Part 2: Effectiveness 91

4 So what's so special about randomisation? 93
JOS KLEIJNEN, PETER GØTZSCHE, REGINA A KUNZ, ANDY D OXMAN, IAIN CHALMERS

5 Cochrane and the benefits of aspirin 107
PETER ELWOOD

6 Social work: beyond control? 122
GERALDINE MACDONALD

Part 3: Efficiency 147

7 Health economics: has it fulfilled its potential? 149
ALAN MAYNARD, TREVOR A SHELDON

Part 4: Equity 167

8 Beyond effectiveness and efficiency . . . lies equality! 169
ALAN WILLIAMS

9 Equitable distribution of the risks and benefits associated with medical innovations 184
WILLIAM SILVERMAN

Part 5: Evolution 195

10 Large-scale randomised evidence: trials and overviews 197
RORY COLLINS, RICHARD PETO, RICHARD GRAY, SARAH PARISH

11 The Cochrane Collaboration 231
IAIN CHALMERS, DAVID SACKETT, CHRIS SILAGY

12 Improving the reporting of randomised controlled trials 250
DAVID MOHER, JESSE BERLIN

13 Exploring lay perspectives on questions of effectiveness 272
SANDY OLIVER

Cochrane's obituary 292

Index 295

Contributors

Jesse Berlin
Associate Professor of Biostatistics
Center for Clinical Epidemiology and Biostatistics
University of Pennsylvania School of Medicine
Philadelphia
USA

Michael Burr
Senior Lecturer
Centre for Applied Public Health Medicine
University of Wales College of Medicine
Cardiff
UK

Iain Chalmers
Director
UK Cochrane Centre
NHS Research and Development Programme
Oxford
UK

RHL Cohen
Formerly Deputy Chief Medical Officer and Chief Scientist
Department of Health and Social Security
London
UK

Rory Collins
Professor of Medicine and Epidemiology
Clinical Trial Service Unit and Epidemiological Studies Unit
Nuffield Department of Clinical Medicine
University of Oxford
Oxford
UK

Richard Doll
Emeritus Professor of Medicine
Clinical Trial Service Unit and Epidemiological Studies Unit
Nuffield Department of Clinical Medicine
University of Oxford
Oxford
UK

Peter Elwood
Honorary Professor
Centre for Applied Public Health Medicine
University of Wales College of Medicine
Penarth
UK

Peter Gøtzsche
Director
Nordic Cochrane Centre
Rigshospitalet
Copenhagen
Denmark

Richard Gray
Professor of Medical Statistics and Director
Clinical Trials Unit
University of Birmingham
Birmingham
UK

Julian Tudor Hart
Formerly General Practitioner
Glyncorrwg
South Wales
UK

Etienne Gubéran
Formerly Médicin du Travail
Geneva
Switzerland

Jos Kleijnen
Director
Dutch Cochrane Centre
Department of Clinical Epidemiology and Biostatistics
University of Amsterdam
Amsterdam
The Netherlands

Regina Kunz
Assistenzaerztin
Department of Endocrinology and Nephrology
University of Berlin
Berlin
Germany

Sarah Parish
Senior Research Fellow
Clinical Trial Service Unit and Epidemiological Studies Unit
Nuffield Department of Clinical Medicine
University of Oxford
Oxford
UK

Richard Peto
Professor of Medical Statistics and Epidemiology
Clinical Trial Service Unit and Epidemiological Studies Unit
Nuffield Department of Clinical Medicine
University of Oxford
Oxford
UK

André Rougemont
Professor and Director
Department of Community Health and Medicine
Geneva University Medical School
Geneva
Switzerland

David Sackett
Former Chair, Cochrane Collaboration Steering Group
General Physician and Director
NHS R&D Centre for Evidence Based Medicine
Nuffield Department of Clinical Medicine
University of Oxford
Oxford
UK

Trevor A Sheldon
Director
NHS Centre for Reviews and Dissemination
University of York
York
UK

Chris Silagy
Chair, Cochrane Collaboration Steering Group
Director, Australasian Cochrane Centre
Professor and Head
Department of General Practice
The Flinders University of South Australia
Adelaide
Australia

Geraldine Macdonald
Archie Cochrane Research Fellow, Green College, Oxford
Professor of Social Work and Applied Social Studies
Centre for Professional Studies
University of Bristol
Bristol
UK

Alan Maynard
Professor of Economics and formerly Director
Centre for Health Economics
University of York
York
UK

Gordon McLachlan
Formerly Secretary
Nuffield Provincial Hospitals Trust
London
UK

David Moher
Assistant Professor
Department of Medicine, Epidemiology and Community Health
University of Ottawa
Ottawa
Canada

Sandy Oliver
Honorary Visiting Fellow, UK Cochrane Centre
Research Officer
Social Science Research Unit
University of London Institute of Education
London
UK

Andy Oxman
Co-editor, Cochrane Collaboration *Handbook*
Director
Health Services Research Unit
National Institute of Public Health
Oslo
Norway

William Silverman
Archie Cochrane Fellow, UK Cochrane Centre, 1994
Formerly Professor of Pediatrics
Columbia University
New York
USA

George Davey Smith
Professor of Clinical Epidemiology
Department of Social Medicine
University of Bristol
Bristol
UK

Hugh F Thomas
Honorary Archivist, Cochrane Archive
Epidemiologist
MRC Epidemiology Unit (South Wales)
Penarth
UK

Kerr L White
Formerly Deputy Director for Health Sciences
Rockefeller Foundation
New York
USA

Alan Williams
Professor of Economics
Centre for Health Economics
University of York
York
UK

Foreword

On 20 March 1972, Archie Cochrane, Director of the British Medical Research Council's Epidemiology Unit, gave a lecture in Edinburgh entitled "Effectiveness and efficiency: random reflections on health services". The lecture was based on a monograph which had been commissioned by the Nuffield Provincial Hospitals Trust, which had awarded Cochrane its 1971 Rock Carling Fellowship. The radical critique of health and social services presented in Cochrane's monograph had a substantial and lasting impact both within and outside the United Kingdom. He highlighted the absence of an adequate knowledge base for much of the care provided, and made a strong case for the evaluation of new and existing forms of care in controlled trials.

The present book is being published to celebrate the 25th anniversary of the publication of Cochrane's Rock Carling monograph. It opens with some personal reminiscences of the man by his medical contemporaries—Richard Doll, Kerr White, and Dick Cohen. Gordon McLachlan goes on to note that Cochrane's initial presentation of the lecture in Edinburgh was far from perfect; but Hugh Thomas, André Rougemont, and Etienne Gubéran reflect on the important impact of the published version of the lecture in English and other languages. After these brief remembrances, contributions to the book have been grouped to reflect five themes relevant to Cochrane's interests—epidemiology, effectiveness, efficiency, equity, and evolution.

This commemoration of Cochrane and his work charts some achievements during the past 25 years. As Cochrane would have expected, however, all of the contributions to the book also present challenges for the present and for the future. Much health and social care has yet to be evaluated; and much practice has yet to be changed to reflect the existing knowledge base. Cochrane might have found most challenging the opening and closing chapters in the book. In these, Julian Tudor Hart and Sandy Oliver, respectively, suggest that researchers and health professionals will serve public interests more effectively when they come to regard lay people as "coproducers" of the knowledge needed for effective and efficient promotion of their own and the public health.

This theme represents as radical a challenge today as Cochrane's monograph has done for the past 25 years. Some rather perverse incentives drive the choice of questions addressed in many of today's controlled trials, and the priorities of researchers cannot be assumed to be the same as the priorities of those using the health services. To what extent are researchers addressing genuinely important uncertainties about the effects of health and social care in terms that are meaningful to those who use these services? On the 50th anniversary of *Effectiveness and Efficiency* it should be possible to assess the extent to which these new challenges have been taken seriously by researchers and health professionals.

Alan Maynard
University of York

Iain Chalmers
UK Cochrane Centre

Acknowledgements

The authors gratefully acknowledge the support and funding from the Nuffield Provincial Hospitals Trust during the writing and publication of this book.

The editors wish to express their gratitude to Basil Haynes and Alex Stibbe for helping to prepare the book for publication.

Introductory Reminiscences

Archie Cochrane's legacy: an American perspective

KERR L WHITE

Archie Cochrane was both an icon and an iconoclast. In the United States his recognition as an epidemiological icon only recently has reached the stature his seminal contributions to the improvement of health services deserve. This has been achieved largely through the expanding impact of the Cochrane Collaboration.[1–3] But the long delay in recognising the central importance of Archie's message may well reflect the unfortunate tendency among too many American medical academicians to think that all good ideas arise from within its boundaries and, often, shortly after they take office. History, especially medical history, is not one of our profession's strong points. Archie himself has testified that by nature he was iconoclastic. Usually he seemed to revel in the notion as he made his thrusts with gentle scepticism, a touch of humour, and by asking penetrating questions with a twist of feigned innocence that in the United States is often referred to as a "country boy" manner.

My first encounter with Archie was in 1960 during a visit to the Pneumoconiosis Research Unit at Cardiff when his Medical Research Council (MRC) Epidemiology Unit was emerging as a separate entity. The visit was urged by Professor Jerry (JN) Morris, then Head of the MRC Social Medicine Research Unit at the London Hospital, with whom I was spending a sabbatical year. As Archie acknowledges in his autobiography Morris had recommended him to Charles Fletcher, the first director of the Pneumoconiosis Unit.[4] My notes of the visit recorded four principles that Archie vigorously expounded and that later I was able to pass on to students and colleagues in teaching and research: (1) the necessity of calibrating, refining, pretesting, and standardising survey instruments as carefully as one did other measurement instruments; (2) the necessity for identifying and measuring observer error and other forms of bias whether, for example, in surveys of occupational, nutritional, and social histories, the reading of ECGs and chest radiographs, or the recording of blood pressure; (3) the value of the private census of a population defined by geography or other geopolitical jurisdiction as the universe from which to draw series of small but adequate samples with extremely high response rates (95% or better); and (4) the feasibility of randomising defined populations and institutions, as well as individuals.

There was one point, however, on which we differed. When Archie inquired about my activities I expressed an interest in employing epidemiological concepts and methods to the evaluation of what we then called "medical care". I distinctly remember my disappointment when he dismissed the notion that medical care research could or should use epidemiological principles. He saw the application of the latter to the study of environmental and social factors in the genesis of a wide variety of diseases but was quite disdainful of the notion that health services themselves could be investigated directly. Clearly his interests broadened and his priorities changed in the 1960s. For this he credits generously the influence of several colleagues including Julian Tudor Hart, Ian Higgins, Jerry Morris, Bill Miall, Estlin Waters, and Jean Weddel.

My next encounter with Archie was at an early meeting of the International Epidemiological Association (IEA) on the island of Korčula close to Dubrovnik in 1961. From then on we met at IEA meetings every three years or so and I followed his work in the literature. In 1973 Gordon McLachlan, at that time secretary of the Nuffield Provincial Hospitals Trust (NPHT) whom I also first met in 1960, sent me a copy of *Effectiveness and efficiency.*[5] As were many others, I was delighted with both the style and substance of his arguments and examples. Archie's slim volume seemed the ideal vehicle for helping our academic colleagues in the United States to appreciate the central importance of fundamental questions that Sir William Petty asked in the 17th century and Florence Nightingale asked in the 19th! At the time we were not making too much headway in the United States, or at Johns Hopkins either for that matter, where in 1964 I founded a Department of Health Care Organisation (now called Department of Health Policy and Management). The problems we encountered with many fellow clinicians were similar to those experienced by Archie, only more so.

Having been elected in 1974 to the Council of the United States National Academy of Sciences' newly established Institute of Medicine (IOM), I was in a strategic position to start introducing representatives of the American academic medical establishment to the prospects of evaluating health services. As chairman of the nominating committee that year I successfully sponsored Gordon McLachlan for IOM membership in the hope of expanding the Institute's vision and awareness of the initiatives the NPHT was taking in sponsoring health services research. I learned from Gordon that Archie shortly would visit the United States. Accordingly we invited him to Johns Hopkins in May of that year. He gave a delightful talk reminiscing about his war experiences, the evolution of his research ideas, and of his Epidemiology Unit. Among his numerous pithy examples were his recounting of the ludicrous vitamin B12 story (the amount of B12 prescribed in Britain's National Health Service was 8.6 times the amount that reasonably might have been expected). Archie's remarks were presented in his usual low key, quizzical manner laced with considerable scepticism but little cynicism. Unfortunately, all too few of Hopkins' leading clinicians attended his talk or the following luncheon where the group was regaled with further gems from Archie's rich experience in challenging what he referred to as the "God complex" besetting all too many medical academicians.

During IOM Council meetings I argued that health services research could save money by dissuading physicians and others from employing useless interventions. The resultant savings would provide more money for research into the fundamental causes of disease. Some of my colleagues listened and a few thought well of such ideas. To better acquaint both them and the wider academic medical community with these ideas Archie Cochrane's book seemed the ideal vehicle. I persuaded the IOM Council to purchase (or perhaps Gordon McLachlan donated) at least 100 (perhaps 200) copies of *Effectiveness and efficiency* to distribute free at the IOM annual meeting in 1974; all were taken quickly. I am sure that other copies of Archie's classic trickled across the Atlantic but I like to think that this distribution helped to disseminate his message more rapidly than otherwise might have been the case.

In 1976 Archie and I were guests at several institutions in New Zealand and on one occasion we both addressed a meeting at Wellington Hospital. Not wishing to startle unduly the staid group of white coated clinicians I tempered my message slightly by stating, instead of 10–15%, that only between 15–20% of physicians' interventions were supported by objective evidence that they did more good than harm. In mid-sentence Archie suddenly called out: "Kerr, you're a damned liar, you know perfectly well that it isn't more than 10%!" We were probably both correct and may well have used the same study for our observations (funded, I believe, by Gordon McLachlan and the NPHT). My figures came from a two week survey in 1963 by 19 general practitioners "representing almost every partnership and practice in a northern (British) industrial town". All recorded the "intent" of each prescription written. Those for proprietary drugs with "specific" benefit were 9.3%. Another 22.8% were considered to be of "probable" benefit, 27.2% of "possible" benefit, 28.2% were "hopeful", and 8.9% were regarded as a placebo; 3.6% were "not stated". Distributions for non-proprietary drugs were similar.[6]

At subsequent IEA meetings Archie and I met from time to time but perhaps the best testimony I can offer to his extraordinary influence was our initiative at the Rockefeller Foundation to spread his gospel more widely. Archie had been the recipient of a Rockefeller Foundation fellowship to the United States in 1947. Three decades later, based on many of the principles that Archie espoused, the Foundation established the International Clinical Epidemiology Network (INCLEN). Almost two decades since its inception INCLEN consists of five clinical epidemiology units in 27 medical schools in China, India, south east Asia, Latin America, and Africa. Each of the units is staffed by five or six young clinicians with a Master of Science degree in clinical epidemiology after training at one of our five "western" university training centres. They work with two health statisticians, a health economist, and a social scientist, all similarly trained.[7] These groups conduct randomised controlled trials and population based surveys, and increasingly influence educational, local, and national health priorities. Some of these units—for example, the Centro Cochrane do Brasil—have links with the Cochrane Collaboration and the future may bring more. Many of us believe that Archie would be pleased that his legacy lives on in the developing world as well as in the so-called developed world. All medical venues have a long way to go before Archie would be satisfied fully but global implementation of his ideas is well underway.

1 Warren KS, Mosteller F. *Doing more good than harm: the evaluation of health care interventions.* New York: Annals of the New York Academy of Sciences Publishers, 1993.
2 Bero L, Rennie D. The Cochrane Collaboration: preparing, maintaining, and disseminating systematic reviews of the effects of health care. *JAMA* 1995;275:1935–8.
3 Taube G. Looking for evidence in medicine. *Science* 1996;272:22–4.
4 Cochrane AL, Blythe M. *One man's medicine: an autobiography of Professor Archie Cochrane.* London: British Medical Journal Memoir Club, 1989.
5 Cochrane AL. *Effectiveness and efficiency: random reflections on health services.* London: The Nuffield Provincial Hospitals Trust, 1972.
6 Forsyth G. An enquiry into the drug bill. *Med Care,* 1963:1;10–16.
7 White KL. *Healing the schism: epidemiology, medicine, and the public's health.* New York: Springer-Verlag, 1991.

A reminiscence of Archie Cochrane

RICHARD DOLL

Archie and I were near contemporaries. Born nearly four years before me he qualified as a doctor two years later, partly because his preclinical studies involved the natural science tripos in Cambridge and a double first in this led him to work for a DPhil (a project he abandoned after one year because he thought it too trivial), partly because he spent two and a half years in Germany, Austria, and the Netherlands under the tutelage of Theodor Reik as Reik fled from the Nazis, and partly because he broke his clinical studies to serve for a year in a field ambulance unit in support of the international brigade in the Spanish civil war. We met on his return from Spain while Archie was still a clinical student at University College, as a result of our common interests in support of the Spanish government, opposition to Fascism, and enthusiasm for some sort of national health service. The friendship we struck up then was cemented by our wartime experience and reinforced by our postwar interest in the environmental causes of disease, methods of epidemiological research, and the practice of randomised controlled trials.

On the outbreak of war, our paths separated but they met again in January 1941 when we found ourselves members of a 50 strong body of medical reinforcements aboard a troopship bound for Egypt. We sailed in a convoy from Greenock and it took us six weeks to reach Port Said via the Cape of Good Hope with only one day ashore at Durban. Time hung heavily on board and after all our money had been lost to Australian troops, the men playing two up and the officers chemin de fer, there was little left to do, except to organise concert parties and play bridge. As far as I could make out, Archie and I were the only officers who spent any time trying to learn Arabic—Archie from a large tome that began with the Arabic script and me from the Berlitz paperback *Teach yourself Arabic in three months*.

On arrival in Egypt our paths separated again. I went to a small hospital in Cyprus and he went to a general hospital between Cairo and the Suez

Canal. He had not been there long, however, before he was asked to volunteer for a post with a commando regiment, which included 70 Spanish refugees from the civil war who had eventually, after many vicissitudes, enlisted in the British Army, and he always thought he was asked to join them because he was the only medical officer in the Middle East who spoke Spanish. The regiment was sent to Crete where he was captured by the invading Germans and he spent the last four years of the war as medical officer, and sometimes officer in charge, of large prisoner of war camps in Greece and Germany. I wrote to him periodically during his captivity, but had little contact with him after our return to the United Kingdom until he was appointed to the staff of the Medical Research Council's Pneumoconiosis Research Unit near Cardiff in 1948.

From then on we met regularly and whenever Joan (my wife) and I had reason to visit Cardiff we visited him and sometimes stayed with him at Rhoose Farm House and admired the garden he had created and his collection of Phormiums, which rivalled the national collection at Connington. On one occasion he told me how he had teased the cardiological members of a committee that had been set up under Lord Platt to advise on the ethics of conducting a controlled trial of the value of the then relatively new coronary care units. Archie and Gordon Mather, a cardiologist at Bristol, wanted to conduct a trial in which selected patients would be referred at random to a coronary care unit or for continued care by a general practitioner, but this was bitterly opposed by the cardiologists with whom he worked. The Platt Committee ruled that the trial was ethical but the Cardiff cardiologists still would not cooperate and the trial had to proceed in Bristol, Exeter, Plymouth, and Torquay alone. After it had been running for some months Archie had to report the interim results to the Platt Committee and I continue in the words of his autobiography:

> "The results at that stage showed a slight numerical advantage for those who had been treated at home. I rather wickedly compiled two reports: one reversing the number of deaths on the two sides of the trial. As we were going into the committee, in the anteroom, I showed some cardiologists the results. They were vociferous in their abuse: 'Archie,' they said, 'we always thought you were unethical. You must stop the trial at once.' I let them have their say for some time and then apologised and gave them the true results, challenging them to say, as vehemently, that coronary care units should be stopped immediately. There was dead silence and I felt rather sick because they were, after all, my medical colleagues."[1,2]

Some years before this incident, while still at the Pneumoconiosis Research Unit, Archie was found to have a small epithelioma on the back of his right hand, almost certainly the result of repeated exposure to ionising radiations when he was in charge of patients with tuberculosis in the prisoner of war camps in Germany and had had to carry out many radiological examinations under primitive conditions. The epithelioma was removed; but Sir Harold Himsworth, the secretary of the Medical Research Council, was worried and advised him to see a specialist in London. A small gland was discovered in Archie's right axilla and he was advised to have it removed by a distinguished surgeon. I visited Archie in hospital after the operation and found him utterly miserable. The surgeon had just told him that his axilla was full of cancerous tissue, that he had done his best to excise it but that he might not have been able to remove it all. It subsequently turned out that the pathologist could find no evidence of cancer in any of the excised tissue and the experience left Archie with a contempt for surgeons who were prepared to break bad news on the basis of a clinical impression, but probably also helped him to take so calmly the really bad news, some 30 years later, that the surgeon had not been able to remove all traces of a carcinoma of the colon.

Archie's final illness dragged on with recurrent acute episodes over four years, but in between his general health was good and a year before he died he attended the party that Joan and I gave in Green College to celebrate the 50th anniversary of our medical qualification. Shortly before this, he had consulted Richard Peto and me about the disposal of the large sum that he expected to be realised by the sale of the works of art that he had collected when he set up home in Rhoose Farm House. He had appreciated the quality of several artists' work at a time when they were relatively unknown and the paintings and statues had increased enormously in value. He wanted the money to be used for research into the epidemiology of AIDS, which, at the time, had been inadequately funded, and he wanted to avoid having it diminished by inheritance tax. This we advised him was quite simple to arrange. All he needed to do was to leave it to some academic institution recognised for charitable purposes, such as Green College, and send a separate note to the institution expressing the hope that the legacy would be used for the purpose he had in mind. We heard no more about the proposal until after Archie's death, when, to our surprise, he was found to have left a half share in the residue of his estate to Green College, without expressing any wish as to how it should be used.

I last saw Archie a week or two before he died, when I visited him in his nephew's house in Dorset, where he was being lovingly looked after. We talked, as might be expected, about controlled trials and particularly about the enormous contribution that Peto and Collins had made by demonstrating the practicability of conducting trials on a large enough scale to show conclusively the value of treatment for common conditions, even if they had only moderate effects. For such treatments were more likely to be introduced than treatments that had a dramatic effect and they would save more premature deaths than would be saved by a treatment that cured all cases of a relatively uncommon disease. Both of us, we found, had changed our minds on many things since our student days, but not on our humanist philosophy of life and death.

1 Cochrane AL, Blythe M. *One man's medicine: an autobiography of Professor Archie Cochrane.* London: British Medical Journal Memoir Club, 1989.
2 Mather HG, Morgan DC, Pearson NG, *et al.* Myocardial infarction: a comparison between home and hospital care for patients. *BMJ* 1976;i:925–9.

Archie Cochrane: an appreciation

DICK COHEN

Archie was a very dear friend of mine and of my wife's for more than 60 years. I think anyone who has read his autobiography and particularly the story of his life as a POW from Salonica to Wittenberg will have realised that his was a character of rare nobility.

When in the early 1960s George Godber asked Max Wilson and me to develop a programme of health services research we were well aware that our first task was to persuade a sceptical scientific community that such work was worthwhile and that support emanating from a government department would not seriously damage their health. So we set out to enlist the help of the MRC where I had been working for the previous 14 years and turned first to Archie who was an old friend of both of us and whose credentials for independence, honesty, and high standards were unlikely to be challenged. And he, after a good look round and out of the kindness of his heart and a burgeoning interest in the problems of the health service, took us under his wing and gave us unstinting support from then on.

This was the time of the first rather uncritical wave of enthusiasm for mass screening in all its forms and Archie, Max, and I were all serving on a Nuffield Provincial Hospitals Trust (NPHT) committee which Gordon McLachlan had set up with Tom McKeown as chairman to consider its potentialities and problems. This was a fortunate conjunction for it was Archie's work on glaucoma in south Wales, together with parallel work which we were supporting at the Institute of Ophthalmology in London, that enabled the Ministry to make a reasoned response when the clamour arose, orchestrated by the then medical correspondent of *The Times* and backed by letters from 100 MPs in one week, for the introduction of a nationwide glaucoma screening service.

From then on Archie became steadily more and more involved in NHS problems and the Epidemiology Unit of which he was director broadened to include virtually any aspect susceptible to randomised controlled trial, a technique of which Archie had become a passionate advocate. This diversion of his interests was not altogether welcome to his masters at the

MRC and one of his proposals received this answer: "Archie, I have no criticism of your protocol and I am sure it would be very useful but it's not quite the sort of thing the MRC does". Archie of course, as always, went his own way and all turned out well and in due course led to an award by the NPHT of a Rock Carling Fellowship and to the publication of *Effectiveness and efficiency*, which certainly to its author's surprise and perhaps also to Gordon's, became an almost instant best seller. These "random reflections" broke new ground, with a fresh and arresting message which articulated and brought to topical debate ideas that must have been simmering unrecognised beneath the surface of many minds in many countries.

Archie had greatly longed for some memorable achievement that would leave a name behind him and this commemorative volume would have made him proud and happy. But, in his lifetime, though he enjoyed the celebrity and the opportunities it opened, he remained on guard against being kidnapped by flattery into the ranks of the great and good, where he didn't really belong, and turned into a pillar of the Establishment. For the truth is he preferred the underdog; overdogs he associated with humbug and pomposity, two failings he particularly detested. Bias in all its manifestations he hated even more. In the ordinary affairs of life, but never in science, he could be as biased as anyone else, though he tried not to be, for he was by nature hot headed and readily indignant. As he got older he enjoyed parodying himself and I was once rung from his hospital bed in Edinburgh and asked if I thought it would be legitimate for him to complain that the hospital had been unable to provide him with *The Times*. "Why ever not?" "Well, you see when I was in the Middlesex I never asked them for *The Scotsman*". In science, however, bias was anathema to him. He never forgave it and where he scented it he could be formidable. Once when he was acting as statistical watchdog on our behalf on a committee supervising a clinical trial he went so far as to set a trap to test the intellectual honesty of its members about whom he felt suspicious.

Archie's experiences as a young man had led him to reject all hypotheses, however attractive, that could not be validated, so randomised controlled trials when they came on the scene were a godsend, so to speak. Naturally, Bradford Hill was his great hero (he thought Nye Bevan and Bradford Hill had done more for British medicine than anyone else in his lifetime) and nothing gave him greater pleasure as first president of the new Faculty of Community Medicine than to confer on Bradford Hill its first honorary fellowship. Sometimes Archie and I used to play a game in which we awarded a Bradford to the specialty that had been most honest during the year and a wooden spoon to the one which had been least. The results will remain confidential until 2001.

Archie's approach to people was unusually direct and immediate. He could not be bothered with preliminaries but went straight to the point he wanted to talk about. Thus, at the lunch party he gave at The Ritz to his own family and mine on the day he went to the Palace to receive his CBE, he said to my son (whom he hadn't seen since childhood) as they sat down together at table: "Does King's still regard kindness as the second of the two cardinal virtues [truth was the first], as they did in my day?" There was no mistaking that this was a serious question requiring a serious answer.

His own kindnesses were legendary. Whether you were a young Soviet pilot prisoner of war dumped on him without warning, moribund and screaming, or a scarcely known great aunt slowly starving herself to death, or a student with an unwanted pregnancy you could be sure of all the practical help within his power and of being treated with imaginative insight and a sensitive respect for human dignity.

But if I were asked to choose one scene that would best convey the unique flavour of Archie's personality, it would be none of these but rather the "curious sherry party" he gave for all his available relatives at which he gave a short lecture on porphyria and its implications for them all and followed it by distributing DIY kits and requesting samples of urine and faeces. It's so sensible and practical and at the same time so trusting and somehow comical. In the end he seems to have discovered the great grandfather who was the original source and to have traced and examined by DIY kit 152 out of his 153 widely scattered living descendants—152 out of 153—that was the standard that Archie had always set himself for all his work.

Archie and the Nuffield Provincial Hospitals Trust

GORDON McLACHLAN

Although I had heard of Archie from George Pickering, Chairman of the Trust's Medical Advisory Committee, who was vastly amused by and an admirer of his radical outlook, I first met Archie in the mid-1960s when we assembled a group of epidemiologists, not all medical, under the chairmanship of Tom McKeown to look at the question of the validation of a range of screening procedures currently in vogue. Apart from the improvement in health care, we found we had a common interest in rugby football.

His appointment to the 1971 Rock Carling Fellowship and the subject, were in effect complementary to and a development of the theses of effectiveness in services in the Report of the Screening Group, *Screening in medical care*.[1] Archie not infrequently and often to the merriment of many in the group, harped on about the need for randomised controlled trials in clinical issues, which was a new theme to me, astonished as I was as the study proceeded with the failure of a number of screening tests to pass the validation criteria. Indeed randomised controlled trials are mentioned specifically in one of the essays of which Archie was coauthor.[1] In the preface to the collection, Lord Cohen of Birkenhead rammed home the lessons of the study when he drew attention to the lack of "intelligence" machinery for "controlled clinical research".

John Brotherston was a sitting-in observer of the group (he could not be a full member because of his position as chief medical officer in Scotland) and in 1970 as a member of the Rock Carling Panel pressed successfully for Archie's nomination. I say "pressed" for it must be recalled that Archie was regarded as somewhat of a maverick in those days. John was one of the three friends mentioned specifically by Archie in the introductory chapter of the monograph[2] together with Dick Cohen and Max Wilson both of whom were members of the Screening Group.

In the interest of historical accuracy I felt bound to deny the impression given in the original notice about Archie's Rock Carling Fellowship that the undoubted influence of his monograph started with his lecture introducing it in Edinburgh. As was stated in all the monographs published, the Fellow is appointed with the specific commission not for a lecture but to write a monograph, to be "introduced by a public lecture to be given at a recognised medical teaching centre in the United Kingdom".

In fact, Archie's lecture in Edinburgh University was a near disaster for the presentation was awful and dismaying to the Nuffield contingent which included Norrie Robson, the principal of the University and the chairman of the Trust, Bill Williams, who used to class it as the worst Rock Carling lecture at which he had been present. I recall the Nuffield contingent maintaining stiff upper lips in the face of the Scots medical establishment's raised eyebrows. I see from my notes that I felt he had clearly not prepared a formal lecture ("*dirty scraps of paper*"). Part of the reason was that he was uneasy about the inclusion in the monograph of the first two chapters which his "young men" (unidentified, but presumably who worked with him in Cardiff), felt were "not scientific". He had produced the manuscript for the monograph very late the previous year, and had had second thoughts about the first two chapters by the time he originally raised this question with me at the International Epidemiological Association meeting in Primosten in Yugoslavia in August. I felt that he would be wrong to expunge these since they above all established him as a sensitive human being, not just someone thinking in purely scientific terms. Applying the "Nelson Touch" (euphemism for a fib) I told him it was too late since I had sent the manuscript to the printer before I had left London. I may say, Archie's own version of the case of the first two chapters[3] is a great joke in the McLachlan household since my wife, who was actually in Primosten with me at the crucial time, can hardly believe that anyone who knows us could possibly think that she took the fateful decision! As for the title I don't recall a problem. What we wanted for each of the publications in our burgeoning publication list, was a pithy title plus a subtitle to put it into perspective. After the Edinburgh debacle I insisted on getting an advance copy of the lecture from future Fellows on the excuse that I needed it for the press release.

The rest is history not I fear yet altogether based on the facts, but the success of both *Screening* and *Effectiveness and efficiency* owes a lot to the Americans who were the major buyers and who picked up the messages of both and pushed them hard for their own purposes. The director of the American Government's Health, Education and Welfare (HEW) Health Services Research Division, the steering group of which was chaired by Professor Kerr White of Johns Hopkins University, once told me the circulation of the low key *Screening in medical care* was used extensively in

HEW, the Office of Management and Budget, and the General Accounting Office—the main policy departments concerned with health care—and its financing was used to halt a lot of costly pie-in-the-sky nonsense from the hi-tech aristocrats aching to get into the health scene, who were very much in the ascendancy in the United States, after the moon landings.

With a foot in both American and British health services research camps (I was a consultant to the American Hospital Association's Hospital Research and Education Trust from 1964, and elected to membership of the Institute of Medicine from 1974) I had some knowledge of how these publications were hailed. I reckon that the prime mover in the recognition of the importance of *Screening* and *Effectiveness and efficiency* on both sides of the Atlantic was Kerr White whose stimulation of the theses of validation of effectiveness and efficiency of care in the United States had a reactive effect in the United Kingdom. British visitors to various institutions in the United States used to ask me on their return about *Effectiveness and efficiency*, even before Alan Williams in York took up the theme here on the economic side.

Archie used to drop in on me frequently to complain that I had disturbed his real research because he felt that he had to go to take the lead in seminars (he excelled in discussion groups of the seminar sort) in various universities in the United States. I took that with a fair number of pinches of salt for he loved expounding the gospel in the knockabout mode of the seminar; and had quite a following as a result.

In the meantime, however, with its translation into many languages, he was getting even more uneasy about the original monograph; and after we transferred the copyright to him, he banned further reprintings beyond the two paperbacks I had arranged before surrendering the copyright. The Americans were still asking for copies and once I tried unsuccessfully to discourage a request from one university to produce 500 photographed copies of one of the paperback reprints by demanding an exorbitant copyright fee on Archie's behalf, which to my surprise was paid to him. He did eventually agree to write an updated version for one of the prestigious university presses but never got round to completing it.

Archie's book was very important and the association of randomised controlled trials with his name provides an icon for "intelligence" gathering for health services policies although its real strength is in its reference to clinical applications: but I hope well-intentioned people will not go too far. I was at a forum not so long ago where there was great enthusiasm for the messages in the book if no great caution about what is involved, and I could feel Archie's Celtic uneasiness sweep all over me. It was clear to me that many of the most enthusiastic contributors to the debate, concerned with health services improvement to a man (and woman), had not read the book closely with all its reservations. I only hope that there will not be in time too great a spoiling reaction by somebody deconstructing the original in pursuit of fame, or a PhD!

1 Nuffield Provincial Hospitals Trust. *Screening in medical care: revising the evidence*: Oxford: Oxford University Press, 1968.
2 Cochrane AL. *Effectiveness and efficiency: random reflections on health services*. London: The Nuffield Provincial Hospitals Trust, 1972.
3 Cochrane AL, Blythe M. *One man's medicine: an autobiography of Professor Archie Cochrane*: London: British Medical Journal Memoir Club, 1989.

"What have Communism and Catholicism against randomised controlled trials?"

ANDRÉ ROUGEMONT, ETIENNE GUBÉRAN

> "Another very different reason for the relatively slow use of the randomised controlled trials in measuring effectiveness is illustrated by its geographical distribution. If some such index as the number of randomised controlled trials per 1000 doctors per year for all countries were worked out and a map of the world shaded according to the level of the index (black being the highest), one would see the United Kingdom in black, and scattered black patches in Scandinavia, the USA, and a few other countries; the rest would be nearly white. It appears in general it is Catholicism, Communism, and underdevelopment that appear to be against randomised controlled trials. In underdeveloped countries this can be understood, but what have Communism and Catholicism against randomised controlled trials? Is authoritarianism the common link, or is Communism a Catholic heresy?"

Archie Cochrane's observation in *Effectiveness and efficiency* that culture might be important in influencing the acceptability of his ideas brings to mind the critical reception doctors of the Faculty of Medicine of Paris gave to William Harvey's notions about the circulation of blood. It may be that experiment in the practice and art of medicine and the organisation of health services is a particularly British cultural characteristic. Whether or not that is so, cultural barriers seem sometimes to have prevented people understanding the importance of Archie Cochrane's ideas.

Some years after the publication of *Effectiveness and efficiency*, a friend of Archie's, Giulio Maccacaro, suggested that an Italian translation of the book should be included in Feltrinelli's new series *Medicina e Potere*, for which he was the series editor. Unfortunately, although an excellent professional translator produced what was—in linguistic terms—a flawless translation, it was rejected by Feltrinelli's publishing committee as quite unreadable!

It was against this unpromising background that, as French speaking doctors deeply committed to Archie Cochrane's ideas, we offered to try to bring his analyses and suggestions to life within our "Latin" culture. We believed that, rather than a simple translation of *Effectiveness and efficiency*, a culturally appropriate adaptation was required. We were encouraged in this undertaking both by Archie himself, who went over the whole manuscript with us during our two long visits to Rhoose Farm House, and by Gérard Horst, philosopher and chronicler for the French newspaper *Nouvel Observateur*, who assured us that the results of our efforts would be published by Editions Galilée.

This is not the place to describe in detail the problems that confronted us. Suffice it to say that, to find French equivalents for simple but new scientific and other concepts was a hard task. And when Archie suggested formulations in French which he intended should bring smiles to the lips of our readers, we often had to point out that, in our language, they were more likely to bring readers close to tears. We found ourselves in a situation not unlike that which prompted Archie to note that, in the prisoner of war camp in Salonica where he was the only doctor, "it was bad enough being a POW, but having me as your doctor was a bit too much!" For him, it must have been bad enough trying to ensure that his ideas were faithfully rendered in French, but having us as his translators must also have been, at times, "a bit too much!"

Happily, events and good nature—in short, everything that came to the assistance of Dr Cochrane in the camp in Salonica—helped us in our rather rash undertaking. Once our efforts had been approved by Archie and Gérard Horst, publication of *L'inflation médicale*,[1] with an introduction by Louis Massé retracing Archie's adventures in the Welsh coalfields and a preface by J P Dupuy and S Karsenty, proceeded relatively rapidly. The book received good reviews in *Le Monde* and *Le Nouvel Observateur.* Indeed, one piece of evidence that our efforts to bridge the cultural divide had been relatively successful was that Feltrinelli simply had our French text translated into Italian and published on the spot as *L'inflazione medica*.[2] This too achieved only critical acclaim.

L'inflation médicale probably arrived on the francophone medical market about 20 years too early. The odds are that a straight translation of *Effectiveness and efficiency* into French or Italian today would be much more successful: there are now many books written by and for doctors which reflect Archie's ideas, such as that recently published by Domenighetti *et al.*[3] Indeed, the Centro Cochrane Italiano and the Centre Cochrane Français are testimony to his influence in Italy and France. We should not leave you with the impression, however, that Archie had no French forerunners in the promotion of controlled experiments to assess the effects of interventions. More than 100 years ago, in a chapter entitled *Certainties* in his *Philosophical dialogues*,[4] Ernest Renan wrote:

> "Even in the event that the mass of a population believed they had experienced the efficacy of prayer, it would prove nothing. The Carthaginians claimed to have experienced the same efficacy and were wrong since their gods (as everyone today will admit) were powerless.
>
> The statistics would be easy enough. In a time of drought, twenty or thirty parishes in the same region would have processions to bring on rain; twenty or thirty would have none. By keeping careful records and by working with a large number of cases, it would be easy to see whether the processions had any effect—whether the parishes which organised processions were more blessed than the others, and whether the quantity of rain with which they were blessed was proportional to their fervour.
>
> One could renew the experiment in a thousand ways. One could fill two rooms with children suffering from the same illness, taking precautions to avoid all fraud in the distribution. Religious people would be allowed to bestow supposedly miraculous medallions on the children in one group, and children in the other group would receive nothing; and it could be observed whether an appreciable difference had been produced. But this has never been done, and all sensible people will grant me, I trust, that if one were to attempt it, the result would be a foregone conclusion."

1 Cochrane AL. *L'inflation médicale*. Paris: Galilée éd, 1977. (French version by A Rougemont and E Gubéran of *Effectiveness and efficiency.*)
2 Cochrane AL. *L'inflazione medica*. Milano: Feltrinelli editore, 1978.
3 Domenighetti G, *et al. Consommation chirurgicale en Suisse et comparaison avec la France*, Lausanne; Réalités sociales éd, 1996.
4 Renan F (1823–92). *Dialogues philosophiques*. Paris: CNRS ed, 1992:92.

Some reactions to *Effectiveness and Efficiency*

HUGH F THOMAS

Archie Cochrane was genuinely surprised at the media interest in his monograph *Effectiveness and efficiency: random reflections on health services.*[1] The examples he used of ineffective, unproved, and occasionally harmful treatments, and wide variations in medical practice, were not new but their collection together in a single volume presented an articulate challenge to the modern medical establishment. His main message, which he considered the logical outcome of his observations on current medical practice, was the importance of the randomised controlled trial to evaluate all health measures the benefits of which were not clear.

The book appeared at a time when there was growing concern in many countries about rising health care expenditure and the increase in expensive medical technology. Health services research in Britain owes much to the ideas of wartime operational research and it is interesting that a 1962 Nuffield report[2] on the subject, which was held in the MRC Epidemiology Unit library, contains a short section headed "Effectiveness and efficiency". It may, consciously or unconsciously, have provided Cochrane with a title, although it was one which he claimed not to have liked.[3] The intended audiences for the book were medical students and non-medical intellectuals.[3] The following examples of references to the monograph show that it was read by a wide range of people in the United Kingdom and abroad. The local south Wales press was quick to appreciate the significance of the new book. A commentator in the *Western Mail* wrote on the day of publication[4] that Cochrane "continues his uncompromising role as maverick of the medical world with the publication of his provocative views on much clinical treatment". He continued "The randomised controlled trials procedure was developed 20 years ago to help the health service ensure treatment was effective. Dr Cochrane believes it has to be used far more than at present . . . In a sense, he considers that much of the problem of ineffective treatment has arisen from an unconscious conspiracy between the patient who longs to be cured and the doctor anxious to help." It was this latter theme that was taken up in some national headlines—"Dying to help" said the *Guardian*[5] and the *Sunday Times*[6] report and interview was headed "The wishful thinking that guides doctors".

While both articles mention randomised controlled trials, it was the apparent failure of medicine that struck the feature writers—"From his reflections it's little short of astonishing that any of us get to stop off at all between the service and the funeral fires".[5] *The Economist*[7], true to its name, headed its review "Too free" and concluded, after noting the main plea for greater use of the randomised controlled trial, "Dr Cochrane does not ask for more money for the health service. He establishes a strong case for saying that enough could be found to reduce the inequality between its curing branch and its caring one (geriatrics for instance) if effective therapy were deployed to the right people in the right place at the right time." Thus in addition to describing ineffectiveness and inefficiency within the health service, Cochrane was also seen to be drawing attention to inequality.

Although Cochrane was concerned that he may have been too hard on his medical colleagues, whom he greatly respected, the immediate and later responses to his book were generally positive. A "constructive attack" was how Colin Dollery, the *British Medical Journal* reviewer described the book.[8] He supported the call for randomised controlled trials but emphasised that doing good trials required a lot of sustained effort. The *Lancet* review was also favourable—"Some writers make health services research sound dull; not so Professor Cochrane. He presents a well ordered case clearly and entertainingly. He provokes, but does it so nicely that he will win friends not lose them."[9]

The editor of *The Practitioner*[10] suggested that Cochrane "has achieved a well earned reputation for being one of the hardest hitters of Aunt Sallys in the medical profession." Describing the 1972 Rock Carling monograph as a book which should not be ignored and is a joy to read, he suggested that the sooner it became compulsory reading in the medical corridors of power the better. The only predominantly critical review of the book considered that Cochrane was hostile to the social sciences.[11] This criticism was challenged by Cochrane[12] and Dixon,[13] and in his defence Cochrane pointed out that his unit had been among the first to recruit a sociologist into epidemiological research. This subject is discussed elsewhere in this book (see chapter 6). Archie Cochrane chose to give his Rock Carling lecture at Edinburgh as it was the closest suitable location to his birthplace in the Scottish lowlands. He was therefore quietly pleased to receive from his sister a cutting from the local Galashiels newspaper reporting the publication of his book and his inauguration as the first president of the Faculty of Community Medicine. The short report was titled "Gala Professor Makes His Mark in the Medical Field" and concluded, "As a Borderer, he's certainly done the area proud." Cochrane's monograph has often been cited in books and journals over the past 25 years. A variety of books, selected from the shelves of local medical libraries, illustrate how Cochrane's monograph has been interpreted.

In 1975 Ivan Illich published his famous work, *Medical nemesis—the expropriation of health*[14] and cited Cochrane's book to contradict "the dangerous delusion that contemporary medicine is highly effective". The following year Thomas McKeown's Rock Carling monograph *The role of medicine—dream, mirage or nemesis?*[15] supported Cochrane's emphasis on the need for critical appraisal of medical measures but further argued that external influences and personal behaviour were the predominant determinants of health.

Senior figures in the medical establishment discussed the criticisms of Cochrane, Illich, and McKeown. Sir Douglas Black, the chief scientist to the Department of Health and Social Security and president of the Royal College of Physicians, sought to challenge some of the views of sociologists and economists but acknowledged "that it would indeed be hard to find more engagingly written monographs on a medical theme than the Rock Carling lectures respectively of Cochrane and McKeown."[16] Three years later Black chaired a committee examining inequalities in health, whose findings (commonly known as the *Black Report*[17]), referred extensively to Cochrane and McKeown.

The 1977 Rock Carling monograph *Research in medicine—problems and prospects*[18] was written by Sir Andrew Watt Kay, a leading academic surgeon and chief scientist to the Scottish Home and Health Department. He gave examples of several (unreferenced) medical evaluation studies prior to 1972 and thereby suggested that Cochrane's priorities for research in the general applied area were recognised and had been fulfilled before Cochrane promoted them. But he wrote "The very considerable impact of Archie Cochrane's Rock Carling monograph reveals, however, that the medical profession and many medical scientists required his advocacy". Watt Kay nevertheless expressed reservations about the tedium, lack of stimulation, and cost of a long term evaluation programme and the ability of the medical profession to rigorously implement the results ("On the basis of past experience my serum hope level is at a dangerously low level").

The 1978 Rock Carling monograph—*The end of an age of optimism—medical science in retrospect and prospect*[19]—was written by Colin Dollery, professor of clinical pharmacology at the Royal Postgraduate Medical School, University of London. He considered a number of charges made against modern medicine. He summarised Cochrane's charge as "gullibility" and gave a "guilty" verdict with the sentence of "compulsory retraining in the design of experiments and interpretation of evidence. Forbidden to make therapeutic claims for five years".

In the early 1980s Cochrane's work was quoted by several major critics of modern medicine. A lawyer, Ian Kennedy, gave the 1980 Reith lectures entitled "*The unmasking of medicine*".[20] He described *Effectiveness and efficiency* as a seminal book and echoed Cochrane's concern that randomised controlled trials were much neglected. In *The diseases of civilisation*,[21] Brian Inglis, a journalist and author, gave only qualified support for randomised controlled trials but endorsed Cochrane's criticisms of medical screening.

Cochrane's ideas continue to reach a large group of social science and health science students as an abridged extract on randomised controlled trials from the monograph is included in *Health and disease: a reader*,[22] an Open University set book. The reader, which also includes extracts from Illich and McKeown, was first published in 1984, with seven reprints, and a second edition in 1995 was reprinted within the year.

Although books which quote *Effectiveness and efficiency* cannot be identified using conventional medical literature searches, it is possible to study journal articles that include the monograph in their references. Two Spanish workers examined English language citations in the Social Science and Science Citation Indexes between 1972 and 1988.[23] They found 596 articles, including 253 from western Europe, 234 from North America, 20 from Oceania, and 16 from Africa. The main types of journal in which they appeared were medical (275), public health (177), and health service administration (105). Although the examples of medical practice which Cochrane described were taken from the British health care system the issues that he identified struck a chord with many overseas. Eli Ginzberg, a leading American health policy researcher, observed:

> "Our British cousins remind us now and again that there is an alternative to the Teutonic tradition that long ago captured the American scholarly world. The majority of qualified scholars in the United States believe that of all the work written in the last decade, the one that may yet have the most influence on health policy is AL Cochrane's 80 odd pages on *Effectiveness and efficiency: random reflections on health services.*"[24]

A British review assessing the most influential medical books, by decade, also chose the monograph as the most important in the 1970s.[25] Translations of the book were made into Polish, French, Italian, and Spanish with translators usually being personal friends whom Cochrane had met either in this country or when lecturing abroad. Most found some difficulty in translating the finer distinctions of the text and also had to provide some explanation of the British health and social service system.

There can be little doubt that *Effectiveness and efficiency* has had influence in the corridors of power. In the United Kingdom, Elston[26], writing in 1991, suggested that the works of McKeown, Cochrane, and Illich "created a climate in which questioning of medicine's use of resources could become a more legitimate activity for politicians. We may now be seeing the effect of the percolation of these academic ideas to a receptive political audience". The effects of British National Health Service reforms over the past decade have been the subject of considerable debate. It is probably too early to make an objective assessment, which must await a postmillennial successor to Cochrane. However, the recent health service changes have addressed issues which Cochrane considered such as length of stay, place of treatment and the scientific basis of therapy, including evidence from randomised controlled trials. The Cochrane Collaboration, with its international framework, is supported as part of the NHS Research and Development Programme and is an enterprise of which he would have been proud.[27]

Professor Charles Fletcher in the 1972 Rock Carling Monograph *Communication in medicine* made an important point.

> "The consumer's view must be clearly expressed in relation to the important questions concerning the appropriate allocation of resources within the health services discussed by Cochrane in last year's Rock Carling monograph. . . . There is also a need to develop methods for evaluating the effectiveness and value of different kinds of medical care. In all such judgements the consumer's point of view, and not just the doctor's interest, must be paramount."[28]

Cochrane's 1972 *Sunday Times* interview also included predictions, such as the movement of the centre of gravity of medicine from the hospital to the community, associated with a rise in the importance of the GP in relation to the consultant, which have been partially fulfilled. I only knew Archie Cochrane for the last 15 years of his life when he was retired but still active in research both as an epidemiologist and research committee chairman. By nature he was kind, considerate, and approachable, especially to young researchers and students, and offered constructive advice when asked. He did not reject or apologise for his privileged background but freely acknowledged the benefits of having a private income. Lack of financial worries or daily family commitments may have contributed to his ability to devote so much time and emotional energy to research but these were combined with an intellect and application which few of us have but most of us recognise. It was his unique mixture of the radical and the establishment that was appealing. He was, I believe, aware that by criticising medicine from within its ranks he could potentially lose friends and make powerful enemies. But he was prepared to take the risk and it paid off. Almost all who have read *Effectiveness and efficiency* see within it a powerful logic. Archie Cochrane never claimed that the randomised controlled trial was the only way to do research but he considered it one of the best in a health service in which he identified ineffectiveness, inefficiency, inequality, and increasing cost. In 1978 the Office of Health Economics sponsored a symposium on *Medicines for the year 2000* at the Royal College of Physicians in London.[29] It was at that meeting that Cochrane called for a critical summary by specialty or subspecialty, updated periodically, of all relevant randomised controlled trials. At the same meeting Sir John Butterfield, regius professor of physic at Cambridge, spoke of "the recent assault on modern medicine's reputation by Illich, McKeown, and Cochrane, but," he continued, "the medical profession, like the great amoeba it is, absorbs important ideas and changes. It does not despair or die. I believe good professions must breed elements of self criticism, be outraged by the "pups" they spawn, react to them, albeit slowly, sit up, bandage the corporate ego, convalesce, rehabilitate, and move on again, though in a different way." It is difficult to consider the 62 year old Cochrane as a "pup" and yet he had a vitality and originality, which combined with wide experience in peace and war, produced a book that has influenced the direction of medicine and benefited the profession and those it serves.

1 Cochrane AL. *Effectiveness and efficiency: random reflections on health services*. London: Nuffield Provincial Hospitals Trust, 1972.
2 Davies JOF, Brotherston J, Bailey N, Forsyth G, Logan R. *Towards a measure of medical care—Operational research in the health service: a symposium*. London: Nuffield Provincial Hospitals Trust, 1962 (p xii—foreword by Gordon McLachlan).
3 Cochrane AL, Blythe M. *One man's medicine: an autobiography of Professor Archie Cochrane*. London: British Medical Journal Memoir Club, 1989:236–7.
4 Anonymous. Round the world. *The Western Mail* 1972, March 21.
5 Shearer A. Dying to help. *The Guardian* 1972, March 21.
6 Silcock B. The wishful thinking that guides doctors. *The Sunday Times* 1972, March 19.
7 Anonymous. Too free? *The Economist*, 1972, March 21: 28.
8 Dollery C. Constructive attack [book reviews]. *BMJ* 1972;**2**:56.
9 Anonymous. Effectiveness and efficiency [book reviews]. *Lancet* 1972;ii:668–9.
10 Thomson WAR. Welsh professor's antidote for health service failures. *Western Mail* 1972, April 6.
11 Anonymous. Review: Cochrane's glance at sociology. *Community Medicine* 1972;**128**:128.
12 Cochrane AL. Disappointed but open-minded on sociologists' contribution to solving the problems of the NHS. *Community Medicine* 1972;**128**:192.
13 Dixon PN. Critical scrutiny essential to NHS. *Community Medicine* 1972;**128**:192.
14 Illich I. *Medical nemesis—the expropriation of health*. London: Calder and Boyars, 1975.
15 McKeown T. *The role of medicine—dream, mirage or nemesis*? London: Nuffield Provincial Hospitals Trust, 1976.
16 Black D. *Cui Bono (The Harveian Oration)*. London: Royal College of Physicians, 1977.
17 Department of Health and Social Security. *Inequalities in health (chairman: Sir Douglas Black)*. London: DHSS, 1980.
18 Kay AW. *Research in medicine—problems and prospects*. London: Nuffield Provincial Hospitals Trust, 1977.
19 Dollery C. *The end of an age of optimism—medical science in retrospect and prospect*. London: Nuffield Provincial Hospitals Trust, 1978.
20 Kennedy I. *The unmasking of medicine*. London: Allen and Unwin, 1981.
21 Inglis B. *The diseases of civilisation*. London: Hodder and Stoughton, 1981.
22 Davey B, Gray A, Seale C, eds. *Health and disease: a reader*. Buckingham: Open University Press, 1995.
23 Alvarez-Dardet C, Ruiz MT. Thomas McKeown and Archibald Cochrane: a journey through the diffusion of their ideas. *BMJ* 1993;**306**:1252–4.
24 Ginzberg E. *The limits of health reform—the search for realism*. New York: Basic Books Inc, 1977:4.
25 Anonymous. Classic of the decade—1970s. *BMJ* 1990;**301**:762.

26 Elston MA. *The politics of professional power: medicine in a changing health service*. In: Gabe J, Calnan M, Bury M, eds. *The sociology of the health service*. London: Routledge, 1991: 58–87.
27 Editorial. Cochrane's legacy. *Lancet* 1992;**340**:1131–2.
28 Fletcher C. *Communication in medicine*. London: Nuffield Provincial Hospitals Trust, 1972.
29 Teeling-Smith G, Wells N, eds. *Medicines for the year 2000*. London: Office of Health Economics, 1979.

Part 1
Epidemiology

1: Response rates in south Wales 1950–96: changing requirements for mass participation in human research

JULIAN TUDOR HART,
assisted by GEORGE DAVEY SMITH

Introduction

In a very subordinate capacity, I worked with Archie Cochrane for about 12 months in 1960–1, at the Medical Research Council's Epidemiology Research Unit (which then operated alongside the Pneumoconiosis Research Unit at Llandough) and in the field in the Rhondda Fach.[1] We continued a disputatious friendship until Archie died in 1988. I knew and worked with most of those in the field and office teams who obtained and processed data, including Hugh Bates, Tom Benjamin, Gwilym Jonathan, Fred Moore, Diana Seys-Prosser, and Mary Thomas; some important other players in and around the Rhondda coalfield, including Dr Morley Davies (then Medical Officer of Health), Dr Frank Jarman (Archie's coauthor of the original Rhondda Fach tuberculosis survey), Dr Phillip D'Arcy Hart (who laid foundations for the Pneumoconiosis Research Unit in the late 1940s), Dai Dan Evans of the National Union of Mineworkers, who moved the NUM into action in support of the Rhondda Fach studies, and the Union's then Education Officer (now Professor) Ron Frankenberg, who was a link between the Union and the MRC.

Hugh Bates, Frank Jarman, and Dai Dan have all died, but in preparing this paper myself and my wife Mary Thomas (one of Cochrane's field team) interviewed all the others, as well as surviving ex-miners who were respondents in the studies, contacted through a letter in the *Rhondda Leader*, Trefor Stanley Jones of Maerdy, and Merlin Thomas of Porth.

In writing this chapter I decided to concentrate on just one aspect of Archie's work, the interface between his research unit and its study population as recalled by him and his coworkers and observed by me in 1960–61, and thereafter to track experience of applying essentially the same techniques to a similar neighbouring community over the following 30 years, which has endured much the same social changes as the Rhondda Fach. This work gave a good underview of field epidemiology, but not much of an overview of this form of research as a whole and internationally. George Davey Smith has supplied this important additional perspective.

Cochrane's rigour and response rates

In 1952, when Archie's first Rhondda Fach study hit the medical public,[2] the rigour of his approach set an entirely new standard for population research. As he said in that paper, prevalence rates for lung tuberculosis based on open access to mass radiography plus wartime poster and radio campaigns had rarely led to more than 30% of adults having their chests *x* rayed. In one leap, the Rhondda Fach study raised this to 92% for men and 86% for women among all the 19 218 adults living in that narrow, winding, blood and spit soaked valley. Response for miners was 98%, and for ex-miners 95%, and similar rates were achieved subsequently in the Cynon Valley and in a Rhondda Fach follow up study in 1953. The consequently much higher prevalence rates for recognised tuberculosis had a big impact on medical thought at the time, and were the main subject of editorial comment.

With the humility of a true scientist, Archie drew attention to even higher response rates, up to 99%, in earlier German and Scandinavian literature, but none of these had defined or cross checked their target population with anything like Archie's rigour. He set a new gold standard which others from then on had to emulate, when 60% response had been generally considered good enough for previous epidemiological or sociological work. Almost a decade later, the classic study of cardiovascular epidemiology in Framingham, Massachusetts, was retrospectively claimed in 1980 to have achieved a 69% response.[3] Reading the original papers it seems likely that the true initial response rate was less than this. The conclusions drawn from all subsequent Framingham follow up studies were limited by this initial weakness.

Archie was extremely self critical about quality of observations and measurements, with an initial presumption of substantial error, originating from his own prison camp experience of chest radiography. He systematically sought and measured his own errors in all his work. This was a very unusual attitude at that time, when perfection was the presumed state of all good doctoring. Comparing digit preference in the Rhondda Fach studies of arterial pressure[4] published three years before the Framingham study even began, with those subsequently found in the raw data of the Framingham study itself[5] differences are equally striking.

These large differences in methodological rigour arose not from differences in professional skills or devotion, but from important differences in the social base and historical context of these two studies, including the recent birth of the National Health Service in the United Kingdom and persistence of medical trade in the United States, and their consequences for medical and mass culture. These have important lessons for epidemiological research today and in the future.

Order effects

There were particular reasons why a very high response rate was important for the original Rhondda Fach study. Jethro Gough had suggested that progression of simple pneumoconiosis to progressive massive fibrosis (PMF) was caused by an interaction between retained coal dust and tuberculosis.[6] Archie's eventual aim was to test this by virtually eliminating sources of tuberculous infection in the Rhondda Fach, identifying sputum positive cases and removing them to hospital, and then comparing progression of simple pneumoconiosis to PMF in the Rhondda Fach, and in the neighbouring Cynon Valley, a control population in which no special measures had been taken to reduce tuberculosis infectivity.[7] To have any hope of finding a significant difference in progression of PMF, there had to be a large difference in tuberculosis infectivity between the test and control valleys. Despite a 60% reduction in infectious tuberculosis in the Rhondda Fach by 1953, there was also a rapid though smaller fall in the Cynon Valley because of the unanticipated advent of effective antibiotics. Nor was any significant difference found in the attack rate of PMF, because of an unexpectedly rapid fall in dust levels in both valleys after nationalisation, with renewed investment in modern equipment. Initially, however, Archie had exceptional reasons for seeking an exceptional response.

He certainly appreciated more general reasons why response rates were important for all studies. Non-respondents are always a selected group, their non-response depending more on choice than chance. These choices may lead to variable but often large effects from order of coming up in relation to detectable pathology. In the first Rhondda Fach study, the earliest respondents had an above average prevalence of tuberculosis; they included disproportionate numbers of sick people who wanted diagnosis and treatment. Then came the mass of respondents, with average avidity for chest *x* rays and below average prevalence of tuberculosis. Finally, among the most reluctant respondents and non-respondents, there was again excess prevalence, because this group included disproportionate numbers of sick people who denied their illness and did not want their fears confirmed. Archie dealt with this original and important theme in 1954,[8] but later it seemed to drift out of sight. It may be more obviously important to the increasing proportion of community generalist clinicians who accept responsibility for identifying still massive unmet needs in their registered populations,[9] and for incomplete delivery of care, which remains the normal state of all health services,[10] than it now seems to some epidemiologists. The effect has recently been dramatically illustrated by Tin, *et al* in a follow up study of the late effects of births at less than 32 weeks gestation, with a sevenfold greater prevalence of severe disability in the last 6% of respondents.[11]

Archie's team routinely visited people up to six times in their own homes before accepting refusal as final. Some of these most reluctant recruits were bizarre, or would seem so to people without experience of contacting 100% of virtually any population. Driving through the Rhondda Fach 10 years later, visiting participants in a study of tuberculin sensitivity in relation to

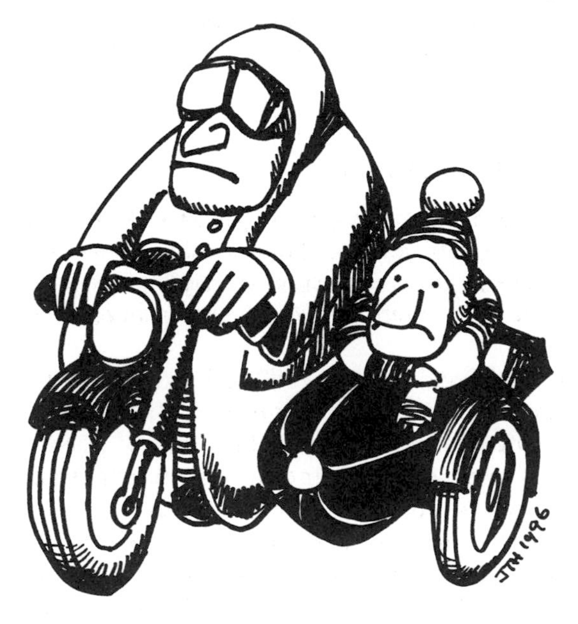

FIG 1.1

progressive massive fibrosis, I passed an extraordinary sight, a very large and determined lady driving an Ariel Square-4 motorcycle combination (figure 1.1). She wore a leather aviator's helmet and was wrapped to the ankles in a vast leather coat; in the sidecar, a contented face sat like a pumpkin, framed above by a woollen bobble cap and below by a scarf.

According to Fred Moore, this couple were discovered in the first Rhondda Fach survey. The woman agreed to have her own chest *x* rayed, but was unwilling for her husband even to get out of bed, let alone leave the house. She explained that in 1943 Dr Frank Jarman had found a spot on his lung during a mass *x* ray screening at work. He was told to go home and rest in bed until space in a hospital could be found. No letter ever arrived, so he stayed in bed for the rest of the war and another five years of peace. The MRC team eventually persuaded her to let him have another chest *x* ray, the spot had gone, and the only problem was his return to normal life, a task for which Archie rightly accepted responsibility. Ten years later the motorcycle combination, in which the quasi-invalid cautiously took the air, was still the best anyone could achieve.

Specific sequences of response obviously depend on local cultures and the subject studied, but if this entails stigma, or has a reputation as untreatable, the same U-shaped pattern of initial avidity and terminal denial is likely. For example, this was certainly true of breast cancer in the elderly, and can be anticipated for alcohol problems, AIDS, or incontinence. In such cases even very high response rates may conceal a small group of sick non-respondents, leading to substantial error in estimates of prevalence and community needs.[12]

We never used Alsatians

The Rhondda Fach study began in January 1950, with an intense bombardment of the target population, using every weapon available over the next eight months, so that when the mass miniature *x* ray units began to operate in September, rapid and economic flows could be guaranteed.

In the 1950s the Rhondda Valleys still had a vigorous social, intellectual, and political life, within a socialist *cum* syndicalist tradition which made fiercely independent local union lodges more powerful than local government, and both seem in some ways more important than national government.[13] Each of the eight small towns in the Rhondda Fach had its own large workmen's hall and library, as well as at least three or four social clubs. On a big night (and an opportunity to hear and question a research doctor *was* a big night) each of these would hold at least two or three hundred men (almost none of the clubs then admitted women). Archie must have given at least 30 short lectures of this kind, explaining the nature of the study and what people would be asked to do, and answering questions on a wide range of subjects from his audience. These lectures were organised, chaired, and backed up by local support committees in each town organised by the National Union of Mineworkers (NUM), with lodges in each of the four pits then operating. These committees also helped to distribute leaflets and posters. Rhondda women always supported their men in either promoting or resisting social changes affecting the common interest, so when the NUM endorsed the campaign, this was enough to ensure good response from most of them. The then numerous chapels of many rival sects trailed a long way behind this almost entirely male NUM culture, but in the 1950s probably provided the main direct access to women. Chapel preachers supported the campaign, and so did Methodist Women's Guilds. There was also good coverage by the local press and BBC radio (mass television came later, with the coronation in 1953).

This heavy artillery ensured successful invasion, but secure occupation of ground gained depended on hand to hand combat at the pithead, on the doorstep, and eventually in garden sheds, gents' urinals, gatherings for illegal street betting, or anywhere else recalcitrants might hide. Archie was every inch an officer and gentleman, but his experience as a prisoner of war had made him more streetwise than most patricians of his generation, and Rhondda people readily assimilated foreigners if they seemed to be on their side. Most of his field team was recruited locally, from men who shared the local culture, its occupational experience, and in some cases its pathology. Gwilym Jonathan and Tom Benjamin had both survived cavitated lung tuberculosis, and Hugh Bates was already breathless with advanced PMF.

The ends to which these field staff worked were well defined as percentage responses in the high 90s, and they were never allowed to forget them. The means used to attain these figures seem to have been left almost entirely to the discretion of fieldworkers themselves. However they were obtained, the quality of the data was beyond reproach. Because the original Rhondda Fach studies used the whole population rather than random samples, there was no way fieldworkers could make life easier by knocking at number 56 Prosser's Terrace if they had a refusal at number 55, thus systematically biasing data away from difficult people or people with difficulties. This eliminated a major source of error for researchers tempted to rely on market research agencies instead of developing, maintaining, and paying for their own field teams. As experience of the Heartbeat Wales questionnaire surveys showed, such agencies not only produce results of poor quality, but hopeless response rates around 60%.[14] These response rates have to compare with rates ranging from 82% to 100% (mean 93.4%) in Archie's unit in the Rhondda Fach and his successors in Caerphilly in 22 studies from 1960 to 1995.[15]

Cochrane's workers acquired a ferocious avidity for accurate data at almost any cost, either to themselves or their participating subjects. As Archie's principal Aide de Camp Fred Moore wrily remarked, "We never used Alsatians". Field staff were driven by intense pride in the quality of their work, which in turn depended on having been given excellent and practical initial training, frequent feedback on their achievement, full autonomy in how they performed their work within the limits set by study design, and a strong sense of personal participation in the advance of medical knowledge.

This proper sense of their own importance was reinforced by Archie's decision to include his most important but formally unqualified field workers and data managers as coauthors of his published work. Starting in 1956, of the 56 multiauthor papers he published over the next 30 years, 30 included one or more of his ancillary or technically unqualified field staff as coauthors. A fair rule of thumb for who should or should not qualify as coauthor of a research paper, is competence to give an interesting lecture on an important aspect of the work performed to a peer audience. Strictly applied, this might leave too many published papers without any authors at all, but it would not have excluded any of Archie's fieldworkers. All of them could have given an interesting and entertaining lecture on some important aspect of the work to which they had contributed, which would have left a peer audience better educated and informed. It is disappointing that so few researchers have chosen to follow Archie's lead in this respect, acknowledging what is often the hardest work only in small print at the end of their papers, and sometimes not at all.

This sense of personal responsibility, of scientific knowledge as a high calling, and of the sometimes apparently trivial data they were gathering as important steps toward that knowledge, all far outweighed the weaknesses Archie had as a team leader, which chiefly derived from his great personal wealth and generosity. This sometimes put him in a no win situation, occasionally impaired the stability of his team, and may have perpetuated the tendency of the entire MRC scientific staff in those days to retain a whiff of aristocratic dilettantism. However, in the general social atmosphere of the time, this was relatively unimportant. His field workers were Marine Commandos, expected and allowed to win any way they could, for whom nothing was impossible.

By common consent, Gwilym Jonathan and Hugh Bates were the most popular and effective of the early Rhondda Fach fieldworkers. They were naturally friendly, and Gwilym had large reserves of irresistible charm. Hugh had a huge local reputation as a champion boxer, was a strong Union man (and communist), and had a disarmingly direct manner. In pursuit of the last few reluctant respondents, he was the ultimate weapon. He would make his way into pithead baths, grope his way through the steam, find his nude target, and then, in a comradely but forceful way, give him a brief public lecture on his duties to his own health, the honour of his family and community, and to science and mankind.

Achieving and maintaining response rates in Glyncorrwg

At the end of 1961 I left Archie's unit to resume general practice and set up my own unit in Glyncorrwg, over the mountain from the Rhondda Fawr and socially similar to the Rhondda Fach, though more isolated. Mary Thomas worked in Archie's Rhondda Fach unit from 1961 to 1963 as a field assistant. We married in 1963 and she eventually led the Glyncorrwg research team. On a miniature scale, the Glyncorrwg unit provided both clinical care for about 2000 people, and made them available

Response rates in Glyncorrwg research studies

Year	Target group	Subject	Response (%)
1968	All aged 20–54	Distribution of arterial pressure[17]	98
1975	Random sample aged 3–70	Early morning urine organic acids[18]	98
1976	Random sample aged 40–70	Stools ×2 for bile acids and fat splitting bacteria[19]	80
1977–81	All newborn	Monitoring of arterial pressure age 0–11	98
1978	All over age 5	Questionnaire and interview on urine incontinence[20]	98
1981	Offspring of parents in top and bottom tertiles of distribution of arterial pressure	Seven consecutive 24 hour urine collections[21]	87
1986	All men aged 45–64	Coronary risk factors including venepuncture[22]	82
1987	1986 cohort as above	Randomisation to warfarin or placebo for at least five years	87

for recruitment to epidemiological research, with an enumerated population updated weekly, first on a card index, later on computer. Population screening (or case finding) began in 1968, and from 1970 to the present day this cumulative data set of a widening range of variables provided material for a steady stream of publications, including one estimating long-term health outputs from this style of anticipatory personal whole-population care.[16] The box shows the response rates achieved in our larger studies.

Glyncorrwg response rates of 80–98% were therefore comparable with those in the Rhondda Fach, and were maintained around this level for over 20 years, although unlike all but the first of the Rhondda Fach studies, most of ours had repeatedly to recruit entire age and sex groups of the population rather than random samples, because of the small numbers available. Our population was therefore more intensively used, with potentially greater difficulties for maintaining participation.

In Glyncorrwg we initially used essentially the same methods of recruitment as Archie had done in the Rhondda Fach: public meetings with collective explanation and discussion of the aims and methods of proposed studies, followed by individual explanation and recruitment. For longer studies, for example the trial of low dose warfarin for primary prevention of coronary thrombosis beginning in 1986 and due to finish in December 1997, we organised annual meetings of participants to report progress in the trial as it extended throughout the United Kingdom. We took full advantage of our influence over the population gained through providing care, limiting such pressure mainly by our own experience of the point at which pressure became counter-productive in a population we knew we would continue to need. This judgement was assisted by a patients' committee elected from a public meeting in 1974, which had from then on a consulting role before any research design was finalised.

Using these techniques we attained and maintained high response rates, with levels of compliance which are even in retrospect astonishing. Our sodium studies entailed collecting whole urine outputs over seven consecutive days, therefore including work and leisure time, in a population nearly all of whom were manual workers. We had men working 60 feet above the ground on scaffolding, we had men working 600 feet underground at the coalface, we had women working in a furniture factory where nobody could have any secrets, we had men and women living it up at the clubs over the weekend, and we had teenagers in school whose entire lives revolved around avoidance of social isolation and ridicule. All these had to use urine containers throughout the day, and to eat food tasting like cotton wool. Despite all this we had an 87% initial response rate and 63.6% dietary compliance (24 hour urine sodium <100 mmol and >40 mmol difference between periods on placebo and taking "slow sodium").

Our local consultant chemical pathologist had advised us that in his experience with individual patients motivated by concern for their own health, complete samples of urine were difficult to achieve even over 24 hours. This seems to be one of many examples confirming that collective shifts in behaviour to conform with newly perceived group norms may be easier than individual shifts to protect personal health.

The warfarin trial entailed firstly, identification in the top quintile of coronary risk, a potentially threatening experience; and then randomisation to rat poison or placebo, with nearly 12 years of venepunctures every three months and a then unknown risk of iatrogenic bleeding. Our early admission that warfarin was also used to kill rats was fortunate; the Blaengwynfi rodent officer became one of our participants—never imagine your patients won't know what you're up to. So great were the demands we made on our trial participants that when we, and Dr John Davies' practice in Midsomer Norton, undertook the pilot studies for this project (later extended to over 100 practices throughout the United Kingdom in the MRC General Practice Research Framework (GPRF)), the main question we had to answer was not how to do such a trial, but whether it was feasible. However, 82% of men in our target age group agreed to screening for categorisation of risk, and 87% of those identified in the top quintile of risk were still in the randomised treatment phase 18 months later. Recruitment throughout the GPRF began in 1987, and the trial will finish in December 1997, with about 40 000 person-years of experience. The overall national response rate for screening was 65.7%, and 52.1% of those in the top quintile of risk entered the treatment phase.[23]

Randomised controlled trials for the 21st century: rising demand, more exacting supply

Randomised controlled trials with positive results (and therefore published), fully meeting modern criteria, were born in 1948,[24] the same year as the National Health Service (NHS). Although such trials have grown almost exponentially in both size and number ever since, less than half of all treatments in widespread use have ever been evaluated with the rigour possible only by this means.[25] Trials for important treatments which may be linked, positively or negatively, with significant but infrequent harmful events, may require millions of participants observed over several years. The MRC GPRF now includes 6.49 million people, 10.7% of the United Kingdom population, and 900 practices, 8.1% of all practices.[26] Pilot studies are in progress for a major randomised controlled trial of hormone replacement therapy (HRT) planned to contribute 18 000 women to an international trial including 34 000 women, to measure effects of HRT on coronary heart disease, stroke, osteoporotic fractures, breast cancer, Alzheimer's disease, and autoimmune disease.[27]

The need for participants in randomised controlled trials has risen, but their recruitment is almost certainly more difficult, at least in the sense that researchers will have to do a lot more listening and explaining to carry public opinion with them. There are as yet no clear trends in response rates in major United Kingdom community based studies, although there is some evidence from the Paisley-Renfrew study that response rates are rising even in younger age groups. However this may be, high rates certainly cannot be taken for granted. They may depend on public attitudes associated with a National Health Service hitherto perceived as a practical expression of social solidarity rather than a business. If so, this perception is a threatened asset.

Pilot studies for the GPRF HRT trial showed a response rate of only about 50% for screening, and 33% for entry to the trial, with another 18% of these dropping out within three months, reaching 35% by three years.[28] Ominously for the future, higher social class and greater personal commitment to self care were associated with lower response rates.[29] All the early Rhondda Fach studies showed similar trends, with better educated people having lower response rates. According to folk wisdom, better education and rising social class are associated with less social solidarity, or in liberal terminology, less altruism; in a market economy, as things seem to get better, people seem to get worse.

Although this common belief probably has some truth, our guess is that this all too obvious historical process is far more complex than it appears. Experience in Glyncorrwg suggested that education itself had a positive association with response, but perceived social status seemed often to have a negative association, although even this was inconsistent. Far more certainly, better educated people are more critical, and today more than ever before, want full explanations and opportunity for considered choice before signing consent forms. Although the design of randomised controlled trials performed in the 1950s and 1960s might get past an ethics committee even today, the real quality of consent obtained from participants would have to be much higher to achieve anything like the responses won in the Rhondda Fach. Although the average quality of explanations by researchers of the risks and potential benefits of trials has probably always been better than explanations by surgeons and physicians of the risks and potential benefits of treatments, all have remained within the same cultural pattern, with progress coming at least as much from rising expectations of patients as from less condescending professionals.

Randomised controlled trials developed when NHS patients were generally uncritical supplicants, and doctors knew best. We are now well into an age in which patients are increasingly seen, and see themselves, as consumers. A purely consumer role for patients is in our opinion ultimately compatible only with medical trade, not with medical science, but even for professionals who understand this, growing consumerism is what we now have, and will for the immediate future have to be taken into account as a new factor affecting recruitment to randomised controlled trials.[30]

Such problems can to some extent be evaded by using workplace populations, in which response rates range from 100% to as low as 30%, depending at least in part on whether non-participation is perceived as a breach of work discipline. Such populations cannot be fully representative of the whole communities from which they are drawn, so conclusions from them may not be easily applied to common practice. We are unconvinced by claims that with randomisation and good follow up of respondents response rates are no longer important.[31]

The high response rates obtained in the Rhondda Fach, and later by others working in similar apparently uncritically cooperative populations, tend to be seen as impossible to achieve in supposedly more sophisticated community based populations today. If this is true, the much larger trials we need will either not be performed at all, will have to make do with much lower response rates, will use unusual populations unable to refuse participation, or we shall have to start paying participants. This last solution entails large additional costs, erodes other motives for participation, may distort results by introducing new sources for potential bias, and is a one way road from which it would be hard to return. We know from colleagues in the United States that for several years past, it has been impossible to contemplate any major epidemiological study that makes important demands on participants, without paying them to take part.

Agreeing to be researched upon is little different from agreeing to give one's blood, both depending on gift relationships[32] in a society perceived as mutually dependent, at least in the final analysis. In New Zealand, where privatisation of the blood donor service is now being considered, 345 consecutive donors were questioned with a 98% response. Over half were opposed to profits being made from blood, 71% were concerned about blood quality in a commercialised service, 41% would no longer give blood if profits were made from selling blood products, and 10% were reconsidering giving blood because market competition had been imposed on the New Zealand health service.[33] Although the question seems not to have been asked, it seems unlikely that their motivation would be improved by payment, or that people so obtained would be safer donors.

Simply to get good response rates, and regardless of any loftier motives, it seems wise to exempt participation in research from all commercial considerations of any kind, however illogical this may appear to health economists, and likewise the entire institutional package of population based research, to which commercial concepts like intellectual property can only be damaging. At a time when at least one MRC unit has found itself compelled to accept funding from the British American Tobacco Company,[34] the possibility of a slide toward the attitudes and techniques of market research has to be taken seriously.

Social factors influencing response rates: compensation for pneumoconiosis and access to care

Before dismissing the high response rates of the Rhondda Fach and similar studies as dependent on social factors now obsolete or destroyed, we should look more carefully at what these factors were.

Discussing his high response rates in the first Rhondda Fach studies, Archie wrote:

> "... the chief reason for our success in examining such a high proportion of the population was that we were working in an area profoundly affected by pneumoconiosis, whose worst effects the scheme was designed to mitigate. We had the enthusiastic support of the NUM ... and we persisted in visiting the lapsees in their homes until we were faced with a firm and immovable refusal to be *x*-rayed."[2]

After interviewing even a few surviving participants in those studies, we have no doubt about the thoroughly material basis for mass support. A small minority of grossly lung damaged men with proved and gross exposure to silica rock dust were eligible for compensation for silicosis from the early 1930s, but the reality of serious disability from retained coal dust, and particularly from PMF, was denied by employers and by the medical establishment[35] until the war suddenly made coal, and therefore miners, valuable again. After 15 years of unemployment at or over 50% of the male population of working age in the Rhondda valleys, in 1940 the wartime government sent a Medical Research Council team led by Philip D'Arcy Hart to discover the effects of large scale mechanisation in the 1930s, which had hugely increased dust levels. He found an epidemic of PMF.[36] Serious investment in dust control began with nationalisation of the industry in 1947, and coalworkers' pneumoconiosis became a compensable disease in 1948.

For the first time, pneumoconiosis panels were set up to provide machinery for identifying men with the disease. By 1950 these panels were beginning, rather uncertainly, to operate, but miners suspected that they might not be wholly independent from management even in the newly nationalised industry, headed as it was by Lord Hyndley, the biggest of the old south Wales coal owners. Many had recourse to Dr Harper, a private medical practitioner with an *x* ray machine, who would, for a fee, provide his own opinion, but his independence was equally if not more doubtful;

people who buy information tend to be given what they want. The NUM understood that the Rhondda Fach study, and subsequent follow up studies, would provide opportunities for state of the art and truly independent radiology, and perhaps for access to other high quality independent medical advice.

Altruism, solidarity, and moral benefits

This in no way conflicts with the equally strong commitment of the NUM, and the self educated men who led it, to the cause of medical science, the growth of human knowledge, and a better future for the human race. The conflict between altruism and self interest perceived from their life experience by liberal employers, was generally absent from the life experience of coal miners. For them, the need for solidarity was a fact of life, painfully learned through generations of experience; although some who tried to rise on the backs of others had always succeeded, most had always failed. Solidarity for occupational lung damage to be compensated was of the same nature as solidarity for it to be understood and prevented. Either way, solidarity was a material force with a material basis, and if participation in research seemed likely to result in gain, in either money or health or a combination of the two, this would benefit both people today, and their future descendants. For mining communities, solidarity and altruism were interchangeable terms without contradiction. Cui bono? A similar though perhaps less obvious basis for two entirely different views exists today, and deserves to be borne in mind for recruitment design.

Without paid participants, randomised controlled trials generally cannot be associated with cash benefits, and this was never a factor in any of our studies in Glyncorrwg, or most studies in the Rhondda Fach after the 1950s. There were other material benefits, more relevant than ever to motivation of participants today, when recruitment has become more urgent and difficult. The greatest of these was simply access to better medical care.

Participation in trials, whether as test cases or controls, almost invariably brings material benefits to participants, measurable as reduced mortality or morbidity or just feeling good. These benefits rise with compliance, whether in the test or control group.[37] Reasons for this consistent finding are complex. It is pleasant to believe that simply sharing in the pride and dignity of serious attempts to extend knowledge for the common benefit of mankind, a special kind of Hawthorne effect,[38] possibly related to the antidepressant effects of confiding relationships[39], may have some measurable effect on health. Far more certainly, trial participants meet health professionals with much more time to talk and listen, and a more rigorous and self critical attitude to diagnosis and treatment, than they are likely ever to have experienced before. From participation in trials they learn about the real, unmechanistic nature of human biology, the real limits to current knowledge, and the foundation of science on doubt; this also is both a personal and community gain.

These gains occur whether or not research staff have any overt clinical responsibility for trial participants. Patients in randomised controlled trials get advice and access to care outside official trial designs, because clinicians in trials are usually much better resourced, particularly in time, than those providing routine care in most working class communities, and because both patients and health professionals understand that a trade off, state of the art advice for participants on almost any problem they have, is implicit in any trial that really cares about high response. Indeed, for some trials conducted in populations with usually poor access to care, the results are impossible to explain otherwise than through effects of quid pro quo advice of this kind, rarely included in published reports.[40,41]

There were many examples of this in the early Rhondda Fach studies, where the population had access to personal care of generally low quality. While I worked there in 1961, I augmented my miserly income from the MRC by acting as locum tenens for two local practices. In Mardy I saw about 30 patients each morning, did 12 to 15 home visits, and then saw another 30 in the evening. In Ferndale I saw about 60 in the morning, did over 20 home visits, and then saw another 60 in the evening. These practices each served about the same population (about 3000 patients). The difference in workload was mainly because a receptionist was employed in Mardy who prescribed and certified unfitness for work for many of the supposedly straightforward chronic cases, getting the doctor to sign blank prescriptions and sickness certificates before each session. This was both dangerous and illegal, but was customary practice to which I conformed. Welsh Health Authorities at that time evidently turned a blind eye, knowing that if they enforced the law, they would lose even the doctors they had. There was some visible tightening up by the Welsh Office in the late 1960s, when recruitment to general practice improved after the new GP contract of 1966.

Participants in the Rhondda Fach studies looked for, and generally received, medical advice on a much wider range of social and clinical problems than trial designs required or were designed to accept. Because few researchers had any general practice experience, they most probably underestimated the importance of this subordinate part of their work, but it was very important to patients, and remembered by them to this day. The wife of one man investigated for PMF in one of the early studies told us of their child, a frail and emaciated girl who could be persuaded to eat only by scattering bread on the pavement outside their terrace house, where she would pick it up and eat it because the roaming sheep and lambs (characteristic of all mining villages in those days) did the same. Archie had her chest *x* rayed, found evidence of a large septal defect, and got her referred to a teaching hospital where open heart surgery had just come to birth. One generous act of that kind would, in the Rhondda, be known everywhere within days, and probably had more effect on response than any amount of arm twisting.

A periphery of excellence?

Toward the end of 1961, I suggested to Archie that if the Rhondda Fach population was to have a long term future as target for a succession of randomised controlled trials with continuing high response rates, this trade off between participation in trials and material gains from better medical advice needed to be institutionalised, by getting a primary care base which could develop as a periphery of excellence both for primary care and for research. This would be a counterpart to the teaching hospitals tradition, centres of excellence which offered poor people state of the art hospital care by specialists, in return for being taught and experimented upon.

At first he was enthusiastic, suggesting that as soon as a Rhondda Fach practice fell vacant, I should take it over as an MRC salaried clinician, responsible for continuing care in a research population. To reach anything like the numbers needed for research of the sort then being undertaken by the MRC, this population would have to expand rapidly to at least 10 000. This was close to the entire Rhondda Fach population at that time (which had fallen since 1950, mainly by outmigration), so everything would depend on how this new unit related to surrounding established providers. For this problem Archie's solution was simple: the MRC's good young doctor would drive out the established bad old doctors. As soon as the word spread that a doctor was available who actually took people's clothes off to examine them, did blood tests, and gave them an average 10 minutes instead of two, patients would flock out of the established practices and join our outpost of medical science. We would recruit more progressive young doctors, and the old men would evaporate.

In those days I was a naive romantic with much yet to learn of the street wisdom necessary for survival in the valleys, but even I was not ignorant enough to believe that any plan of this sort could end other than in tears. Archie had little respect for clinicians, and none at all for those at the bottom of the heap, operating a primary care service resourced only from their own pockets, in which the clinical poverty of the doctors matched the material poverty of their patients, both of them victims of circumstances which neither controlled.[42]

Archie evaded this dilemma by ignoring it, substituting one of his own invention: that I was by nature a doer and committed evangelist, rather than an observer and objective analyst. He believed that good clinicians came from the first category, medical scientists from the second, and young doctors ambitious to serve had to choose which of these mutually exclusive roles they were best suited to pursue. Our disagreement was not, as he suggested in his autobiography, about speed, it was about direction.[43]

In practice, if not in rhetoric, population based research still depended on doing things to people (including local medical professionals) rather than with them. It was already clear that this sort of research would in future come to depend entirely on the intelligent participation of informed participants as coproducers. If we needed more or less captive populations for this sort of research, it could be done only in association with, and limited by, more or less captive doctors, whose first responsibility would be to act as advocates for that population, with research requirements strictly subordinated to immediate care needs and popular expectations.

There are many reasons why by the late 1960s epidemiological research moved away from the Rhondda Fach, to be resited in Caerphilly. The South Wales MRC Epidemiology Unit was finally wound up in 1996, with no definite plans to continue a cumulative data base spanning several generations, integrating information from the entire range of human biology, including its sociology and anthropology. Though the most important of all research opportunities, population-based studies of the human genome, have been undertaken in Caerphilly[44,45] and there have been recent attempts to integrate this research with the tasks of patient care, the concept of a periphery of clinical and research excellence was not pursued in the 1970s, before research in general passed into the ice age, and will be more difficult to launch in the new climate. As for service development, Cardiff University projects like Teamcare Valleys were not sustained long enough to sink real roots into the valley communities. The two vocational training schemes based at Neath and Merthyr Tydfil, which had previously provided occasional recruits to Valleys general practice, collapsed soon after the NHS market reforms. All the former mining valleys of south Wales are now a disaster area for recruitment and retention of general practitioners.

The present state of social medicine

In retrospect, the Rhondda Fach studies of the 1950s were a high point in epidemiological thought and action. Since then there have been big advances in methodology, but in social conception it has been in many ways a long, deceptively painless retreat.

Development of meta-analyses was obviously a step forward, in that they can make some agreed sense out of an excess of small projects, to supplement a still inadequate number of studies planned from the beginning to provide sufficient person-years to give plausible results. But meta-analyses may also take us three steps back: they reduce those able to form consensus to a handful of non-clinicians with hyperspecialised statistical skills[46,47]; the growing number of meta-analyses could conceal a decline in the number of truly original source studies; and they perpetuate obsolete, fragmented research effort, when our main thrust should be to integrate the tasks of clinical medicine, teaching, and research in a growing proportion of all units of the NHS, so that medical practice not only uses science as and when this is convenient, but becomes itself an integral part of science, subject to the same rigour, mutual criticism, and willingness to admit limitations.

In the 1950s, where Departments of Social Medicine existed at all, that is what they were called. Both the few barely funded pioneers who believed in social medicine, and the many wealthy and powerful reactionaries who opposed it, were not afraid to use plain words with clear meanings. The less value laden term "epidemiology" arrived in the 1960s, as commitment to social ideas gave way to the allegedly more powerful, less judgemental calculations of value free methodology.

The trouble with reducing a scientific philosophy to a technical instrument is that it can then be used for any purpose by anyone with enough money to pay for it. That seems to be the state we are now in, a possibility derided by Archie in his lifetime, but which he would scarcely deny now. Brecht's Galileo foresaw a future in which, because of his failure to stand up to organised superstition, scientists would become "a race of intelligent dwarfs, who could be hired for anything". That is not a bad description of some developments today which like to trace their origins to *Effectiveness and efficiency*, and were anticipated when that mould-breaking work first appeared.[48]

Of course, that is an incomplete view of the United Kingdom epidemiological scene. It leaves out a huge expansion in quantity, and above all, a rise in quality of recruitment of participants for randomised controlled trials. Like similar improvements in the quality of consultation and clinical decisions, which increasingly respect the intelligence and opinions of patients, more trials have stopped paying lip service to informed consent, and begun to make this a reality. We suspect that this has less to do with medical or academic conscience, or even with ethics committees, than with changes in social attitude in the population as a whole. Some of the social assumptions on which the NHS was based, feudal survivals in no way essential and indeed a serious obstacle to its future progress, have almost disappeared. We no longer have mature men and women willing to be treated like children, or grateful for almost nothing in return for the privilege of being used by medical science. Our populations assume that the NHS is their own, they and their parents and grandparents paid for it, and it no longer belongs to doctors or to politicians. There have been some changes toward selfishness, asking "What's in it for me?"; but overwhelmingly, people still ask the entirely necessary, proper, and reasonable question "What's in it for us?", an entirely different concept. And we now have a generation of young doctors, particularly those entering general practice, prepared to take time and trouble to answer that question.

Eight preconditions for high and sustained response rates

Practical experience of achieving and maintaining high response rates over many years indicates eight rules of behaviour for people who design and run randomised controlled trials using the general population.
These are:

- Respect
- Comprehensibility
- Continuity
- Concern
- Contract
- Captivity
- Feedback
- Shared experience

• The school and university experience of doctors generally provides a poor foundation on which to build *respect* for the brains of their patients or potential participants in controlled experiments. Having been selected over and over again for the particular academic aptitudes and social disabilities usually required for examination success, it is hard for doctors to learn that for almost all other purposes, most of their patients are not less intelligent than themselves, just less informed. Given encouragement, both patients in consultation and participants in trials ask simple but important questions about diseases and their treatment which come very close to our own ultimate aims; why her but not me, why some cells but not others, how much of so and so is enough to cause such and such, and so on.[49] The aims, design, and methods of randomised controlled trials, including the social ethics and logical justification of randomisation itself, must be fully explained to potential participants, preferably in groups as well as individually, and time must be set aside for this.

• If the aims or methods of a study cannot be made *comprehensible* to virtually all participants, it is unlikely that researchers themselves fully understand them, or that the experimental design is sound. Ability to describe a specialised subject to non-specialists is a good test of real comprehension and of an important research question.

- *Continuity* of staffing is essential, to build cumulative mutual respect between staff and participants.

- Staff must have time and referral pathways through which to demonstrate *concern* for participants in material ways. If participants think that research staff may be able to help them about other problems apparently unrelated to the main theme of a project, their choice of adviser must be respected, and often leads to better information directly relevant to assessment of more centrally relevant data.

- Researchers must ensure that the *contract* they offer participants will actually operate throughout the trial, on the original terms. For example, pilot projects may entail many more years of participation in an experiment, than the main cohort has to endure.

- *Captive* patients are obviously easier to recruit to trials and to follow up. This means not only institutional captivity, but the concern felt by all patients that if their doctor asks them to do something, they are under some pressure to comply, including fears that if they do not, their future relationship may suffer. So great may this pressure be that Ann Cartwright has gone so far as to recommend that clinicians generally should not be involved in recruitment of their own patients to trials.[50] I think that the answer to this is that these doctors must be as captive to their patients as the patients are to their doctors. However casual or ephemeral doctor-patient relationships may become in the current worldwide retreat to shopkeeping for doctors and consumerism for patients, the relation between researchers and their trial participants must entail a continuing responsibility and concern to face all the consequences personally. If, and only if, this is done, I see no ethical problem for primary generalists recruiting of participants from their own populations.

- The birth and first year or so of any project tends to be a honeymoon, in which everyone at all levels seems convinced that their project will be a milestone on the road toward greater knowledge. Five years later and perhaps halfway through a major prospective trial its main authors have moved on to a new romance, all too often leaving their field staff and participants almost completely uninformed about the progress of the project, or about other researches which may cast a different light on the hypothesis under test. Frequent *feedback* at every stage of a project is an essential part of real respect for participants and field staff, all too often neglected or done casually and unimaginatively. This should include reporting back final results personally and collectively to field staff and participants.

- So far as possible, researchers and their entire teams should subject themselves to the processes they intend to inflict on participants, so that respondents are offered an at least partially *shared experience*, a long and honourable tradition in human experiment. This is always possible at least in part, and during pilot trials to develop a feasible design it should be mandatory. In many trials it should be possible for at least some of the research team in appropriate age and sex groups to enter the sampling or randomisation process, and become trial participants themselves. Our team in Glyncorrwg followed this rule in all trials, and always learned from the experience, often in unpredicted ways.

If these eight lessons have really been learned, we suspect that ethical questions will increasingly take care of themselves. Ethics committees today usually include people with real experience of having to make the choices they criticise in others, but they often underestimate the willingness and intelligence of the general population, and may underestimate the new relationships possible if research is conducted within continuing primary care, with professionals acting as informed advocates for their patients, with the skills required for care of populations merged with those required for personal care,[51] and patients encouraged and helped to advance from a consumer to a coproducer role.[52] This is so different from the circumstances and social relationships of hospital based clinical research[53] that although ethics committees will probably still be needed as ultimate arbiters, their composition and assumptions need to change as participants in trials are encouraged and allowed to become more participative.

In these new and still rapidly shifting circumstances, the real rate limiting factor on what is tolerable for patients, with informed hindsight as well as speculative foresight, will become what experienced participating populations agree to tolerate when fully informed, within a continuing relationship in which researchers and participants must live with the consequences of their joint decisions. Researchers who stay in one place and so far as possible share the experience of trial participants will become informed advocates for their patients first, and will subordinate research demands to this higher priority. If they do not, response rates will fall and the population will, as a site for epidemiological research, become exhausted and barren. Whether this would eventually have happened in the Rhondda Fach, had the MRC unit continued to observe and experiment on its population to ever higher standards of quality while leaving primary medical care to its own squalor, will never be known, because work was transferred to Caerphilly.

Requirements for a mass research facility in the NHS

By creating registered populations given health care free at the point of use on a solidarity principle, with patients retaining the habits of sharing, mutual support, and respect for medical professionals as their helpers rather than their exploiters, the NHS also created a huge potential research facility. This was recognised by the multinational pharmaceutical industry, which by the 1960s habitually referred to "the British facility", in contrast with the United States, where fee chasing on one hand and consumerism on the other were creating adversarial relationships that drove randomised controlled trials first to indigent populations, then to paid participants.

Fully to develop this huge opportunity, research would have to base itself where community based populations actually are, registered in primary care. There have been many obstacles to this development, and it has taken a long time to clear them away, not least because so many have an interest in pretending they do not exist. Inspired lone researchers in general practice, legendary figures like William Mackenzie and Will Pickles, do not provide useful models for the mass research required for randomised controlled trials. We need not a few exceptional doctors doing exceptional things to the small numbers of patients they have available, but numerous small teams each doing generally commonplace things at an exceptional standard of quality, with usually small numbers screened and sampled from literally millions of people, adding their work to planned multicentre designs with truly professional statistical and logistic support.

This mythology of lone genius, with research as an exceptional activity rather than a routine necessity, has been our main obstacle. If primary care is to mean anything more than sitting in a doctor's shop waiting for customers to define your work for you, if a primary care led NHS is to be anything more than painless political rhetoric, we have to define the work of each practice not only by responding to existing demand (although that must come first) but also by identifying the health needs of our communities. Some of this work will already have been done, other people's data on expected prevalence which in the absence of local data, we must assume to prevail locally, at least as an order of magnitude; but no practice can know what local needs actually are, or devise intelligent strategies for meeting them, without some sort of organised local enquiry. Little can be done to improve care without some measure not only of what is already being done, but also of what is not being done.[10] The agenda for the present generation of entrants to primary care is that every practice must learn to become both a teaching practice and a research practice.[54] This may seem irrelevant to the development of general practitioners as entrepreneurs in the current fashion, whether in corner shops or supermarkets, but all the evidence we have confirms that an entrepreneurial role is itself irrelevant or perhaps inimical either to improving health care for the whole population, or to advancing research. If competition in the NHS really is replaced by cooperation, without any restoration of pre-reform droits de seigneur for doctors, and if patients are at last encouraged to accept a role as coproducers of health rather than consumers of care, we are on the eve of great change, and we need to get ready for it.

The MRC general practitioner research framework (GPRF)

Serious primary care based research must be conducted in networks, in which the only exceptional practices will be pilots for larger studies, and must be backed by professional epidemiologists, statisticians, and a wide range of other experts. There is no way the Royal College of General Practitioners (RCGP) can provide such a network, such a range of expert backup, or people with truly professional experience of conducting large multicentre randomised controlled trials. There have been many excellent individual researchers in United Kingdom general practice, and there have been some important multicentre studies, such as the long series of national morbidity surveys from the RCGP's Birmingham Unit, or the oral contraceptive studies from its Manchester Unit, but the problems presented by these activities were simpler by an order of magnitude than those already met and overcome by the MRC's low dose warfarin trial, or those that will certainly be met in its HRT study. In the present climate of competitive bidding for scarce funding, resource-hungry institutions of all kinds may be tempted to tender for tasks far beyond their capacity to perform.

Responsibility for primary care based research cannot be left to leaders of the general practitioner establishment whose eminence derives from entirely different qualities. Nor can it be left to leaders of the MRC establishment without experience of providing primary care, who have in the past selected GP advisers for their diplomatic rather than imaginative qualities or research productivity. Despite this caveat, the MRC GPRF already provides most of the material framework we need for an intelligent mass research policy, even if it occasionally needs a stiff dose of social imagination.

The MRC GPRF will become the main base for future research in all aspects of social medicine on a mass scale. It was created as a vehicle for the MRC randomised controlled trials of treatment for mild to moderate hypertension.[55,56] Recruitment to research studies in general practice tends always to be biased in favour of practices with lower workload, lower morbidity, and lower event rates, because GPs working without these conditions seldom wish to add to their burdens. To reduce costs in the

MRC study, an early decision was taken to confine recruitment to practice populations of 10 000 and over. The predictable (and predicted) consequence was an even greater bias toward large partnerships in market towns with generally affluent populations, which were pleasant to work with and minimised logistic problems during the initial period of data collection. When it came to follow up, however, event rates were much lower than they would have been if more industrial and postindustrial practices had been included, and inevitably there were doubts about whether its conclusions could be accurately applied to such populations.

Providing it is remembered, this fundamental error is not likely to be repeated, and the MRC Epidemiology and Medical Care Unit has worked, and is still working, hard to obtain more balanced and representative, as well as larger, populations for the GPRF, by actively seeking more practices in less affluent areas. In doing this, the MRC will acquire energetic young GPs with their own forceful views on the wider nature of mass research. We are likely to see bolder and more imaginative inputs from GP advisers, and more ideas from below at annual GPRF research meetings.

Ironically, perhaps the best opportunity of this kind may arise in the south Wales valleys of which Archie's Rhondda Fach is the epicentre, because collapse of recruitment and retention of entrepreneurial GPs is for the first time compelling government and opposition parties, and even the BMA, to take a salaried primary care service seriously. If, and only if, such a service defines its aims in terms of health outputs rather than process, allows its health workers to pursue these aims in their own way, and guarantees this clinical autonomy by supporting close links with university departments so that salaried service really does for the first time provide protected time for personal and team development, we might realise the full potential of the changes pioneered by Archie Cochrane in the Rhondda Fach.

Epidemiology is participative democracy in action

As Archie was one of the first to appreciate, though not in these precise terms, epidemiology is by its nature democratic: one person, one vote; every vote is valuable, each vote is equal. This is so even though researchers can, for a short time, obtain apparently good results by authoritarian methods. Authoritarian research, which may obey the letter of ethical rules but is in practice interested only in getting signatures to legalise veterinary human experiment, is soon self limiting, because nobody will submit to such studies a second time.

Patients who participate in randomised research are examples par excellence of transition from consumer to coproducer status, the key to any effective and affordable national health service anywhere. The new attitudes to science that they will learn from this experience, and will communicate to their families, friends, and communities, will help the public generally to adopt the doubts of human biology and discard the certainties of mechanical engineering as their conceptual model for medical science. They will learn that good medical practice depends as much on knowledge of limitations as on specialised competence, that science is about limited doubt rather than boundless certainty, that most important medical decisions have to be made on incomplete evidence, that much if not most of that evidence must come from patients, and that most things we cannot yet do will one day be done not by paying huge fees, but by processes of discovery to which all should contribute.

We have our own measure of democracy. People enjoy it to the extent that the decisions ruling their lives are taken by people who share the consequences. Archie would have agreed with that.

Acknowledgements

Preparation of this paper would not have been possible without help from former office and field staff of the MRC Epidemiology Unit in South Wales: Tom Benjamin, Gwilym Jonathan, Fred Moore, Diana Pritchard (*née* Seys-Prosser) and Mary Thomas; and from surviving participants in the 1950 Rhondda Fach studies, Trefor Stanley Jones and Merlin Thomas. We are particularly grateful to Professor Graham Watt for very helpful amendments to the text, and for other advice from Dr Morley Davies, retired Medical Officer of Health for Rhondda, Professors Leon Eisenberg, Victor Hawthorne, Bill Silverman, and Paul Wallace, and Dr Hugh Thomas.

1 Hart JT, Cochrane AL, Higgins ITT. Tuberculin sensitivity in coal workers' pneumoconiosis. *Tubercle (Lond)* 1963;**44**:141–52.
2 Cochrane AL, Cox JG, Jarman TF. Pulmonary tuberculosis in the Rhondda Fach. *BMJ* 1952;ii:843–53.
3 Dawber TR. *The Framingham study: the epidemiology of atherosclerotic disease.* New York: Harvard University Press, 1980.
4 Miall WE, Oldham PD. Factors influencing arterial pressure in the general population. *Clin Sci* 1958;**17**:409–44.
5 Anderson TW. Re-examination of some of the Framingham blood pressure data. *Lancet* 1978;ii:1139–41.
6 Gough J. *Proceedings of a conference on silicosis, pneumoconiosis, and dust suppression in mines.* London: HMSO, 1947:7.
7 Cochrane AL, Miall WE, Clarke WG, Jarman TF, Jonathan G, Moore F. Factors influencing the radiological attack rate of progressive massive fibrosis. *BMJ* 1996;i:1193–9.
8 Cochrane AL. The detection of pulmonary tuberculosis in a community. *Br Med Bull* 1954;**10**:91–5.
9 Hart JT. Rule of halves: implications of underdiagnosis and dropout for future workload and prescribing costs in primary care. *Br J Gen Pract* 1992;**42**:116–19.
10 Hart JT. Measurement of omission. *BMJ* 1982;**284**:1686–9.
11 Tin W, Fritz S, Wariyar U, Hey E. Incomplete follow-up studies of neonatal outcome underestimate the prevalence of disability among survivors. 1997 (in preparation).
12 Cartwright A. *Health surveys in practice and in potential: a critical view of their scope and methods.* London: Tavistock Publications, 1981:160.

13 Williams C. *Democratic Rhondda: politics and society 1885–1951*. Cardiff: University of Wales Press, 1996.
14 Nutbeam D, Smith C, Murphy J, Catford J. Maintaining evaluation designs in long term community based health promotion programmes: Heartbeat Wales case study. *J Epidemiol Community Health* 1993;**47**:127–33.
15 Thomas H. Three decades of occupational health research in South Wales. *Occupational and Environmental Medicine* 1996;**53**:141–2.
16 Hart JT, Thomas C, Gibbons B, *et al*. Twenty five years of audited screening in a socially deprived community. *BMJ* 1991;**302**:1509–13.
17 Hart JT. Semicontinuous screening of a whole community for hypertension. *Lancet* 1970; ii:223–7.
18 Chalmers RA, Hart JT, Healy MJR, Lawson AM, Watts RWE. Urinary organic acids in man III: quantitative ranges and patterns of excretion in a normal population. *Clin Chem* 1976;**22**:1292–8.
19 This was a pilot study for what later became a major nationwide study in the MRC general practice research framework, relating fat splitting faecal anaerobic bacteria to subsequent large bowel cancer. So far as I know (in October 1996) results have not yet been published.
20 Thomas TM, Plymat KR, Blannin J, Meade TW. Prevalence of urinary incontinence. *BMJ* 1980;**281**:1243–5.
21 Watt GCM, Foy CJW, Hart JT, Bingham G, *et al*. Dietary sodium and arterial blood pressure: evidence against genetic susceptibility. *BMJ* 1985;**291**:1525–8.
22 Meade TW, Wilkes HC, Stirling Y, *et al*. Randomized controlled trial of low dose warfarin in the primary prevention of ischaemic heart disease in men at high risk: design and pilot study. *European Heart J* 1988;**9**:836–43.
23 Zhurie R. Thrombosis prevention trial. *General Practitioner Research Framework (GPRF) Newsletter* issue 3, July 1996:4–5.
24 Medical Research Council. Streptomycin treatment of pulmonary tuberculosis. *BMJ* 1948;ii:769–82.
25 Smith R. Where is the wisdom . . .? The poverty of medical evidence. *BMJ* 1991;**303**: 798–9.
26 *General Practitioner Research Framework (GPRF) Newsletter* issue 3, July 1996:2.
27 Wilkes HC, Meade TW. Hormone replacement therapy in general practice: a survey of doctors in the MRC's general practice research framework. *BMJ* 1991;**302**:1317–20.
28 Vickers M. Long-term randomised controlled trial of hormone replacement therapy. *GPRF Newsletter* issue 3, July 1996:10.
29 Welton M. Patients' willingness to enter a clinical trial and impact of a placebo arm upon intention. *GPRF Newsletter* issue 3, July 1996:5–6.
30 *Report on workshop on patient preferences and randomized trials*. Oxford: UK Cochrane Centre, 1994.
31 Peto R. Clinical trial reporting. *Lancet* 1996;**348**:894–5.
32 Titmuss RM. *The gift relationship: from human blood to social policy*. London: George Allen and Unwin, 1970.
33 Howden-Chapman P, Carter J, Woods N. Blood money: blood donors' attitudes to changes in the New Zealand blood transfusion service. *BMJ* 1996;**312**:1131–2.
34 Carnall D. Medical Research Council unit takes tobacco cash. *BMJ* 1996;**313**:577.
35 Meiklejohn A. The development of compensation for occupational diseases of the lungs in Great Britain. *Br J Ind Med* 1954;**11**:198–212.
36 Hart PD'A, Aslett AE. *Special Report Series No 243*. London: Medical Research Council, 1942.
37 Hart JT, Dieppe P. Caring effects. *Lancet* 1996;**347**:1606–8.
38 Roethlisberger FJ, Dickson WJ. *Management and the worker*. Boston: Harvard University Press, 1939.
39 Brown GW, Davison S, Harris T, *et al*. Psychiatric disorder in London and North Uist. *Soc Sci Med* 1977;**11**:367–77.
40 Hypertension Detection and Follow up Program Co-operative group. Five-year findings of the HDFP. I. Reduction in mortality of persons with high blood pressure, including mild hypertension. *JAMA* 1979;**242**:2562–71.

41 Hypertension Detection and Follow-up Program Co-operative group. Five-year findings of the HDFP. II. Mortality by race, sex and age. *JAMA* 1979;**242**:2572–7.
42 Hart JT. *A new kind of doctor: the general practitioner's part in the health of the community.* London: Merlin Press, 1988.
43 Cochrane AL, Blythe M. *One man's medicine: an autobiography of Professor Archie Cochrane.* London: British Medical Journal Memoir Club, 1989:162–3.
44 Mattu RK, Needham EWA. DPL variants at the LPL gene locus associated with angiographically defined severity of atherosclerosis and serum lipoprotein levels in a Welsh population. *Arterioscler Thromb* 1994;**14**:1090–7.
45 Mattu RK, Needham EWA, Galton DJ, *et al.* DNA variant at the angiotensin-converting enzyme gene locus associates with coronary artery disease in the Caerphilly heart study. *Circulation* 1995;**91**:270–4.
46 Rosendaal FR. The emergence of a new species: the professional meta-analyst. *J Clin Epidemiol* 1994;**47**:1325–6;1331–2.
47 Cook DJ, Guyatt GH. The professional meta-analyst: an evolutionary advantage. *J Clin Epidemiol* 1994;**47**:1327–9.
48 Hart JT. An assault on all custom: Cochrane's "effectiveness and efficiency". *Int J Health Serv* 1973;**3**:101–4.
49 Cromarty I. What do patients think about during their consultations? A qualitative study. *Br J Gen Pract* 1996;**46**:525–8.
50 Cartwright A. *Health surveys in practice and in potential: a critical view of their scope and methods.* London: Tavistock Publications, 1981.
51 White KL. *Healing the schism: epidemiology, medicine and the public's health.* New York: Springer-Verlag, 1991.
52 Hart JT. Clinical and economic consequences of patients as producers. *J Public Health Med* 1995;**17**:383–6.
53 Silverman WA. *Human experimentation: a guided step into the unknown.* London: Oxford University Press, 1985.
54 Hart JT. Opportunities and risks of local population research in general practice. In: Gray DJP, ed. *Forty years on: the story of the first forty years of the Royal College of General Practitioners.* London: RCGP, 1992:199–204.
55 Peart WS, Miall WE. MRC treatment trial for mild hypertension. *BMJ* 1979;**2**:48.
56 Medical Research Council Working Party. MRC trial of treatment of mild hypertension: principal results. *BMJ* 1985;**291**:97–104.

2: Cochrane and the benefits of wine

RICHARD DOLL

Introduction

Archie Cochrane, whose life we commemorate in this book, was a close friend for over 50 years. I first met him in 1938, when he returned to his clinical studies after serving for a year with a field ambulance unit sponsored by the British Committee for Spanish Medical Aid in support of the democratic government forces in the Spanish civil war—a unit in which he was the only member with neither religious nor political affiliation—and I saw him regularly thereafter until shortly before his death. His name is now indelibly linked with the conduct of randomised controlled trials; but it is as an epidemiologist that I believe he would have liked to be primarily remembered. If I had ever had any doubts about this, they would have been dispelled recently when I read the chapter that Cochrane had added to the 1989 edition of his book *Effectiveness and efficiency.*[1] For in it, he said that one effect of the publication of the first edition had depressed him, because "the medical world forgot my work on pneumoconiosis and common diseases in the Rhondda Fach. I did my best work there and I am sorry to see it forgotten." I make no apology, therefore, for interpreting my remit to give the fourth Archie Cochrane Lecture* (the basis for this chapter) on the theme of effectiveness and efficiency so broadly that I can use it to examine the evidence for the specific effectiveness of wine as a prophylactic against ischaemic heart disease; for it was the epidemiological observations that he inspired that led to the proposition that the negative association between deaths from ischaemic heart disease and the consumption of alcohol was wholly attributable to the beneficial effect of consuming wine.[2]

---

* Delivered at Green College, Oxford, on 21 March 1996.

Cochrane's ecological observations on mortality and wine

The idea that wine might have a specific effect independent of its content of ethanol arose from the results of his attempt to dissect out the social and environmental factors that determined total mortality in developed countries. For this purpose, Cochrane and his colleagues[2] had studied first the total mortality experience of countries with a gross national product exceeding $2000 per caput in 1949 and with a population of more than 2 million, adding in only the Republic of Ireland, with a gross national product per caput of $1949, separating Scotland from England and Wales, and excluding Japan, because of the possible influence that genetic factors might have had in determining much of the difference in mortality between Japan and the other countries under investigation.

For these 18 countries, Cochrane and his colleagues examined the correlations between age-specific total mortality rates up to 65 years of age in 1970 with 17 health service, dietary, and economic indices. This led to nothing of great interest—except perhaps for one finding that intrigued him and which he used to tease self-satisfied members of the medical establishment: namely, the finding of a close **positive** correlation between infant and childhood mortality and the number of doctors per 1000 population. Despite attempts to explain the association in terms of other variables he was unable to make the anomaly go away and neither he, nor anyone else to my knowledge, has been able to explain it.

A subsequent examination of the correlation of these 17 indices with the principal cause-specific mortality rates rather than with total mortality was scientifically more promising.[3] The most interesting findings were the correlations for ischaemic heart disease at 55–64 years of age, which are shown in table 2.1. One was the strong **negative** correlation with the consumption of alcohol ($r = -0.70$ for men and -0.58 for women) which was independent of, and almost as strong as, the **positive** correlation with the predictive index for the effect of different combinations of dietary fat given by Keys' equation[4] ($r = 0.70$ for men and 0.69 for women). Though not anticipated, the correlation with alcohol was not surprising; but it was surprising that it should have been entirely explained by the correlation with the consumption of wine.

A U-shaped relationship between the total mortality and the consumption of alcoholic beverages had been reported by Pearl 50 years before from the data of the Metropolitan Life Insurance Company of New York[5] and many studies had subsequently suggested that there might be a negative association between ischaemic heart disease and the consumption of alcoholic beverages in general (though the implication had seldom been taken seriously). Cochrane's group, however, was the first to suggest a

TABLE 2.1—*Correlation between certain variables and mortality from ischaemic heart disease in men and women aged 55–64 years*

Variable (per caput)	Correlation coefficient	
	Men	Women
Gross national product	−0.17	−0.26
Cigarettes	0.28	0.44
Saturated fat	0.64	0.62
Keys' predictive fat index	0.70	0.69
Alcohol	−0.70	−0.58
Wine	−0.70	−0.61
Beer	0.23	0.31
Spirits	−0.26	−0.32

After St Leger *et al.*[2]

specific effect for the consumption of wine. Coming from a Scottish Presbyterian family it was, perhaps, natural for him to ask his Welsh non-conformist colleague, Dr Hugh Thomas, where the verse in the bible was to be found that recommended a modicum of wine. It was, Thomas said, "1. Timothy ch 5, v 23: Be no longer a water drinker, but use a little wine for thy stomach's sake." "Well", said Archie "it should have been heart, but I suppose they didn't have much knowledge of anatomy in those days." (HF Thomas, personal communication.)

Cochrane and his colleagues were well aware of the potential pitfalls of ecological studies and they noted that the observations of Yano *et al*[6] on a cohort of Japanese men had suggested that beer might be equally effective. They were, therefore, restrained in their conclusions. If, however, wine had a specific protective effect, it might be due to constituents other than alcohol. Wines, they noted, were rich in aromatic components and other trace compounds that give them their distinctive characters and it might be to these that we should look for the beneficial effect of wine on risk. One possibility that attracted Cochrane was that the copper content of red wine might be important. This, he thought was suggested by the literature and according to his colleague, Thomas (personal communication), he could see some logic in it, as the DHSS subcommittee on back pain, which he had chaired in 1976, had found that the few sound randomised controlled trials of treatment indicated that wearing a copper bracelet was beneficial and I happen to know that he had, in fact, taken to wearing one himself. Such ideas, Cochrane and his colleagues recognised, were speculative and wine drinking might be of no greater significance than its reputed indication of a relaxed way of living.[2] What they firmly believed, however, was that their evidence and that from other studies justified an experimental approach.

An initial step, they suggested "would be to examine the effect of alcohol and, in particular wine on blood lipids, platelet aggregation, and on such other blood constituents as may plausibly be involved in the pathogenesis of atheroma." Then, if the results were sufficiently promising, they would hope to see the conduct of randomised controlled trials of the preventive or therapeutic effects of moderate wine consumption. Even such a staunch advocate of randomisation as Cochrane recognised, however, that the conduct of such trials would (I quote) "pose severe ethical and practical difficulties" and they have never been carried out. Should, however, research lead to the conclusion that wine contained a specific constituent protective against ischaemic heart disease it would, he thought, be almost a sacrilege that the constituent should be isolated, for the medicine was already in a highly palatable form.[2]

Cochrane's findings, interesting as they are in retrospect now that the evidence for a beneficial effect of alcoholic beverages on the risk of ischaemic heart disease is widely accepted, attracted little attention at the time and what attention they did attract was wholly critical. McMichael, the leading cardiologist of the day, attributed the findings to flaws in the comparability of death certificates,[7] on the grounds that the French attributed death to myocardial infarction only if it occurred shortly after the event, while deaths that occurred later were attributed to ischaemic heart disease in other countries but to myocarditis in France. This difference, however, had already been allowed for by Cochrane, who had shown that the negative correlation was unaltered by the exclusion of France or by the addition of the category of "other diseases of the heart" to the French data for ischaemic heart disease.[2,8] Others suggested that the results could be explained by confounding with the consumption of garlic,[9,10] some unknown geographical factor related to latitude,[11] or with dietary fats[12] despite the fact that the correlation had been found to occur independently of Keys' predictive index of fat consumption.[2]

The prophylactic value of alcoholic beverages

For 10 years little further interest was shown in the subject. The harmful effects of alcohol were so many and so obvious, both medically and socially, that national policies for improving public health throughout the world uniformly stressed the desirability of reducing per caput consumption and held total abstention to be the medical ideal. Gradually, however, the evidence for a beneficial effect of alcohol became too hard to resist; in particular, that the risk of ischaemic heart disease and, to a less extent, the risks of death from other vascular diseases and from all causes were truly lower in men and women who drank small quantities of alcohol than in total abstainers and that this was not due to confounding with other factors.

In many studies, ex-drinkers and lifelong non-drinkers had been classed together as non-drinkers and it was possible to argue, as Shaper *et al* did for many years,[13] that the higher mortality in non-drinkers than in light drinkers was due to a high mortality in ex-drinkers, who were at high risk because of the amount they had drunk in the past or because they had given up drinking specifically because of developing disease. This view was not tenable, however, when studies that distinguished between lifelong non-drinkers and ex-drinkers regularly showed J-shaped or U-shaped mortality curves, not only for ischaemic heart disease but also for mortality from all causes. An example is provided by the observations of Klatsky *et al*[14] on 20 000 men and women who had health examinations in a prepaid health plan in California and were subsequently followed up for eight years, which

TABLE 2.2—*Relative risk of death compared with risk in lifelong abstainers*

Drinking category	Relative risk*		
	Coronary artery disease	Cerebrovascular disease	All causes (2430)
Abstainers (lifelong)	1.0	1.0	1.0
Ex-drinkers	1.0	1.0	1.1
Drinkers:			
Occasional (>monthly)	0.8	0.8	0.9
1–2/day	0.6	0.8	0.9
3–5/day	0.6	0.7	1.0
≥6/day	0.8	1.4	1.4

* Adjusted for age, sex, smoking, and nine other "risk factors".
After Klatsky *et al.*[14]

are summarised in table 2.2. Similar J-shaped or U-shaped curves have also been found in large studies limited to men initially free from major disease, as is shown by the results for death from ischaemic heart disease in our study of 12 000 middle aged and elderly British doctors, 5000 of whom had had no vascular disease on entry[15] and whose mortality showed the same pattern, and for total mortality in the massive American Cancer Society's study of 277 000 men aged 40–59 years.[16]

The general pattern is, I think, incontrovertible. The increasing mortality with amount drunk observed in the ascending limb of the curve after standardisation for smoking is contributed to by many causes about which there is no argument—that is, a few deaths attributed directly to alcoholic psychosis and dependence, a much larger number attributed to hepatic cirrhosis, cancers of the oral cavity, pharynx, oesophagus, larynx, and liver, some cardiomyopathies, haemorrhagic stroke, and nearly all the major external causes of injury and poisoning including suicide. The decreasing limb, in contrast, results chiefly from the relationship with ischaemic heart disease and cerebral thrombosis; but other vascular diseases may also contribute to it, as may some infectious diseases,[17,18] cholelithiasis,[19–21] and non-insulin dependent diabetes mellitus,[22,23] and an increased mineral density of bone may counteract some of the risks of injury.[24]

The decrease with the amount drunk cannot plausibly be explained by confounding, at least in so far as it results from a decreasing risk of thrombotic vascular disease, as the factors that are known to increase the risk of this type of disease are either independent of alcohol consumption (such as body mass index and, over the range from zero to moderate consumption, systolic and diastolic pressure) or are positively associated with alcohol consumption, such as smoking and a high fat diet with little fruit and green vegetables[25] while socioeconomic factors, which could have influenced the results of some studies, cannot have done so to any material extent in the case of the relatively homogeneous British doctors.[15] A beneficial effect on vascular disease is moreover physiologically plausible—as will be discussed later—and the observed relationship is most economically explained by cause and effect, an explanation that has been accepted by the independent group of scientists who were contracted by the European Office of the World Health Organisation to prepare a report on alcohol and public policy.[26]

Many questions, however, are unanswered, some of which are important. One is the level of consumption at which the minimum mortality is obtained. Another is the variation in the balance of risk with sex and age, and a third is the difference, if any, between the effect of different types of alcoholic beverage—beer, spirits, and wine.

Optimum level of consumption

Twenty nine studies that related total mortality to alcohol consumption were reviewed by Poikolainen in 1995.[27] Over half described findings in United States populations and the majority of those that provided quantitative data reported that the minimum occurred with one drink a day. One reported the minimum at a lower level[28] and several reported it at higher levels, the highest being five drinks a day in a study in Italy.[29] Changing habits and random errors will have blurred the differences between the alcohol consumption groups, so that the true differences in risk associated with the regular consumption of different amounts may well be substantially greater than those recorded[30] and systematic errors could have diminished the true differences even further. Some heavy drinkers are likely to have underestimated the amount they drink and so also are moderate and light drinkers in societies in which the consumption of alcohol may be disapproved. Surveys have regularly shown that consumption reported by individuals underestimates sales figures by 30 to

80%[31–33] and American epidemiologists, in my experience, have been unanimously of the opinion that members of the American public would generally underestimate their consumption in response to questionnaires. There is, therefore, a strong case for thinking that the level associated with the minimum mortality could be more accurately reflected by the two to three drinks a day recorded for British doctors than the one and a half British drinks a day recorded in the massive study carried out by the American Cancer Society (actually recorded as one drink a day[16] as the American "units" of alcohol are 50% greater than the British). Much of the difference recorded could, however, be attributable to differences in age distribution of the people observed, which have not been taken into consideration and could have a substantial effect, as is shown later.

Variation with sex and age

For women the optimal level may be associated with a smaller consumption than for men, not only because of their smaller size, but also because of their lesser risk of ischaemic heart disease and greater susceptibility to liver damage and perhaps also because small amounts of alcohol may increase the risk of breast cancer. In compensation, however, women are less prone to death from violence and poisoning and cohort studies consistently show a lower total mortality in women who drink small amounts of alcohol than in abstainers.[34,35]

For young adults there is very little evidence, but the low ratio of the number of deaths from coronary heart disease to the number from external

TABLE 2.3—*Ratio of deaths from ischaemic heart disease and violence in developed countries with market economies by sex and age*

Age (y)	Ratio of deaths in 1990	
	Males	Females
30–44	0.24	0.16
45–59	1.8	1.3
60–69	5.7	5.2
70 and over	9.0	9.9

After Murray and Lopez.[36]

injury and poisoning at young ages,[36] shown in table 2.3, suggests that alcohol is unlikely to produce any reduction in the annual risk of death until about 45 years of age. The only study of younger men that I have found showed an increasing linear relationship between alcohol and total mortality rates at all levels of consumption.[37] The process of vascular degeneration starts, however, at young ages and it may be that moderate drinking in early adult life slows the process and contributes to the benefit in middle age. This, however, is speculative and has yet to be shown.

At the other extreme of life, when vascular disease is pre-eminent, the evidence is clear. In a small study of men aged 65 years and older in Massachusetts,[38] there was a significant reduction in mortality with levels of consumption up to 34 g ethanol a day (corresponding to about 28 British units a week) as there was in British doctors at ages 55 to 70 years and at ages 75 years and over[15]—although the minimum mortality in the older group was observed with smaller quantities (8–14 units a week) than in those whom we may describe as being of late middle age. Plato, it seems, knew something that was subsequently forgotten, for, according to Montaigne writing in 1595, he forbad the use of wine by children before they were 18 and intoxication before the age of 40.[39] "But", I quote "after they have passed that age he orders them to take a pleasure in it ... intoxication being, he says ... calculated to put heart into the elderly."

Specific benefits of different beverages

For the practice of public health the third outstanding question is the one that so interested Cochrane—namely, the relative effect of the different types of alcoholic beverage. Perhaps surprisingly, there have been relatively few case-control and cohort studies that have sought information about it, despite the need, in all but the most exceptional circumstances, to obtain information about risk in people whose individual exposure is known before a causal relationship can be deduced. It is not an easy subject to study, however, as so many people drink different types of alcoholic beverage at different times. In most studies people have, therefore, been characterised solely according to the frequency with which they drank alcohol or, if they drank regularly, according to the number of standard size drinks or grams of ethanol they consumed on average each day. Investigators who have tried to study the differential effect of different types of drink have had to be satisfied with classifying drinkers according to their preferred beverage, and have often compared drinkers of one type of beverage with a combined group of abstainers and people who drank only other types of beverage.

Epidemiological evidence

Four studies have reported wine to be much more beneficial than other beverages. In one, Grønbaek *et al*[35] examined the mortality of some 13 000 Danes aged 30–79 years, who had responded to a questionnaire, out of an age-stratified but otherwise random sample of the population of a sector of Copenhagen in the late 1970s. Individuals were characterised according to whether they never or hardly ever drank either beer or wine or spirits or, if they did drink any one of the three beverages, whether they drank it monthly, weekly, or daily and, if daily, the number of such drinks they consumed on average each day. Those who reported more than five drinks a day of any one type were excluded. Others were then followed up to the beginning of 1978—that is, for 10–12 years—and their mortality from different causes examined. The relative risks of death from all causes in individuals drinking different amounts of each of the three types of beverage were compared with the risks in those who never or hardly ever drank that particular type. The results were standardised for smoking, but not for education, income, or body mass index, which were found not to have had any significant effect on the results. The trends for the three types of drink were very different. With wine, the relative risk decreased progressively to 0.5 for those drinking three to five glasses a day, with an even greater decrease to 0.4 for death from cardiovascular and cerebrovascular disease. With beer there was a smaller decrease to 0.7 for vascular deaths and little or no change in total mortality. With spirits there was no reduction in vascular deaths and little or no difference in total mortality apart from a statistically significant increase of 34% at the highest level of consumption.

The results of the other three studies that found wine to be the most effective type of drink are summarised in table 2.4 in comparison with

TABLE 2.4—*Relative risks of morbidity or mortality according to preferred beverage*

Study	Relative risk in drinkers of		
	Wine	Beer	Spirits
(*a*) Grønbaek *et al*[35]	0.5	0.9	1.1
(*b*) Dean *et al*[40]	0.5	1.0	1.0
(*c*) Rosenberg *et al*[41]	0.4	0.8	0.9
(*d*) Klatsky and Armstrong[42]	(0.7)	(0.9)	(1.0)

(*a*) Risk of death from all causes compared with that in non-drinkers of that beverage.
(*b*) Risk of death from coronary heart disease compared as in (*a*).
(*c*) Risk of myocardial infarction compared with that in abstainers.
(*d*) Risk of death from cardiovascular disease compared with that in spirit drinkers.

those of Grønbaek *et al.*[35] Dean *et al*[40] had carried out a case-control study of men and women who had died from one or other of four common diseases in north east England, which was undertaken primarily to assess the contribution of smoking. Information was, however, also obtained about tea, coffee, and alcohol consumption and about the types of alcohol drunk. Drinking histories were obtained from the relatives of 571 men who had died from coronary heart disease and from household members of about 2500 male controls selected by a random sampling method from electoral registers. Regular wine drinkers were estimated to have only half the risk of death from coronary heart disease of non-wine drinkers, but beer and spirit drinkers showed no comparable reduction at all.

A similar benefit from wine was found by Rosenberg *et al*[41] in a study involving 511 women with myocardial infarction treated in hospital in the north east United States and 899 matched hospital controls. Women whose usual type of drink was wine had a highly significant reduction in relative risk of 0.4 compared with women who never drank, whereas women who usually drank only beer or spirits had relative risks that were not significantly reduced of 0.8 and 0.9. Similar but less sharp differences were recorded by Klatsky and Armstrong[42] in following up for eight years 82 000 men and women who underwent health examinations in a Kaiser Permanente prepaid health plan. Men and women who said that they drank alcohol at least once a month were asked the beverage of their choice. If they drank one type more than one day a week and substantially more often than either of the others they were classed as preferring that type. Cardiovascular mortality in men and women having one or two drinks a day had previously been shown to be about 70% of that in abstainers,[14] and Klatsky and Armstrong[42] then showed that those who preferred wine or beer had relative risks of cardiovascular disease that were, respectively, 70% and 90% of that in those who preferred spirits.

The results of the eight other studies in which comparisons were made between people who drank different types of alcohol cannot be summarised quantitatively in a simple table, as they were presented in such different ways. They are shown qualitatively in table 2.5. In two studies reductions in risk of coronary disease were found to be about equal with wine and

TABLE 2.5—*Relative risks of morbidity or mortality according to preferred beverage*

Study	Relative risk in drinkers of		
	Wine	Beer	Spirits
Stampfer *et al*[43]	⇓	⇓	↓
Friedman and Kimball[44]	⇓	⇓	↓
Hennekens *et al*[45]	⇓	⇓	⇓
Gaziano *et al*[46]	⇓	⇓	⇓
Yano *et al*[6]	↓	⇓	↓
Kozararevic *et al*[47]	↓	↓	⇓
Rimm *et al*[48]	↓	↓	⇓
Salonen *et al*[49]	NA	—	⇓

⇓ substantial reduction; ↓ small reduction; — no reduction; NA = not available.

beer and somewhat less with spirits, but the differences were not significant. One was a four year follow up of 88 000 nurses in the United States aged 34–59 years[43] and the other was a 24 year follow up of 5000 residents of Framingham aged 32 to 61 years who were initially free of coronary disease.[44] Of the remaining six studies, five found reductions in ischaemic heart disease with all three types of beverage, which were equal in two,[45,46] most marked with beer in the one to which Cochrane had drawn attention,[6] and most marked with spirits in two—one in Yugoslavia,[47] and one in the United States.[48] The sixth was carried out in eastern Finland, where too little wine was drunk for useful examination. In this study a substantial reduction was found with spirits but not with beer.[49] To these I can add the preliminary results of the large epidemiological study associated with the ISIS randomised clinical trials of therapies for myocardial infarction, which show a protective effect with wine and beer but not with spirit (S Parish, R Peto, and R Collins, personal communication).

Not all these studies carry equal weight, the numbers of cases varying from 200 to 571 (and to 6000 with the addition of the ISIS study). Nor did all attempt to adjust for social and behavioural factors that might be associated with drinking one or other type of beverage. When such attempts were made the size of the reduction tended to be reduced, but not qualitatively altered. Differences in methodology and in classification of drinkers make a formal meta-analysis of the published data inappropriate, but the sense of the findings is clear: the risk of ischaemic heart disease is reduced with the consumption of small to moderate amounts of alcohol irrespective of the type of beverage in which it occurs. There is some suggestion that in some circumstances the reduction may be greater with wine than with beer or spirits, but the evidence is weak and we need to have much more detailed information than we now have, that would allow adjustments to be made at least for differences in diet, body mass index, education, and smoking habits, which may vary with the preferred beverage.

Another factor that needs to be taken into account, which may be particularly important, as it commonly varies between people who drink different types of beverage, is the pattern of drinking. The physiological effects of ethanol on blood constituents that affect the risk of thrombosis last less than 24 hours, and Jackson *et al*[50] have found that this is reflected clinically in an association between the risk of myocardial infarction and the timing of consumption, a reduced risk being associated with consumption within 24 hours, irrespective of the number of drinks normally consumed per week. Binge drinking, in contrast, is associated with specific harm—not only the risks associated with loss of control of behaviour but also the risk of hypertension. It could be, therefore, that cultural patterns that encourage the consumption of alcohol with meals rather than by itself on isolated occasions may be responsible for some of the national differences that produced the greater negative correlation of ischaemic heart disease with wine than with other alcoholic beverages, which so impressed Cochrane and his colleagues.[2]

Physiological evidence

The physiological evidence to which I referred above would seem overwhelmingly in favour of the simple hypothesis that the benefit is the direct effect of ethanol. Ethanol has been shown to increase the blood concentration of both high density lipoprotein (HDL) cholesterol fractions HDL_2 and HDL_3 and apolipoproteins A-1 and A-2, to reduce the concentration of low density lipoprotein (LDL) cholesterol,[27,51,52] to reduce the aggregability of blood platelets,[53] to decrease the concentration of fibrinogen[54] and to increase the activity of the fibrinolytic system,[55] all of which would tend to reduce the risk of myocardial infarction and vascular disease in general. In contrast to these benefits, moderate amounts of ethanol increase blood pressure, but there seems to be a threshold for this effect at about two American or three British drinks a day.[25,56]

There is, in contrast, no experimental evidence to show that any particular alcoholic beverage has a more beneficial effect on blood constituents or blood pressure than the same amount of ethanol. The idea that antioxidants, or flavenoids, or any other specific constituent of wine has an additional benefit is entirely speculative, as is the idea that red wine is more beneficial than white wine. In the only epidemiological study that I know of that sought to compare the effects of different types of wine, Klatsky and Armstrong[42] found that the relative risk of cardiovascular mortality in those whose preferred drink was wine compared with the risk in people who preferred spirits, was 0.8 if the wine was red and 0.6 if it was some other type. That red wine may indeed be less beneficial is supported by a small experimental study in which 20 men and women with high blood cholesterol levels were divided into two groups. Half drank 6 ounces of a Cabernet red wine a day for four weeks, then no wine for four weeks, and then the same amount of a Chardonnay white wine for four weeks, while the other half followed the same schedule with the timing of the two wines reversed. There were no significant changes in blood cholesterol concentrations, but the blood concentrations of free radicals (which are thought to oxidise LDL) fell by 15% with red wine and 34% with white wine and platelet aggregability fell respectively by 10% and 20%.[57]

Conclusion

I conclude that there is no specific benefit associated with one type of alcoholic beverage, but that the benefit from all types derives from the content of ethanol and that the extra benefit that has been associated with wine in some studies can be accounted for by differences in the pattern of drinking, with wine being characteristically drunk in relatively small amounts most days, rather than in large amounts on one or two days a week.

Implications for public health

The conclusion that a certain amount of alcohol can have a beneficial effect on personal health, decreasing mortality from some major conditions to such an extent that it more than compensates for an increased mortality from other conditions, greatly complicates the formation of public health policy. Before a beneficial effect was appreciated, policy could, and generally did, aim to discourage drinking altogether. Policies aimed solely at reducing heavy drinking had little success and the most effective means of reducing alcohol abuse seemed to be a policy aimed at reducing the average amount consumed by the population as a whole, something that could readily be achieved by increasing taxation.

Precisely what public health policy should now be, will not be the same in all communities, for the importance of vascular thrombosis, which may be alleviated by alcohol, and of trauma, which may be increased by it, vary enormously not only with age and sex but also from one country to another.

TABLE 2.6—*Ratio of deaths from ischaemic heart disease and violence (less war) in different populations by sex*

Population	Ratio of deaths in 1990	
	Males	Females
Developed countries:		
Market economies	2.7	5.2
Former socialist	1.8	10.0
India	1.3	1.3
Other Asia and islands	0.87	2.6
Middle East	0.75	1.6
China	0.40	0.48
Sub-Saharan Africa	0.17	0.47
World	1.0	2.0

After Murray and Lopez.[36]

This is shown in table 2.6 which gives for each sex the variation in the ratio of the number of deaths attributed to ischaemic heart disease and the number attributed to violence in different parts of the world, omitting only deaths attributed to the operation of war. The ratio varies more than 10-fold from the market economies of the developed world (that is, all developed countries other than those in and associated with the old USSR) to the countries of Africa south of the Sahara, from 2.7 to one to 0.17 to one in men and from 5.2 to one to 0.47 to one in women. The balance of benefit and harm from the consumption of alcohol must therefore be very different in different countries and policies that might be good in one country could well be disastrous in another.

But even in the United Kingdom, where the balance of benefit and risk summed over the whole population is strongly in favour of benefit, this is not the only consideration. For policy also has to take into account the effect on other people of intoxication and chronic alcoholism and indeed the effect of drinking quite small amounts in the handling of vehicles and machinery. As I have not attempted to quantify these effects, it would not be appropriate to suggest how national policy in this country should now be formulated in its entirety. I believe, however, that people should be treated as adults and that they should know the facts. These still need to be refined in detail, but in broad outline they are quite clear—that is, that over about 45 years of age some small amount of alcohol within the range of one to three drinks each day is positively good for you, irrespective of the medium in which it is taken.

Envoi

When I chose the benefits of wine as the title of this lecture, I did not expect to conclude that wine was specifically more beneficial than other alcoholic beverages. I chose it, because I wanted to draw attention to Cochrane's work as an epidemiologist and because I thought that Cochrane would have wanted me to discuss some subject of present interest relevant to the practical prevention of disease. Cochrane's observation that wine consumption was negatively correlated in national vital statistics with the mortality from ischaemic heart disease and that wine consumption alone could account for the negative correlation with the consumption of alcohol led to a revival of interest in the possible beneficial effects of alcohol. It has not been possible to prove that alcohol does have such effects by means of a randomised controlled trial, nor do I think that any such trials are likely to be carried out in the future, because of the practical and ethical difficulties to which Cochrane drew attention.[2] The beneficial effect is, however, sufficiently well established for the purpose of prevention without randomised trials, as a result of case-control and cohort studies backed up by the results of the sort of physiological experiments that Cochrane proposed.[2]

That the drinking of wine may be more effective than that of beer or spirits in at least some cultures seems likely; but if it is, its special benefit might well be explained by the customary patterns of drinking, with small amounts of wine being characteristically drunk every day rather than large amounts being drunk on one or two days of the week, and so ensuring that the constituents of the blood that contribute to thrombosis, are continually modified, as is achieved by small doses of aspirin taken on alternate days. We can agree with Cochrane, that the medicine is already in a highly palatable form and no-one should be called on to commit "almost a sacrilege" by trying to isolate a specific prophylactic constituent from wine other than ethanol. We can, however, now give with some confidence the information to our friends that he regretted not being able to give in 1979[2]—namely, that the relative effects of red, white, and rosé wine would all seem to be about equal.

Acknowledgement

I should like to express my thanks to Richard Peto, whose friendship with Archie Cochrane was mainly instrumental in obtaining Archie's generous bequest to Green College, who directed our work on the effect of alcohol in British doctors, drew my attention to the remarkable variation in the ratio of ischaemic heart disease and violent deaths in different countries, and, with Rory Collins, provided me with the facilities to prepare this paper in their department.

1 Cochrane A. *Effectiveness and efficiency: random reflections on health services.* (2nd ed). London: Nuffield Provincial Hospitals Trust, 1989.
2 Cochrane AL, St. Leger AS, Moore F. Health service "input" and mortality "output" in developed countries. *J Epidemiol Community Health* 1978;**32**:200–5.
3 St Leger AS, Cochrane AL, Moore F. Factors associated with cardiac mortality in developed countries with particular reference to the consumption of wine. *Lancet* 1979;i: 1017–20.
4 Keys A, Anderson JT, Grande F. Prediction of serum-cholesterol responses of man to changes in fats in the diet. *Lancet* 1957;ii:959–66.
5 Pearl R. *Alcohol and longevity.* New York: Alfred A Knopf, 1926.
6 Yano K, Rhoads GC, Kagan A. Coffee, alcohol and risk of coronary heart disease among men living in Hawaii. *N Engl J Med* 1977;**297**:405–9.
7 McMichael J. French wine and death certificates. *Lancet* 1979;i:1186–7.
8 St Leger AS, Cochrane AL, Moore F. Ischaemic heart disease and wine. *Lancet* 1979;i: 1294.
9 Slater NGP. Ischaemic heart disease and wine or garlic. *Lancet* 1979;i:1294.
10 Tyrrell M. Ischaemic heart disease and wine or garlic. *Lancet* 1979;i:1294.
11 Segall JJ. Ischaemic heart disease and wine or milk. *Lancet* 1979;i:1294.
12 Rao LG. French wine and death certificates. *Lancet* 1979;i:1187.
13 Shaper AG, Wannamethee G, Walker M. Alcohol and mortality: explaining the U-shaped curve. *Lancet* 1988;ii:1268–73.
14 Klatsky AL, Armstrong MA, Friedman GD. Risk of cardiovascular mortality in alcohol drinkers, ex-drinkers and non-drinkers. *Am J Cardiol* 1990;**66**:1237–43.
15 Doll R, Peto R, Hall E, Wheatley K, Gray R. Mortality in relation to consumption of alcohol: 13 years' observations on male British doctors. *BMJ* 1994;**309**:911–18.
16 Boffeta P, Garfinkel L. Alcohol drinking and mortality among men enrolled in an American Cancer Society prospective study. *Epidemiology* 1990;**1**:342–8.
17 Cohen S, Tyrrell DAJ, Russell MAH, Jarvis MJ, Smith AP. Smoking, alcohol consumption, and susceptibility to the common cold. *Am J Public Health* 1993;**83**:1277–83.

18 Desenclos J-CA, Klontz KC, Wilder MH, Gunn RA. The protective effect of alcohol on the occurrence of oyster-borne hepatitis A. *Epidemiology* 1992;**3**:371–4.
19 Thornton J, Heaton K, Syme S. Moderate alcohol intake reduces bile cholesterol saturation and raises HDL cholesterol. *Lancet* 1986;ii:819–21.
20 Colditz GA. A prospective assessment of moderate alcohol intake and major chronic diseases. *Ann Epidemiol* 1990;**1**:167–77.
21 English DR, Holman CDJ, Milne E, *et al. The quantification of drug caused morbidity and mortality in Australia 1995*. Canberra: AGPS, 1995.
22 Rimm EB, Stampfer MJ, Colditz GA, Willett WC. Prospective study of cigarette smoking, alcohol use, and the risk of diabetes in men. *BMJ* 1995;**310**:555–9.
23 Mayer EJ, Newman B, Queensberry C, Friedman GD, Selby JV. Alcohol consumption and insulin concentrations: role of insulin in associations of alcohol intake with high density lipoprotein cholesterol and triglycerides. *Circulation* 1993;**88**:2190–7.
24 Felson DT, Zhang Y, Hannan MJ, Kannel WB, Kiel DP. Alcohol intake and bone mineral density in elderly men and women. *Am J Epidemiol* 1995;**142**:485–92.
25 Doll R, Peto R, Hall E, Wheatley K, Gray R. Vascular mortality and the consumption of alcohol among male British doctors: effect of confounding factors. *Eur Heart J* 1966 (in press).
26 Edwards G, Anderson P, Babor TF, Casswell S, Ferrence R, Giesbrecht N, *et al. Alcohol policy and the public good.* Oxford: Oxford University Press, 1994.
27 Poikolainen K. Alcohol and mortality: a review. *J Clin Epidemiol* 1995;**488**:445–65.
28 Kivelä S-L, Nissinen A, Ketola A, Punsar S, Puska P, Karvonen M. Alcohol consumption and mortality in aging or aged Finnish men. *J Clin Epidemiol* 1989;**19**:923–30.
29 Farchi G, Fidanza F, Mariott S, Menotti A. Alcohol and mortality in the Italian rural cohorts of the Seven Countries Study. *Int J Epidemiol* 1992;**21**:74–82.
30 MacMahon S, Peto R, Cutler J, Collins R, Sorlie P, Neaton J, *et al.* Blood pressure, stroke, and coronary heart disease. Part 1, prolonged differences in blood pressure: prospective observational studies corrected for the regression dilution bias. *Lancet* 1990; **335**:765–74.
31 Pernanen K. Validity of survey data on alcohol use. In: Gibbens RJ, Israel Y, Kalant H, Popham RE, Schmidt W, Smart RG, eds. *Recent advances in alcohol and drug problems.* New York: Wiley, 1974:355–74.
32 Polich JM. Epidemiology of alcohol abuse in military and civilian populations. *Am J Publ Health* 1981;**71**:1125–32.
33 Simpura J. *Finnish drinking habits: results from interview surveys held in 1968, 1976 and 1985.* Helsinki: Finnish Foundation for alcohol studies, 1987.
34 Garfinkel L, Boffeta P, Stellman D. Alcohol and breast cancer: a cohort study. *Prev Med* 1988;**17**:686–93.
35 Grønbaek M, Deis A, Sørensen TIA, Becker U, Schnohr P, Jensen G. Mortality associated with moderate intakes of wine, beer, or spirits. *Lancet* 1995;**310**:1165–9.
36 Murray CJL, Lopez AD. Global and regional cause of death patterns in 1990. *Global comparative assessments in the health sector.* Geneva: World Health Organisation, 1994.
37 Andréasson S, Romelsjo A, Allebeck P. Alcohol and mortality among young men: longitudinal study of Swedish conscripts. *BMJ* 1988;**296**:1021–5.
38 Colditz GA, Branch LG, Lipnick RJ, Willett WC, Rosner B, Posner B, Hennekens C. Moderate alcohol and decreased cardiovascular mortality in an elderly cohort. *Am Heart J* 1985;**198**:886–9.
39 Montaigne M. Essais de Messire Michel Seigneur de Montaigne Chevalier de l'Ordre du Roy et Gentilhomme Ordinaire de sa chambre. Translated by EJ Trechmann and entitled *The Essays of Montaigne.* Oxford: Oxford University Press, 1595.
40 Dean G, Lee PN, Todd GF, Wicken AJ. *Tobacco Research Council paper No 14, part 1.* London: Tobacco Research Council, 1977.
41 Rosenberg L, Slone D, Shapiro S, Kaufman DW, Miettinen OS, Stolley PD. Alcoholic beverages and myocardial infarction in young women. *Am J Public Health* 1981;**71**:82–5.
42 Klatsky AL, Armstrong MA. Alcoholic beverage choice and risk of coronary heart disease mortality: do red wine drinkers fare best? *Am J Cardiol* 1993;**71**:467–9.

43 Stampfer MJ, Colditz GA, Willett WC, Speizer FE, Hennekens CH. A prospective study of moderate alcohol consumption and the risk of coronary artery disease and stroke in women. *N Engl J Med* 1988;**319**:267–73.
44 Friedman LA, Kimball AQW. Coronary heart disease mortality and alcohol consumption in Framingham. *Am J Epidemiol* 1986;**124**:481–9.
45 Hennekens CH, Willett W, Rosner B, Cole DS, Mayrent SL. Effects of wine, beer, and liquor in coronary deaths. *JAMA* 1979;**242**:1973–4.
46 Gaziano JM, Godfried S, Breslow JL, Hennekens CH, Buring JE. Alcoholic beverage type and risk of myocardial infarction [abstract]. *Circulation* 1995;**92**:(suppl 1):800.
47 Kozararevic D, McGee D, Vojvodic N, Radic Z, Dawber T, Gordon T, *et al.* Frequency of alcohol consumption and morbidity and mortality. *Lancet* 1980;i:613–16.
48 Rimm MJ. Prospective study of alcohol consumption and risk of coronary disease in men. *Lancet* 1991;**338**:464–8.
49 Salonen JT, Puska P, Nissenen A. Intake of spirits and beer and risk of myocardial infarction and death. A longitudinal study in eastern Finland. *J Chron Dis* 1983;**36**:533–43.
50 Jackson R, Scragg R, Beaglehole R. Does recent alcohol consumption reduce the risk of acute myocardial infarction and coronary death in regular drinkers? *Am J Epidemiol* 1992; **136**:819–24.
51 Castelli WP, Doyle JT, Gordon T, Hames CG, Hjortland MC, Hulley SB, *et al.* Alcohol and blood lipids—the co-operative lipoprotein phenotyping study. *Lancet* 1977;ii:153–5.
52 Haskell WL, Camargo C, Williams PT, Vranizan KM, Krauss RM, Lindgren FT, Wood PD. The effect of cessation and resumption of moderate alcohol intake on serum high density lipoprotein sub-fractions: a controlled study. *N Engl J Med* 1984;**310**:805–10.
53 Renaud S, McGregor L, Martin JL. Influence of alcohol on platelet functions in relation to atherosclerosis. In: Pizza G *et al*, eds. *Diet, diabetes and atherosclerosis.* New York: Raven Press, 1986:177–87.
54 Meade TW, Ineson JD, Stirling Y. Effects of changes in smoking and other characteristics on clotting factors and the risk of ischaemic heart disease. *Lancet* 1987;ii:986–88.
55 Hendriks HF, Veenstra J, Wierik EJMV, Schaafsma G, Kluft C. Effect of moderate dose of alcohol with evening meal on fibrinolytic factors. *BMJ* 1994;**308**:1003–6.
56 Criqui MH. Alcohol and hypertension: new insights from population studies. *Eur Heart J* 1987;**8**(suppl B):73–85.
57 University of California, Berkeley. Is only red wine fine? *UC Berkeley Wellness Letter*, February 1996:3.

3: The epidemiology of asthma

MICHAEL BURR

Introduction

Everyone who had the good fortune to work with Archie Cochrane was impressed by his capacity for original thinking. This constantly led him to look at old problems in new ways, to challenge accepted opinions, and to devise fresh lines of approach. He then proceeded to put his ideas into action with immense enthusiasm and energy. There are two techniques for which he will always be remembered as a pioneer who left a permanent impression on medical science, and both have been very useful in clarifying the epidemiology of asthma.

Field epidemiology

Firstly, he demonstrated the value and principles of field epidemiology in the investigation of disease. He undertook large surveys in south Wales and elsewhere, examining the prevalence of coal miners' pneumoconiosis and other diseases. He later wrote, "We tended originally rather to despise cross-sectional studies and to consider them only as base lines for follow up studies. Looking back we probably underestimated them. They have been of considerable value in: (1) defining the size of a problem . . .; (2) establishing average values, for different age-sex groups . . .; (3) comparing the prevalence of the same condition in different areas . . .; (4) producing unexpected associations which start new lines of research; (5) testing the validity of syndromes."[1]

He particularly drew attention to the biases that arise from a low response rate, a defect from which his surveys were notably free: "In general, the acceptance rate is about 98% for surveys completed on "captive populations"; on random samples in the home or for those carried out at a centre in the area, it is 90%, and 88% if the people are examined at a hospital some distance away."

The cross sectional surveys led on to follow up studies in which he endeavoured to obtain information about all the original participants and see all the survivors after intervals of up to 40 years. Again, Cochrane achieved exceptionally high response rates. He wrote, "our follow-up studies have been of value in the following ways: (1) In describing the factors influencing the natural history of a disease or condition . . .; (2) in describing the factors influencing the appearance of a disease . . .; (3) in validating classifications . . .; (4) by random allocation to investigate the effect of varying some factor on the attack rate or progression rate of some disease . . ."[1]

His field surveys of pneumoconiosis and tuberculosis covered other common conditions, including asthma, partly because of "the realization that if you are studying pulmonary disability you must study all common pulmonary and cardiac conditions"[2], and partly out of simple opportunism.

Randomised controlled trials

Secondly, he was a pioneer of what is now called "evidence based medicine", championing the use of the randomised controlled trial. His monograph *Effectiveness and efficiency* dwelt particularly on the value of this technique ("a very beautiful technique, of wide applicability") in evaluating medical evidence. He pointed out that it could be used in a wide variety of situations, by no means limited to comparisons between different drugs, although these have the advantage of allowing a "double blind" design that eliminates some of the possibility of bias. He lamented the way in which medical interventions have become established without a trial being conducted, so that it is then regarded as unethical for a trial to be set up. The only safeguard in his opinion was to randomise the first patient whenever a new treatment was introduced.

The publication of Cochrane's monograph undoubtedly contributed to the recognition of the importance of this technique and enhanced its popularity as a research method. With the rise in the number of published trials it became clear that there was a need for trials to be systematically documented and reviewed, and in consequence the Cochrane Collaboration was set up. Randomised trials dealing with asthma are reviewed by the Cochrane Airways Group.

The measurement of ill health

Cochrane believed that the population survey and the randomised trial were important techniques in the measurement of ill health. "As a medical student I was taught that there was a simple dichotomy between ill and healthy people, and it was not until I started, with my colleagues, measuring the quantitative characteristics of random samples of the people living in the Rhondda Fach and the Vale of Glamorgan, that I learned that there was nearly always a continuum and no dichotomy".[3] He then asked what criteria should determine the point in the distribution that defines ill health, and suggested that for treatable disease it should be the point where treatment begins to do more good than harm. This point can be found only by means of randomised trials applied to persons who occupy regions of the distribution where there is some uncertainty about the value of treatment.

Asthma epidemiology under Cochrane

From 1960 to 1974 Cochrane was the director of the MRC Epidemiology Unit in south Wales. Towards the end of this period a programme was drawn up for work on the epidemiology of asthma, to comprise field surveys and randomised trials. Surveys were conducted in 12 year old schoolchildren and 20–44 year old adults, investigating the relationship between a history of wheezing and diagnosed asthma in these age groups.[4–5] These surveys were repeated 15–20 years later, when it was found that the prevalence of asthma had risen (see below). The randomised trials were set up to test the hypothesis that reducing exposure to the house dust mite would improve the symptoms of asthma in mite sensitive patients. It had been claimed that antimite measures were so effective that a controlled trial was unnecessary and impractical, but under Cochrane's encouragement a series of trials were conducted which showed that much of the supposed benefits were attributable to a placebo effect plus regression to the mean.

Mortality

Although it is a common disease, asthma is seldom fatal; each year it accounts for less than 300 deaths in England and Wales among persons under 35 years of age. Above this age the death rate starts to rise, so that most asthma deaths occur over the age of 65 years. It is more difficult to distinguish asthma from other respiratory conditions in infants and elderly people than in children and young adults, so that comparative studies of death rates tend to focus on people aged 5–34 years. Figure 3.1 shows mortality rates for this age group since 1951. The most striking feature is the sharp rise that occurred in the 1960s. After a few years the death rate declined rapidly to previous levels and has remained fairly constant since then. One curious change (as yet unexplained) is that since the "epidemic"

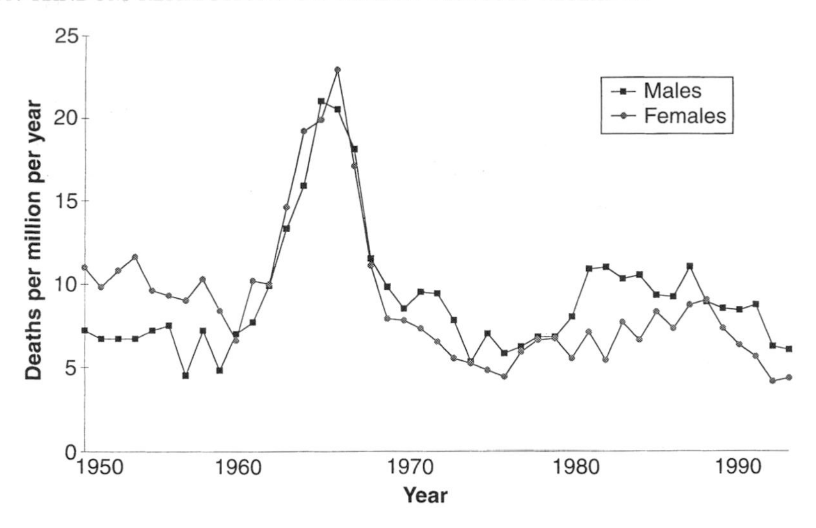

FIG 3.1—*Asthma deaths in England and Wales for persons aged 5–34 years (constructed from data published by the Office of Population Censuses and Surveys).*

the death rate has been higher in males, whereas previously it was consistently higher in females.

There has been some controversy about the cause of this epidemic. It was observed at the time that its onset coincided with the introduction of high dose isoprenaline aerosols, and that the epidemic did not occur in countries where these aerosols were not used. It was therefore suggested that the epidemic was caused by overdosage of sympathomimetic drugs, presumably by means of a cardiotoxic effect. The dangers of overuse were widely publicised, and the asthma death rate then declined. There were, however, some anomalies in the epidemiological evidence that caused some doubt to be cast on this explanation. An alternative hypothesis is that sympathomimetic drugs induce a false sense of security; they may be more effective in relieving symptoms than in overcoming anoxia during a severe attack, so that the patient fails to summon help. Either way, it seems likely that the rise in mortality was attributable (directly or indirectly) to the treatment.

In several other countries the asthma death rate rose more gradually. In New Zealand a second epidemic occurred in the 1970s and 1980s, in which the mortality rate became unusually high. This has been attributed to the use of the β_2 agonist fenoterol, although there is a certain amount of disagreement on the matter. But it is clear that the relationship between benefit and risk is not simple, and it is not always easy to find the point at which treatment begins to do more good than harm. This issue will be dealt with in more detail below.

Prevalence

To measure prevalence it is first necessary to define the condition in question; you cannot count the number of cases until you have decided what constitutes a case. This is rather difficult in relation to asthma. It is no exception to Cochrane's rule that most diseases are at one end of a continuous distribution, so that it is somewhat arbitrary as to where the line should be drawn that separates asthmatics from non-asthmatics. The point at which treatment begins to do more good than harm would be the ideal criterion in clinical practice, but this point is not self evident (see below); furthermore, in epidemiological surveys a "working definition" is needed that is suitable for rapid application to populations. Various tests have been used, including symptom questionnaires, clinical examinations, and bronchial challenge tests. It is difficult to assess the validity of these criteria in the absence of a "gold standard" agreed definition of asthma, and different surveys have used different working definitions, so that their findings cannot easily be compared. The most useful evidence on prevalence derives from the use of the same survey technique in populations in different places or at different times. Certain findings have consistently emerged from prevalence studies. The prevalence is highest in childhood—about 10% of 12 year olds have been diagnosed as asthmatic and have wheezed in the past 12 months. At adolescence it declines and then remains fairly constant during adult life. Virtually all surveys show that the disease is more common in boys than in girls, but the prevalence is roughly similar in men and women. Incidence is highest in children under five years of age, but the disease can begin at any time, even in old age.

Geographical variations

One of the values that Cochrane saw in cross sectional surveys was in "comparing the prevalence of the same condition in different areas and different countries".[1] There is of course a body of data, collected more or less routinely, that might be expected to reflect differences in prevalence: death rates, hospital admissions, general practitioner consultations, prescription data, and certified sickness absence. For various reasons such sources are not a very reliable guide to geographical variations in a condition such as asthma. Most cases are fairly mild, so that the death rate and admissions to hospital do not give any information about most patients with the disease. The use of medical services and sickness absence are influenced by social factors, so that they could show variations between different areas where the prevalence of the disease was really the same. Moreover, since asthma is part of a continuum between health and disease (and is not sharply distinguishable from other diseases), there is a "grey area" of people who would be told that they have asthma by one doctor but not by another, producing artificial differences in prevalence. The only way to be sure of obtaining reliable comparative data is to conduct a survey of the whole population (or a specific age group) in each area, using identical methods. This is a laborious procedure, but it has proved to be of immense value in revealing real differences which suggest lines of investigation into possible causative and protective factors.

One example of this approach is a survey comparing children in different parts of Zimbabwe.[6] Using exercise provocation as an objective test, asthma was found to be equally common in white and black children from the more affluent homes, less common in poor urban black children, and very uncommon in poor rural black children. It seems that the disease is related to urban residence and high living standards but not to ethnic type. Surveys in German children showed a higher prevalence of diagnosed asthma, bronchial hyperreactivity, hay fever, and atopy (as defined by positive skin tests) in west Germany compared with east Germany, although some respiratory symptoms occurred more often in the east. The hypothesis has been put forward that higher living standards in the west promote allergic sensitisation, whereas industrial pollution in the east causes more bronchitis there.[7]

The need for standardised survey methods for identifying asthma has led to the construction of two questionnaires—one for children and one for adults—which are being used in large international surveys, the International Study of Asthma and Allergy in Childhood (ISAAC), and the European Community Respiratory Health Survey. These surveys allow comparisons to be made across a very wide range of countries. With hindsight, it seems strange that it has taken so long for such methods to be devised and become widely accepted; Cochrane drew attention to the need for reproducible questionnaires in 1951,[8] with the result that in 1960 the Medical Research Council issued a questionnaire for chronic bronchitis which has been used internationally since that time. Questionnaires have their limitations, particularly when translated (there is no exact equivalent of the key word "wheeze" in several languages), but they provide a fairly easy way of detecting any obvious differences, which can then be investigated with the aid of objective tests.

Time trends

There is a general impression that asthma is more common than it used to be, or at least that it is diagnosed and treated more often. Schoolteachers remark on the growing proportion of children who bring inhalers to school. Hospital admissions for asthma rose steeply during the 1970s and 1980s, especially for children; they now seem to have stabilised, but at a much higher level than before. Consultations with general practitioners for asthma and prescriptions for antiasthma medications have increased substantially over recent decades.

The important question is whether these trends arise merely from changes in management and diagnostic labelling, or whether there has been a real increase in the prevalence or severity of the disease. Here again, only the field survey can provide the answer. A cross sectional survey of a defined population establishes the size of the problem at one point in time; if it is repeated after a suitable interval in the same area, using exactly the same methods as before, and if on each occasion a high response-rate is achieved, any change in prevalence will be revealed. It is particularly important that the methodology be unchanged, and the temptation to improve on the previous questionnaire or technique must be sternly resisted. One example was the repeat, 15 years later, of a survey originally carried out in south Wales under Cochrane's directorship, which showed a rise in diagnosed asthma and in symptoms suggestive of asthma to about the same extent (5% of all children).[9] On each occasion a simple exercise challenge test was performed, which showed a rise in the proportion of children whose peak expiratory flow rates fell markedly on exercise.

Numerous other repeat surveys (25 at the last count), spanning intervals of 10 years or more, have now been conducted in various parts of the world, and in each case an increase in asthma prevalence has been demonstrated. The methods used have included questionnaires, clinical examinations, and various types of provocation tests; although any one of these studies might be suspected of bias or the play of chance, it is very difficult to see how such explanations could suffice in every case. What is particularly striking is the worldwide nature of the increase: it has been reported in several European countries and in Australia, New Zealand, the United States, Taiwan, Hong Kong, and Japan. Other atopic conditions such as eczema and hay fever seem to have increased over the same period. The cause of the rise in asthma (assuming that it is real) must therefore be something that operates all over the world. The identity of this mysterious factor is much debated, and possible candidates include the following:

(1) *A greater exposure to allergens*—The house dust mite is the major allergen that provokes asthma in many countries, and it is likely that recent changes in housing (central heating, fitted carpets, draught proofing, etc) are favourable to mite infestation. It is rather difficult to obtain evidence on this point, since there have been few surveys of mite concentrations, and in the absence of information about levels in the past it is impossible to know whether they have risen. Two Australian surveys conducted 10 years apart showed a fivefold rise in mite counts and increases in the prevalence of wheeze and of bronchial hyperreactivity,[10] but it cannot be assumed that the same trend has

occurred in countries with very different climates and cultures. Furthermore, it is not obvious how a greater exposure to mites could have caused a rise in the prevalence of hay fever.

(2) *More air pollution*—Although there is no doubt that episodes of severe air pollution aggravate asthma, it is not clear whether the degree of pollution common in western countries has an important effect on the disease. Most forms of pollution have in fact declined in Britain during recent decades, but it is possible that certain pollutants that are increasing (for example, those in vehicle exhaust fumes) exacerbate or even cause asthma.[11] But it is difficult to see how pollution can have caused the rise in asthma in New Zealand or the high prevalence in the highlands of Scotland.[12]

(3) *Better hygiene*—Several surveys have shown a higher prevalence of asthma, hay fever, or atopy in firstborn children than in others, and it has been postulated that infections in early life (which firstborn children are less likely to acquire) protect against allergic disease. There is a certain attraction about the notion of "immunological hooliganism" (the immunological system turning upon itself for want of its natural prey), but the evidence is sparse. If this were the explanation, a clear social class gradient in asthma prevalence might be expected, but no such gradient exists. It is intriguing to speculate what kind of trial Cochrane would have designed to test this hypothesis.

(4) *Diet*—Various theories have been put forward linking the increase in asthma with some dietary change. Mixed feeding in early infancy has been associated with subsequent allergy in some studies but not others. Salt intake is another possibility; it has probably increased in most countries, and salt has been shown to affect bronchial reactivity in some people. Food additives have been suspected of causing allergies, but only a small proportion of asthmatics seem to be sensitive to them.

Causation

The aetiology of asthma may be considered firstly in relation to the factors that decide why one person acquires the disease and another does not, and secondly in relation to the factors that provoke symptoms in patients who are already asthmatic.

Risk factors

The factors that are associated with the acquisition of asthma are detected by cohort studies, those starting at or soon after birth being particularly useful. As asthma is a common disease, with a peak annual incidence of about 1% in children up to the age of 5 years, birth cohort studies yield results in a reasonably short time. A strong hereditary element is nearly always obvious, probably due to a genetic predisposition to atopic disease. Several studies have shown that evidence of atopy (positive skin tests, raised serum IgE, eczema, or hay fever) precedes and predicts the onset of asthma. Other possible risk factors have been suggested by some studies but not confirmed by others; they include low birth weight, maternal smoking, season of birth, bottle feeding in infancy, exposure to the house dust mite, and pet ownership.

Prevention

Although we may never be sure about the reason for the rise in asthma prevalence, and the evidence from cohort studies is somewhat confusing, it is still worthwhile testing hypotheses relating to prevention. As asthma and other atopic conditions run in families, it is fairly easy to identify high risk children even before they are born by obtaining a family history. Potential preventive measures can then be tested in these children by means of randomised controlled trials.

Such trials have been conducted, testing the effect of avoiding various allergens. Most have involved excluding various factors from the mother's diet during pregnancy and lactation and from the child's diet in early infancy. On the whole, these studies have been rather disappointing, perhaps partly because of the difficulty of maintaining compliance. One of the few trials that have shown an effect was conducted in the Isle of Wight and addressed ingested and inhaled allergens.[13] The infants in the intervention group received either breast milk from mothers (who were on an exclusion diet) or an extensively hydrolysed formula; furthermore, their bedrooms and living rooms were subjected to antimite measures, including acaricide treatment. The incidence of asthma was reduced during the first year of life; by the age of two years the reduction in asthma was no longer significant, although there was still a lower prevalence of any allergy in the intervention group. When the children have been followed up for a longer time it will become clear whether allergen avoidance prevented or merely deferred the onset of asthma. The relative value of the dietary restrictions and the removal of mites will need to be investigated in further studies. Meanwhile, a systematic review is being conducted under the auspices of the Cochrane Airways Group to collate the existing evidence from randomised trials, so that a clearer picture should emerge of the value of allergen avoidance in preventing asthma.

Provoking factors

Asthmatic patients know that their attacks are provoked by definite situations, and in most cases they can be shown to be allergic to specific allergens. The relative importance of different allergens can be assessed by the proportion of asthmatics who have positive skin tests to the various extracts. In Britain and many other countries the major allergens are house dust mites, grass pollen, and cats. The effect of eradicating mites from the domestic environment has been tested by randomised trials, which are quite difficult to conduct; if mite allergen can be removed, there is usually an improvement in the patient's condition, but the inconvenience may not be thought worthwhile. It is scarcely feasible to avoid grass pollen, and no-one seems to have tried to set up a trial of cat avoidance—in any case, the antigen is ubiquitous in cat loving populations. Non-allergic provoking factors include respiratory infections, exercise, emotion, cold air, and other irritants.

Natural history

Asthma and other conditions

Cochrane showed the value of epidemiological surveys in testing the validity of syndromes and in validating the classification of diseases. He pointed out that misleading conclusions may be drawn from studies of patients who have been selected by attending clinics; the true relationship between various clinical features can be found only by surveys that provide "a complete unselected population of a particular disease group whose characteristics can then be compared with a proper control group—and by "proper" control group we mean a group, free of the disease in question, of the same age and sex constitution as the group with the disease, chosen by some random process from the same population as that of the diseased group".[2] This issue can be illustrated by the relationship between asthma and other respiratory diseases.

In childhood, there is some uncertainty as to whether asthma should be regarded as distinct from or continuous with wheezy bronchitis. Studies of patients admitted to hospital or attending clinics inevitably omit children with mild symptoms, who form the majority of children who wheeze. To obtain a true picture of the whole spectrum of wheezing disease it is necessary to conduct population surveys. In favour of the view that all wheezing disorders are basically the same condition, an Australian survey showed that, if asthma is defined as wheezing that sometimes occurs in the absence of a cold, wheezy non-asthmatic children are intermediate between asthmatics and non-wheezers in respect of several clinical features.[14] Furthermore, it is not disputed that asthma (however defined) is underdiagnosed, so that many wheezy children would be diagnosed as asthmatic if they were properly investigated. On the other hand, there is some evidence that there are at least two distinct disease entities. In a survey in Southampton, wheeze was not related to bronchial hyperresponsiveness in the absence of atopy, nor to atopy in the absence of hyperresponsiveness, but it was strongly related to the combination of the two.[15] An American cohort study suggested that persistence of wheezing from infancy to childhood is associated with allergy (as shown by serum IgE and skin tests) and maternal asthma, whereas non-persistent early wheezing is linked with maternal smoking and poorer lung function in infancy.[16] It seems likely that asthma has a distinct pathogenesis from other wheezy conditions in childhood, although they are difficult to distinguish in individual patients because both are triggered by respiratory infections.

There is a similar controversy about the classification of chronic respiratory disease in adults. According to the "Dutch hypothesis", asthma, chronic bronchitis, and emphysema should be considered as different expressions of one disease entity, "chronic non-specific lung disease",[17] but outside the Dutch speaking world the opinion has persisted that asthma is quite a distinct condition.[18] Both views are based on population based epidemiological surveys, and it seems strange that the issue has not been resolved after 35 years of applying Cochrane's principles to it. Burrows[19] believes that the apparent conflict of evidence can be explained by differences in the populations in which the surveys were conducted. The Dutch studies were conducted in small towns where heavy smoking was uncommon, particularly among women, so that the relative importance of an "asthmatic constitution" (a predisposition to allergy and bronchial responsiveness) was much greater than in British surveys that included many heavy smokers. Cross sectional and follow up studies in Tucson (USA) suggest that there are at least two different types of chronic airflow obstruction in the local population, one characterised by typical asthmatic symptoms and allergy, and the other (with a much worse prognosis) associated with a history of smoking but not with allergy. Curiously enough, a subject's belief that he or she had asthma was an excellent way of distinguishing the first of these conditions: excluding these subjects from the analysis removed any relationship of forced expiratory volume in one second (FEV_1) to skin sensitivity, eosinophilia, or serum IgE. Similar observations have been made by other investigators.

Course and prognosis

To obtain information about the course of the disease, and the factors that influence it, a prospective study is required. It is important to select a population based cohort so as to represent the whole spectrum of the disease; a group of patients attending a clinic is much easier to identify but will be relatively uninformative about mild asthma. The British National Child Development Study is the follow up of a cohort of all people in Britain who were born during one week in 1958, and has yielded information about the onset and course of asthma by periodic interviews with parents or subjects up to the age of 33 years.[20] Maternal smoking during pregnancy predicted incidence after the age of 16 years more strongly than during childhood. Among children who had asthma or wheezy bronchitis in their first seven years of life, there was a tendency for the disease to remit during adolescence but then to recur after the age of 23 years, especially in atopic subjects and current smokers. Other studies have followed up cohorts of children identified as having asthma or wheezy disease (usually at the age of 7) in population surveys. They tend to show that children with more severe disease and those with other evidence of atopy have a greater risk of asthma in adult life.

Effects of treatment

The treatment of asthma has two main components, comprising "reliever" and "preventer" drugs. The relievers are inhaled bronchodilators, usually β_2 agonists, which are taken when symptoms occur or are expected in the immediate future (for example, if the patient is about to take vigorous exercise). The preventers are antiinflammatory drugs, usually inhaled corticosteroids. Current guidelines advocate the use of both types of drug with the objective of reducing symptoms to the minimum or abolishing them completely. There is no doubt about the effectiveness of these drugs, but anxieties have arisen as to possible adverse effects, and it is not at all clear how to apply Cochrane's criterion of the point at which benefit begins to exceed harm.

So far as the β_2 agonists are concerned, there are two anxieties. One of these relates to a possible cardiotoxic effect and has already been mentioned in relation to asthma mortality. Case-control studies in New Zealand have shown an association between the use of inhaled fenoterol and death from asthma,[21] the mechanism may be a tendency to provoke cardiac arrhythmia in the presence of hypoxaemia. The other anxiety is that these drugs may inhibit the natural antiinflammatory mechanism in the lungs; furthermore, the bronchodilating effect increases the antigen load to the smaller airways.[22] If mild bronchoconstriction is a defence mechanism that reduces the access of antigenic particles to the lower airways, abolishing symptoms may actually be harmful, and there is some evidence to support this view.

Inhaled steroids have short term side effects that are fairly obvious and reversible, such as dysphonia and oropharyngeal candidiasis. There may be chronic effects that are less apparent and more serious. There is a growing body of evidence that bone metabolism is affected, with a consequent loss of bone density and (in children) impairment of growth.[23–24] Whether and to what extent the risk of fractures is raised is unknown, but the possibility cannot be ignored. The incidence of fractured neck of the femur in elderly people is already high and rising; anything that could increase it still further must be taken very seriously. Other potential risks include cataracts and psychiatric disturbances.[23] Repeat prescriptions of inhaled steroids tend to be issued indefinitely, and there is now a cohort of people who have been using these preparations for several years and are likely to continue with them into old age.

There is plainly a need for these potential risks to be investigated so as to relate them to the benefits of treatment. Effects that might appear over the course of a year or two could be examined by means of a randomised controlled trial comparing two principles of asthma management: minimising symptoms *versus* minimising drug usage. This suggestion was once put to a group of general practitioners. They all agreed that such a trial should be done, as long as it was in other doctors' patients. Understandably, they were more nervous about the danger of accusations of neglect than about the possibility of harm caused by treatment. In any case, it would scarcely be feasible to compare longer term risks and benefits in this way. The best approach is probably to utilise existing variations in medical practice, as advocated by McPherson.[25] There is still a considerable degree of heterogeneity in asthma management, and a comparison between the outcomes of different doctors' methods of treatment might be very instructive. It may well be the case that the benefit to the patient of abolishing or minimising symptoms far outweighs any long-term risk, but some attempt should be made to see whether this is really so.

Summary and conclusions

Asthma is a common disease, but most cases are mild, so that only a minority of asthmatic patients attend hospital, and many are not even treated by a doctor. In consequence, the clinical picture can be understood only by means of field surveys in the population at large. Such surveys have been very useful in elucidating the size of the problem, the relationship of asthma to other conditions, and its relative prevalence in different places and at different times. The prevalence has risen in many countries during recent decades, for reasons that are not understood. Geographical comparisons suggest that environmental factors are important, including a "western" lifestyle. Allergy to the house dust mite is a major element in the causation of the disease in Britain.

The treatment of the disease has been transformed by the introduction of antiinflammatory drugs, particularly inhaled steroids, which are very effective in preventing attacks. Relief of symptoms is by means of inhaled bronchodilators. There are still uncertainties about possible adverse effects of both types of drug, particularly when treatment continues over many years.

The possibility of preventing asthma is especially attractive. Children at high risk can be identified by their family history, and there is some evidence that early reduction in exposure to allergens may reduce the incidence of the disease. Further randomised trials are needed to investigate this important issue.

Our knowledge of the epidemiology of asthma derives from the application of the principles of epidemiological investigation set out by Cochrane many years ago, in relation to population surveys and randomised controlled trials. Its advance depends on the continued application of these principles. At present it is particularly desirable to know whether the prevalence is still rising, and what environmental factors are associated with the disease, both geographically and for the individual patient. Associations can then be tested by means of randomised controlled trials to see whether they are causative. Ultimately it may be possible to prevent the disease, at least to some extent.

1 Cochrane AL. Rhondda Fach, south Wales. *Milbank Memorial Quarterly* 1965;**43**:326–31.
2 Cochrane AL. The epidemiology of chronic disease in south Wales. *Proceedings of the Royal Society of Medicine* 1956;**49**:261–2.
3 Cochrane AL. The history of the measurement of ill health. *Int J Epidemiol* 1972;**1**:89–92.
4 Burr ML, Eldridge BA, Borysiewicz LK. Peak expiratory flow rates before and after exercise in schoolchildren. *Arch Dis Child* 1974;**49**:923–6.
5 Burr ML, St Leger AS, Bevan C, Merrett TG. A community survey of asthmatic characteristics. *Thorax* 1975;**30**:663–8.
6 Keeley DJ, Neill P, Gallivan S. Comparison of the prevalence of reversible airways obstruction in rural and urban Zimbabwean children. *Thorax* 1991;**46**:549–53.
7 von Mutius E, Martinez FD, Fritzsch C, Nicolai T, Roell G, Thiemann H-H. Prevalence of asthma and atopy in two areas of West and East Germany. *Am J Respir Crit Care Med* 1994;**149**:358–64.
8 Cochrane AL, Chapman PJ, Oldham PD. Observers' errors in taking medical histories. *Lancet* 1951;**i**:1007–9.
9 Burr ML, Butland BK, King S, Vaughan-Williams E. Changes in asthma prevalence: two surveys 15 years apart. *Arch Dis Child* 1989;**64**:1452–6.
10 Peat JK, van den Berg RH, Green WF, Mellis CM, Leeder SR, Woolcock AJ. Changing prevalence of asthma in Australian children. *BMJ* 1994;**308**:1591–6.
11 Wardlaw AJ. The role of air pollution in asthma. *Clin Exp Allergy* 1993;**23**:81–96.
12 Austin JB, Russell G, Adam MG, Mackintosh D, Kelsey S, Peck DF. Prevalence of asthma and wheeze in the highlands of Scotland. *Arch Dis Child* 1994;**71**:211–6.
13 Hide DW, Matthews S, Matthews L, *et al.* Effect of allergen avoidance in infancy on allergic manifestations at age two years. *J Allergy Clin Immunol* 1994;**93**:842–6.
14 Williams H, McNicol KN. Prevalence, natural history, and relationship of wheezy bronchitis and asthma in children. An epidemiological study. *BMJ* 1969;**4**:321–5.
15 Clifford RD, Howell JB, Radford M, Holgate ST. Associations between respiratory symptoms, bronchial response to methacholine, and atopy in two age groups of schoolchildren. *Arch Dis Child* 1989;**64**:1133–9.
16 Martinez FD, Wright AL, Taussig LM, *et al.* Asthma and wheezing in the first six years of life. *N Engl J Med* 1995;**332**:133–8.
17 Sluiter HJ, Koëter GH, de Monchy JGR, Postma DS, de Vries K, Orie NGM. The Dutch hypothesis (chronic non-specific lung disease) revisited. *Eur Respir J* 1991;**4**:479–89.
18 Vermeire PA, Pride NB. A "splitting" look at chronic nonspecific lung disease (CNSLD): common features but diverse pathogenesis. *Eur Respir J* 1991;**4**:490–6.
19 Burrows B. Epidemiologic evidence for different types of chronic airflow obstruction. *Am Rev Respir Dis* 1991;**143**:1452–5.
20 Strachan DP, Butland BK, Anderson HR. Incidence and prognosis of asthma and wheezing illness from early childhood to age 33 in a national British cohort. *BMJ* 1996;**312**:1195–9.

21 Grainger J, Woodman K, Pearce N, *et al.* Prescribed fenoterol and death from asthma in New Zealand, 1981–7: a further case-control study. *Thorax* 1991:**46**:105–11.
22 Page CP. One explanation of the asthma paradox: inhibition of natural anti-inflammatory mechanism by β_2-agonists. *Lancet* 1991;**337**:717–20.
23 Geddes DM. Inhaled corticosteroids: benefits and risks. *Thorax* 1992;**47**:404–7.
24 Doull I, Freezer N, Holgate S. Osteocalcin, growth, and inhaled corticosteroids: a prospective study. *Arch Dis Child* 1996;**74**:497–501.
25 McPherson K. How should health policy be modified by the evidence of medical practice variations? In: Marinker M, ed. *Controversies in health care policies: challenges to practice.* London: BMJ Publishing Group, 1994.

Part 2
Effectiveness

4: So what's so special about randomisation?

JOS KLEIJNEN, PETER GØTZSCHE,
REGINA A KUNZ, ANDY D OXMAN,
IAIN CHALMERS

Why bother to assess the effects of health and social care?

Human beings have a substantial natural capacity to overcome "dis-ease" in many of its various physical, psychological, and social manifestations, and this is often achieved without any assistance from professionals. This "self healing", restorative tendency can be enhanced by social and psychological factors, such as optimism in the affected person; attention, kindness, and encouragement from others; and physical environments which are conducive to recovery.

In helping people to overcome their "dis-ease", effective professionals exploit the restorative effects of these social, psychological, and environmental aspects of care. This is true for professionals from both conventional and complementary medicine. In addition, professionals usually draw on a range of more specific strategies which are supposed to have or are known to have beneficial effects on the natural histories of the various forms of "dis-ease" which lead people to seek professional help. Although these interventions are offered in good faith, most if not all of them have the capacity for causing inadvertent harm as well as intended benefit. With the best of intentions, professionals offering health and social care have often inadvertently harmed those who have turned to them for help.[1–4] At its most extreme, the harm done has been lethal—by social workers[5] as well as by health professionals.[6] Short of death, the adverse effects of well meant professional prescriptions and proscriptions for care have resulted in much non-lethal morbidity and a good deal of misery.

We believe that people seeking help from professionals have a right to expect that formal measures will be taken to assess the relative merits of the various alternative forms of health and social care on offer, be these radical surgery for prostate cancer or custodial sentences for young offenders.

When is formal assessment of care necessary?

There is increasingly wide support for the principle of reliable assessment of the effects of health and social interventions on outcomes that matter to the people to whom they are offered. Debate continues, however, about the methods of assessment that should be used in implementing this principle in practice.[7] Any attempt to evaluate the effects of professional care must necessarily entail some kind of comparison, even if the comparison is an informal one. Occasionally, the effects of professional interventions are so obvious and dramatic that informal comparisons are an adequate basis for strong causal inferences about the effects of care. When the prognosis of the condition in question is known with great confidence, identifying the effects of professional interventions can be straightforward. Examples include identifying the effects of haemostasis in preventing death from exsanguination, the effects of a sensitive social worker who helps an illiterate person to obtain their entitlements through the social security system, the effect of defibrillation in cardiac arrest, and the effect of hip replacement in osteoarthrosis with severe pain and immobility.

In the more common circumstances when the effects of care are less dramatic, steps must be taken to reduce the likelihood that systematic errors (biases) or random errors (the play of chance) in the comparisons made will lead people to conclude either that a form of care is helpful when it is not, or that it is useless or harmful when the reverse is true. It is because these errors may be dangerously misleading that most countries have national drug assessment procedures intended to help protect the public, and it is becoming increasingly accepted that formal assessment should be extended to other interventions in health and social care to try to ensure that they do more good than harm.

How should groups be assembled for formal treatment comparisons?

One of the most important biases that may distort treatment comparisons is that which can result from the way that comparison groups are assembled.[8,9] Comparison groups can be assembled prospectively or retrospectively, concurrently or at different points in time, and consideration has been given to the extent to which each of these methods is likely to be susceptible to bias. Over 30 years ago, two psychologists outlined a hierarchy of methods for assembling comparison groups, based on the assumed reliability of each for making causal inferences.[10] They placed controlled trials with random assignment to experimental groups at the top of the hierarchy. Below these randomised controlled trials came pretest-post-test comparisons and interrupted time series designs (studies using historical controls). Single group pretest-post-test or post-test only designs (case series or single cases) were judged to provide the least reliable basis for causal inferences. Variations of this basic hierarchy are still being proposed by social and health scientists and drug regulatory authorities.[11–15] Why is it that those who have proposed these hierarchies seem to agree that randomised trials should be regarded as the best way to assemble comparison groups upon which to base causal inferences about the effects of care?

What is special about randomised controlled trials?

The main challenge facing those wishing to assess the relative merits of alternative forms of care is to ensure as far as possible that, on average, the people who make up the comparison groups are comparable in respect of prognosis and responsiveness to treatment. Unless this can be achieved, there is clearly a danger that any observed differences in "outcome" may simply reflect prior differences in the prognoses and therapeutic sensitivity of the people in the comparison groups.

The *only* special claim that can be made for random allocation is that allocation to the comparison groups is unbiased in respect of prognosis and responsiveness to treatment. No other way of creating comparison groups has these properties because it can never be assumed that all factors relevant to prognosis and responsiveness to treatment have been distributed in an unbiased way between the comparison groups. Due solely to chance, there will always be smaller or larger differences of prognosis and responsiveness to treatment; but the larger the size of the trial, the more likely is it that such differences will be trivial.

When random allocation is not used it may be possible to control for differences between comparison groups in other ways—for example, by adjusting for known differences in the analysis. However, this is only possible for factors that are known and measured. Randomisation is the only means of allocation that controls for unknown and unmeasured differences as well as those that are known and measured. Unfortunately it can rarely, if ever, be assumed that all the important prognostic factors are known, and for those that are known difficulties can arise in measuring and accounting for them in analyses. Empirical evidence supports these logical concerns (see tables).

There is consistent evidence from comparisons of randomised and non-randomised trials of the same intervention (table 4.1). These studies indicate important differences in the apparent effects of care in relation to how patients were allocated. It seems that these differences are primarily

TABLE 4.1—*Studies of randomised controlled trials compared with non-randomised controlled trials within specific interventions*

Study	Sample	Comparison	Results
Chalmers *et al*[39]	32 controlled studies of anticoagulation in acute myocardial infarction identified through a systematic search	Randomised controlled trials were compared with CCTs and HCTs on case-fatality rate, thromboembolism rate, and rate of haemorrhages	The largest relative risk reduction for mortality was observed in HCTs (0.42), compared with randomised controlled trials (0.31) and CCTs (0.33). The case-fatality rate was highest in HCs (38.3), compared with RCs (19.6) and CCs (29.2). A similar pattern was found for thromboembolism
Sacks *et al*[40]	Convenience sample of 50 randomised controlled trials and 56 HCTs assessing 6 interventions (treatment of oesophageal varices, coronary artery surgery, anticoagulation in myocardial infarction, chemotherapy in colon cancer, chemotherapy in melanoma, and DES for recurrent miscarriage)	Randomised controlled trials and HCTs were compared on the frequency of detecting statistically significant results ($P \leqq 0.05$) of the primary outcome and reduction of mortality	20% of the randomised controlled trials found a statistically significant benefit from the new therapy, compared with 79% of HCTs. The relative risk reduction of mortality in HCTs *v* randomised controlled trials (HCT/ randomised controlled trials) was 0.49/0.27 (1.8) for cirrhosis, 0.68/0.26 (2.6) for coronary artery surgery at 3 years, 0.49/0.22 (2.2) for anticoagulation in myocardial infarction, 0.67/–0.02 for DES in recurrent miscarriage. Outcomes in the treatment groups were similar in both designs, but outcomes in the control groups were worse among historical controls

(continued)

TABLE 4.1—(*continued*)

Study	Sample	Comparison	Results
Diehl and Perry[41]	19 randomised controlled trials and 17 HCTs for 6 types of cancer (breast, colon, stomach, lung, melanoma, soft tissue sarcoma) identified from the reference lists of two textbooks	RCs and HCs matched for disease, stage, and follow up were compared on survival and relapse free survival	In 43 matched control groups 18 (42%) varied by more than 10% (absolute difference in either outcome), 9 (21%) by more than 20%, and 2 (5%) by more than 30%. Survival or relapse free survival was better in RCs compared with HCs in 17/18 matches

Tables 4.1–4.3 are adapted from Kunz RA, Oxman AD. Empirical evidence of selection bias in studies of the effects of health care: a systematic review. Presented at the Cochrane Colloquium, Oslo, 5–8 October, 1995.
CC = concurrent control; CCT = trial using concurrent controls; HC = historical control; HCT = trial using historical controls; RC = randomised control.

due to a poorer prognosis in non-randomly selected controls compared with randomly selected controls.

The evidence from comparisons across different interventions (table 4.2) is less consistent. This can best be explained by the fact that there are many other factors that could distort or mask an association between randomisation and estimates of the effects of care—that is, there is so much "noise" in these heterogeneous samples of studies that the observed impact of randomisation and other factors on the observed treatment effects is uncertain and difficult to interpret.

Finally, empirical studies that have addressed "allocation concealment" (to prevent foreknowledge of treatment assignment) indicate that it is most likely this feature of random allocation that is crucial in achieving similar comparison groups (table 4.3). When assessing a potential participant's eligibility for a trial, those who are recruiting participants and the participants themselves should remain unaware of the next assignment in the sequence until after the decision about eligibility has been made. Then, after it has been revealed, neither the assignment nor the decision about eligibility should be altered.

It is important to recognise that differences between comparison groups in prognosis, responsiveness to treatment, or exposure to other factors that affect outcomes can distort the apparent effects of care in either direction, causing them to appear either larger or smaller than they are. It is generally not possible to predict the magnitude, and often not even the direction of

TABLE 4.2—*Studies of randomised controlled trials compared with non-randomised controlled trials across different interventions*

Study	Sample	Comparison	Results
Colditz *et al*[42]	113 studies published in 1980 comparing new interventions with old, identified in leading cardiology, neurology, psychiatry, and respiratory journals through a systematic literature search	36 parallel randomised controlled trials, 29 randomised COTs, 3 parallel CCTs, 46 non-random COTs, 5 ECSs, and 9 RRSs were compared on treatment gain (measured by the Mann-Whitney statistic). The relation between quality scores and treatment gains was also examined. The Mann-Whitney statistic is the probability that a patient receiving the new therapy would do better than a patient receiving the old. 0.5 indicates no difference between comparison groups	All but one design had, on average, similar estimates of treatment gain (0.56–0.65). Overall 87% of new treatments were rated as improvements over old, but only in the non-random COTs were patients, on average, significantly more likely to suggest benefit from the new treatment (0.94; P=0.004). Non-double-blinded randomised controlled trials were more likely to suggest a benefit from the new treatment (0.69) than double blinded randomised controlled trials (0.58; P=0.02). Within randomised controlled trials there was not a significant correlation between quality scores and treatment gains ($R = -0.16$; P=0.18)
Miller *et al*[43]	188 studies published in 1983 comparing new interventions in surgery with old, identified in leading surgical journals through a systematic literature search	81 randomised controlled trials, 15 CCTs, 27 ECSs, 91 RRSs, and 7 BASs were compared on treatment gain (measured by the Mann-Whitney statistic). Differences in proportions of treatment success associated with each study design for primary therapy (aimed at the patient's principal disease) and secondary therapy (aimed at complications of therapy) and the relation between quality score and treatment gains were also examined	There was a statistically non-significant trend towards larger treatment gains on new primary therapies in non-randomised controlled trials (0.78 for BASs, 0.63 for ECSs, 0.62 for CCTs, 0.56 for RRSs) compared with randomised controlled trials (0.56). For secondary therapies the treatment gain was similar across all study designs (0.54–0.55) except BASs (0.90). Within randomised controlled trials, there was not a significant correlation between quality scores and treatment gains ($r = 0.04$; P=0.7)

(*continued*)

TABLE 4.2—(*continued*)

Study	Sample	Comparison	Results
Otten-bacher[44]	Sample of randomised controlled trials and non-randomised controlled trials from a systematic search of *N Engl J Med* and *JAMA* (30 articles from each journal, with 50% randomised controlled trials and 50% non-randomised controlled trials) across a variety of medical specialties	Randomised controlled trials were compared with non-randomised controlled trials on treatment effects (measured by standardised mean differences). The standardised mean difference (Cohen's *d* index) estimates the difference between comparison groups in terms of their average standard deviation; for example, a *d* of 0.50 means that 1/2 standard deviation separates the average subject in the two groups	No significant difference was found in standardised mean differences for non-randomised controlled trials (0.23) compared with randomised controlled trials (0.21)

COT = cross over trial; ECS = studies using external controls (from previously published material, often equivalent to historical controls); RRS = study using retrospective review of records ("observational" study); BAS = before and after study. For other abbreviations see table 4.1

this bias in specific studies. However, on average, these differences tend to exaggerate treatment effects and the size of these distortions can be as large or larger than the size of the effects that it is hoped to detect.

What isn't special about randomised controlled trials?

In no respects other than the abolition of bias at the moment of assignment to treatment comparison groups do randomised controlled trials—of necessity—differ from alternative study designs for assessing the effects of health and social care. As with other study designs, the comparison groups in randomised trials may, after the actual moment of assignment to one or other comparison group, differ in ways other than the contrasting forms of care which the study has been designed to compare, and some of these differences may be important in interpreting differences or similarities in the subsequent experiences of the comparison groups.

Researchers using other research designs must also consider eligibility criteria, the size of the comparison groups, outcome measures, subgroup analyses, duration of follow up, blinding of treatment and outcome assessment (whether or not using placebos), and the generalisability of the

TABLE 4.3—*Studies of allocation concealment*

Study	Sample	Comparison	Results
Chalmers *et al*[45]	145 controlled trials of the treatment of acute myocardial infarction, identified through a systematic search	Studies with treatment allocation through non-random assignment, non-concealed random allocation, and concealed random allocation were compared on the frequency of statistically significant ($P \leqq 0.05$) maldistribution of prognostic variables, statistically significant ($P \leqq 0.05$) results, and case fatality rates	There was a 34% maldistribution of prognostic factors in non-randomised controlled trials, 7% in randomised controlled trials with non-concealed allocation, and 3.5% in randomised controlled trials with concealed allocation. 25% of results were statistically significant in non-randomised controlled trials, 11% in randomised controlled trials without concealment of allocation, and 5% in randomised controlled trials with concealed allocation. The average relative risk reduction for mortality was 33% in non-randomised controlled trials, 23% in non-concealed randomised controlled trials, and 3% in randomised controlled trials with concealed allocation. The case fatality rate for the control group was 32% in non-randomised controlled trials; 23% in non-concealed randomised controlled trials, and 16% in randomised controlled trials with concealed allocation. The case fatality rate for treatment groups was 21% in non-randomised controlled trials, 18% in non-concealed randomised controlled trials, and 16% in randomised controlled trials with concealed allocation

(*continued*)

TABLE 4.3—(*continued*)

Study	Sample	Comparison	Results
Schulz *et al*[34]	250 randomised controlled trials from 33 meta analyses from *The Cochrane Pregnancy and Childbirth Database*	The association between four methodological features of randomised controlled trials (allocation concealment, sequence generation, complete follow up after randomisation and double blinding), and treatment effects (measured by the odds ratio) was examined	The treatment effect (odds ratio) was exaggerated by 41% in "randomised controlled trials" with inadequate allocation concealment and by 30% in "randomised controlled trials" in which the adequacy of allocation concealment was unclear ($P<0.001$, after adjustment for other methodological features). The odds ratio was exaggerated by 17% in studies without double blinding compared with studies with adequate double blinding ($P=0.01$). The difference in odds ratios for randomised controlled trials that excluded patients from the analysis compared with randomised controlled trials that did not exclude patients was non-significant (7%, 95% confidence interval −6% to 21%)

For abbreviations see tables 4.1 and 4.2.

results of the comparisons. There are no necessary or inevitable differences between randomised trials and other forms of treatment comparisons in any of these respects.

What shouldn't be special about randomised trials?

> "If you can believe fervently in your treatment, even though controlled tests show that it is quite useless, then your results are much better, your patients are much better, and your income is much better too. I believe this accounts for the remarkable success of some of the less gifted, but more credulous members of our profession, and also for the violent dislike of statistics and controlled tests which fashionable and successful doctors are accustomed to display"[16]

Aspects of the style and content of communication between those providing and those receiving care can influence the effects of care.[17] Over the past three decades, there have been changes in the nature and the content of the interaction between those providing and those receiving care.[18] One of these changes has resulted from externally imposed requirements of professionals to admit their uncertainty about the effects of treatment to their patients, and to provide them with uniform, detailed, and unsolicited information about the alternative forms of care concerned, including details of possible side effects. These requirements about informed consent have been applied selectively, such that they are far more likely to accompany treatments prescribed within the context of randomised trials than they are to accompany prescription of identical forms of care in other kinds of formal treatment comparisons—for example, comparisons using concurrent but non-randomised controls, or care given outside the context of formal comparisons.

Differential imposition of these requirements may result in the psychological effects of care within randomised comparisons being different from those made within other kinds of formal comparisons, particularly if these "setting variables" are effect modifiers of the specific treatments being evaluated.[19,20] In some circumstances, and for some outcomes, a feeling of "specialness" may result from knowing that one is participating in a formal treatment evaluation. This may have beneficial psychological effects, and these, in turn, may be reflected in improved outcome of treatment, even expressed in terms of physical outcomes.[21] In other circumstances, explicit acknowledgement of uncertainty may result in the loss of potentially important placebo effects; indeed, adverse effects of treatment may result from symptom suggestion.

These *de facto* characteristics of treatment comparisons based on randomised groups are not associated with random allocation per se. Rather, they reflect an illogical, externally imposed double standard which results in some patients receiving less information and in different ways than others about the relative merits, demerits, and uncertainties about alternative forms of care.[22] But they may have consequences for the interpretation of the results of formal treatment comparisons. For many people the confident professional certainty which is typical of everyday practice constitutes a more effective form of care than the explicit admission of professional uncertainty that is required of those who are providing care within the context of a randomised trial. The operation of this irrational double standard may result in the psychological effects of care within randomised controlled comparisons being atypical, and thus less generalisable than they might otherwise be.

Limited generalisability due to selected patient populations participating in randomised controlled trials has long been considered an important problem, but the effects on generalisability of different information given to patients in the context of randomised controlled trials compared with daily practice and effects on generalisability of other "setting" factors which influence the expectancy of patients have not received much attention. However, empirical evidence exists demonstrating these phenomena,[20] illustrated by the following examples:

In a randomised trial in general practice, patients presenting with symptoms but no abnormal physical signs, in whom no firm diagnosis could be made, were more satisfied with care and more likely to experience symptomatic improvement after a "positive" consultation (with a confident assurance that the symptoms would disappear in a few days), than control patients who received a "neutral" consultation (in which the doctor admitted that he could not be certain what was wrong or whether his prescribed treatment would have any effect).[23] In another trial, involving women undergoing termination of pregnancy, it was found that, compared with an egalitarian style of consultation, a paternalistic approach not only prompted women to have greater confidence in the physician, but also resulted in them reporting less discomfort during the procedure.[24] Other evidence confirms the importance of psychological and educational factors in mediating the effects of care.[25] The presence of a support person during childbirth, for example, has dramatic effects on the need for analgesics, anaesthetics, episiotomy, caesarian section, and on maternal depression after childbirth.[26]

The extent to which these phenomena compromise the generalisability of results of randomised controlled trials is unknown; but this is certainly an issue which needs to be addressed more actively than hitherto. We believe this should occur at two levels. Firstly, the public must discuss whether continued acquiescence in the double standard currently operated on informed consent to treatment is defensible. We believe that there should be a single standard across the board.

Secondly, researchers must decide how best to design empirical research to assess the effects of the double standard, and of other setting characteristics. This would require, as a first step, more detailed description and reporting of setting and information characteristics in reports of randomised controlled trials.

Discussion

We were prompted to write this article because we were concerned about unfruitful polarisation in current debates on evaluation of interventions, illustrated, on the one hand, by the view that "randomised trials are the only effective way to validate treatment options",[27] and on the other, the rejection of randomised controlled trials, both by social scientists[28–31] and by some medical scientists.[32-33] These polarised viewpoints provide good theatre but a poor basis for making decisions about health and social care. The particular strength of randomisation is the ability to generate unbiased comparison groups. Other research designs are also important, including qualitative research to help elucidate the mechanisms through which interventions may have or fail to have their effects.[34] Those who promote the naive view that randomised trials provide the only secure way of detecting important effects of interventions also overlook the fact that other study designs are often needed to detect rare but important adverse effects of interventions.[35,36] Polemics about the perceived limitations or strengths of randomised experiments are as unhelpful as polemics about the perceived limitations or strengths of any other of the variety of methodological approaches which should be deployed by people seeking valid estimates of the differential effects of health and social care.

We believe that the quality of debate about how to generate reliable comparison groups to assess the relative merits of alternative forms of social and medical care would improve if those involved made greater efforts to seek relevant empirical evidence. We are certainly willing to make a contribution to these efforts. What is clear from empirical investigations is that different ways of generating comparison groups tend to yield different results, and thus different conclusions about the value and safety of health care and social interventions. Studies using strict randomisation to generate comparison groups tend to yield less dramatic estimates of the effects of care than studies using non-randomised control groups.[11,37]

As Susser has pointed out, "Our many errors show that the practice of causal inference . . . remains an art. Although to assist us we have acquired analytical techniques, statistical methods and conventions, and logical criteria, ultimately the conclusions we reach are a matter of judgement."[38] Given that one will always be faced with the need to make judgements in making causal inferences about the effects of health and social care, which logical criteria should we deploy in our attempts to maximise the potential benefits and minimise the potential harm done to people who look to professionals for help?

We are not aware of any empirical evidence which would lead us to reject the hierarchy—with randomised experiments at the top—which has been proposed repeatedly by social and medical scientists over the past three decades. Most drug regulatory authorities established to protect the public interest require evidence from studies which have used random allocation to generate the comparison groups. We endorse the judgement upon which this is based and we believe that those who promote any relaxation of this standard in respect of other forms of health and social care should be required to show how their proposals are more likely to increase the beneficial effects and decrease the harmful effects of well intentioned health and social care. A great deal is at stake—the health and welfare of people who have looked to health professionals and social workers for help.

Acknowledgements

We thank Doug Altman, Clare Bradley, Ann Oakley, and William Silverman for comments on draft versions of this chapter. This does not necessarily mean that they endorse all elements of our analysis and conclusions.

1 Silverman WA. Human experimentation: a guided step into the unknown. Oxford: Oxford University Press, 1980.
2 Fischer J. Is casework effective? A review. *Social Work* 1973;**17**:1–5.
3 Macdonald G, Sheldon B. Contemporary studies of the effectiveness of social work. *British Journal of Social Work* 1992;**22**:615–43.
4 Office of Technology Assessment. *Identifying health technologies that work*. Washington DC: Congress of the United States, 1994:1–308.
5 McCord J. A thirty year follow-up of treatment effects. *Am Psychol* 1978;**33**:284–9.
6 Moore AJ. *Deadly medicine*. New York: Simon and Schuster, 1995.
7 Black N. Why we need observational studies to evaluate the effectiveness of health care. *BMJ* 1996;**312**:1215–18.
8 Ellenberg JH. Cohort studies. Selection bias in observational and experimental studies. *Stat Med* 1994;**13**:557–67.
9 Segelov E, Tattersall MHN, Coates AS. Redressing the balance—The ethics of *not* entering an eligible patient on a randomised clinical trial. *Ann Oncol* 1992;**3**:103–5.
10 Campbell DR, Stanley JC. *Experimental and quasi-experimental designs for research*. Chicago: Rand McNally, 1963.
11 Soumerai SB, McLaughlin TJ, Avorn J. Improving drug prescribing in primary care: a critical analysis of the experimental literature. *Milbank Q* 1989;**67**:268–317.
12 Canadian Task Force on the Periodic Health Examination. The periodic health examination. *Can Med Assoc J* 1979;**121**:1193–254.
13 US Department of Health and Human Services, Public Health Service, Office of the Assistant Secretary for Health, Office of Disease Prevention and Health Promotion, Preventive Services Task Force. *Guide to clinical preventive services*. Baltimore MD: Williams and Wilkins, 1989.
14 Guyatt GH, Sackett DL, Sinclair JC, Hayward R, Cook DJ, Cook RJ, for the Evidence-Based Medicine Working Group. User's guides to the medical literature. IX. A method for grading health care recommendations. *JAMA* 1995;**274**:1800–4.
15 Commonwealth Department of Human Services and Health. *Guidelines for the pharmaceutical industry on preparation of submissions to the pharmaceutical benefits advisory committee*. Canberra, Australia: Commonwealth Department of Human Services and Health, 1995.
16 Asher R. *Talking sense*. London: Pitman Medical, 1972.
17 Luborsky L, McLellan T, Woody GE, O'Brien CP. Therapist success and its determinants. *Arch Gen Psychiatry* 1985;**42**:602–11.
18 Silverman WA, Altman DG. Patients' preferences and randomised trials. *Lancet* 1996; **347**:171–4.
19 Bradley C. Clinical trials—time for a paradigm shift? *Diabet Med* 1988;**5**:107–9.
20 Kleijnen J, de Craen AJM, van Everdingen J, Krol L. Placebo effect in double-blind clinical trials: a review of interactions with medications. *Lancet* 1994;**344**:1347–9.
21 Kramer MS, Shapiro SH. Scientific challenges in the application of randomized controlled trials. *JAMA* 1984;**252**:2739–45.
22 Chalmers I, Silverman WA. Professional and public double standards on clinical experimentation. *Control Clin Trials* 1987;**8**:388–91.

23 Thomas KB. General practice consultations: is there any point in being positive? *BMJ* 1987;**294**:1200–2.
24 LeBaron S, Reyher J, Stack JM. Paternalistic vs egalitarian physician styles: the treatment of patients in crisis. *J Fam Pract* 1985;**21**:56–62.
25 Devine EC, Cook TD. A meta-analytic analysis of effects of psychoeducational interventions on length of postsurgical hospital stay. *Nurs Res* 1983;**32**:267–74.
26 Hodnett ED. Support from caregivers during childbirth. In: Enkin MW, Keirse MJNC, Renfrew MJ, Neilson JP, Crowther C, eds. *Pregnancy and childbirth module of the Cochrane database of systematic reviews*, 1996 [updated 29 February 1996]. Available in the Cochrane Library from BMJ Publishing Group: London.
27 British Medical Association. *Medical ethics today*. London: BMA, 1993:209.
28 Cheetham J, Fuller R, McIvor G, Petch A. *Evaluating social work effectiveness*. Buckingham: Open University Press, 1992.
29 Hunter D. Let's hear it for R&D. *Health Service Journal* 1993;**15**:17.
30 Nutbeam D, Smith C, Calford J. Evaluation in health education: a review of progress, possibilities and problems. *J Epidemiol Community Health* 1990;**44**:83–9.
31 Stecher BM, Davis WA. *How to focus an evaluation*. Newbury Park, CA: Sage Publications, 1987.
32 Charlton BG. Randomised clinical trials: the worst kind of epidemiology? *Nat Med* 1995; **1**:1101–2.
33 Herman J. The demise of the randomised controlled trial. *J Clin Epidemiol* 1995;**48**:985–8.
34 Oakley A. *Social support and motherhood*. Oxford: Blackwell, 1991.
35 Venning GR. The validity of anecdotal reports of suspected adverse drug reactions—the problem of false alarms. *BMJ* 1982;**284**:249–52.
36 Chalmers I. Evaluating the effects of care during pregnancy and childbirth. In: Chalmers I, Enkin M, Keirse MJNC, eds. *Effective care in pregnancy and childbirth*. Oxford: Oxford University Press, 1989:3–38.
37 Schulz KF, Chalmers I, Hayes RJ, Altman DG. Empirical evidence of bias: dimensions of methodological quality associated with estimates of treatment effects in controlled trials. *JAMA* 1995;**273**:408–12.
38 Susser M. Causal thinking in practice: strengths and weaknesses of the clinical vantage point. *Pediatrics* 1984;**74**:842–9.
39 Chalmers TC, Matta RJ, Smith H, Jr., Kunzler AM. Evidence favoring the use of anticoagulants in the hospital phase of acute myocardial infarction. *N Engl J Med* 1977; **297**:1091–6.
40 Sacks H, Chalmers TC, Smith HJ. Randomized versus historical controls for clinical trials. *Am J Med* 1982;**72**:233–40.
41 Diehl LF, Perry DJ. A comparison of randomized concurrent control groups with matched historical control groups: are historical controls valid? *J Clin Oncol* 1986;**4**:1114–20.
42 Colditz GA, Miller JN, Mosteller F. How study design affects outcomes in comparisons of therapy. I: Medical. *Stat Med* 1989;**8**:441–54.
43 Miller JN, Colditz GA, Mosteller F. How study design affects outcomes in comparisons of therapy. II: Surgical. *Stat Med* 1989;**8**:455–66.
44 Ottenbacher K. Impact of random assignment on study outcome: an empirical examination. *Control Clin Trials* 1992;**13**:50–61.
45 Chalmers TC, Celano P, Sacks HS, Smith H, Jr. Bias in treatment assignment in controlled clinical trials. *N Engl J Med* 1983;**309**:1358–61.

5: Cochrane and the benefits of aspirin

PETER ELWOOD

Introduction

There are many facets to the story of aspirin, just as there were many facets to the character of Archie Cochrane. Above all, Archie was an encourager. Had he not encouraged members of his unit to follow new leads, the story of aspirin would have been very different and possibly countless thousands of patients would have been denied its benefits.

The first randomised controlled trial of aspirin in patients after myocardial infarction[1] has perhaps led to greater benefits than any other single study. Furthermore, as this chapter will show, the benefit of aspirin has not been confined to patients after myocardial infarction. The early work on aspirin played a part in the development of "overviews" of evidence, and contributed indirectly to the concept of the Cochrane Collaboration.

Archie loved innovation and however novel an idea, he loved to discuss it. He knew when to employ hyperbole and he would taunt clinicians about their relative ineffectiveness in many conditions, and particularly in the prevention and treatment of coronary thrombosis. He also challenged clinicians for evidence as to the value, or otherwise, of their interventions and in the early days of the development of coronary care units he often debated the balance in their likely merits and demerits. He himself was inventive with regard to possible harmful effects of intensive intervention in patients with an unstable myocardium and he urged that a randomised trial be set up to evaluate the untested coronary care units. He was deeply upset when local colleagues and cardiologists judged that any such trial would be unethical. He did however persuade cardiologists in Bristol, led by Dr Gordon Mather, to set up a randomised trial. Cynic that he was, Archie was delighted when the results favoured treatment at home.[2] It was not the end of that debate, but Archie showed little further interest in that particular topic.

It was in the early days of this debate on coronary care that the suggestion was first made that aspirin might reduce the risk of a coronary thrombosis. Archie was quick of course to recognise the superior merits of prophylaxis, especially in comparison with intensive intervention. Indeed, when he learnt of certain preliminary evidence on aspirin and mortality, he began to taunt cardiologists, warning that "high-tech" coronary care units might well be emptied by the humble aspirin.

Archie and the randomised controlled trial

Above all other strategies in research, Archie loved the randomised controlled trial. He would have randomised every human activity and intervention! In the very early days of his MRC unit he persuaded a sociologist, John Palmer, to set up trials in which school pupils who were late for school, or were caught smoking, were allotted at random to different punishments, or to no punishment.[3] He argued vehemently, but without success, for randomisation of sentences by the courts, and the arguments he used for this have no less validity today. He agreed to pay for an amusing little randomised study which I set up with my children: monitoring the mortality of tropical fish randomised into tanks containing either hard or soft water. The results of this particular trial gave great amusement, the most obvious development being a very marked difference in the population density in the two tanks, which emerged within a few months. This led to the most intriguing conclusion that hard water might be contraceptive. This outcome delighted Archie, but it turned out to be a rather premature judgement when one of the children pointed out that there was a cannibal swordtail in the hard water tank!

Archie often spoke with deep respect of Bradford Hill, attributing to him the introduction of the randomised controlled trial into medicine. On a number of occasions he also expressed gratitude to Peter Armitage who had drawn his attention to what is probably the second published call for a randomised controlled trial (P. Armitage, personal communication), the first having been recorded in Daniel.[4]

> "Let us take out of the hospitals, out of the camps, or elsewhere, 200 or 500 poor people that have fevers, pleuricies etc. Let us divide them into halves, let us cast lots, that one halfe of them may fall to my share and the other halfe to thine. We shall see how many funerals both of us will have. Let the reward of the wager be 300 florens, deposited on both sides." (Van Helmont, 1662)

Despite his enthusiasm for the randomised controlled trial Archie often admitted that he himself had conducted only one controlled trial—a strange statement for the man who, probably more than anyone, has popularised the idea of the randomised controlled trial. His trial must, however, be one of the most remarkable ever conducted and I will never forget having persuaded him to present it at a small local medical meeting I organised in Cardiff. The trial had tested the treatment of famine oedema in men in a German prisoner of war camp in Salonica, by a dietary supplement of yeast. Hearing Archie present this trial for the first time was a most moving experience, his voice almost breaking with emotion as he described the conditions in the camp under which he had had to work. He clearly was helped by having had to talk about the experience and it led to him publishing an account shortly afterwards. My memory is that early drafts of this paper had included the phrase "my only successful clinical trial", but somewhere along the line this phrase was changed to one slightly less humble, and his report eventually bore the title: *Sickness in Salonica: my first, worst, and most successful clinical trial.*[5] Archie was so dismissive of research that had involved any compromise, that the fact that men had been allotted to the treatment groups alternately, and not truly at random, perhaps led him not to use the term "random" in the title, or in the body of the paper.

Archie was indeed inclined to minimise his own work in this kind of way. Yet he was the first to encourage others and he often gave exaggerated prominence to their efforts. It was in such a climate that around 1969 I put forward the idea of a randomised controlled trial of aspirin in patients after myocardial infarction.

The idea was not my own. Each year, and for several years before this a highly inventive and innovative haematologist in Portsmouth, John O'Brien, had written regularly to the journals suggesting that a trial be conducted. O'Brien subsequently became very closely involved in all the work of the unit on haemostatic factors and platelet function. From work on both platelet aggregation and bleeding time tests,[6] O'Brien had generated the idea that aspirin might be protective in a number of thrombotic conditions. In fact he was one of the first, both to call for a trial of aspirin after a thrombotic event such as myocardial infarction[7] and to show that the effect of aspirin on platelet aggregation is the same at low and high dosages.[8] Amongst many other strands in the discussions at that time was an observation by Marjorie Zucker that one of her study volunteers whose blood consistently yielded abnormal clotting results was found to take aspirin regularly.[9] O'Brien was not, however, the only one to call for such a trial at that time. In the United States another haematologist, Harvey Weiss, wrote similar letters to the journals.[10]

As it happens however, both these men had been anticipated by a general practitioner in Mississippi. In a paper on his work, a Dr LL Craven described how he "urged friends and patients to adopt the practice of taking aspirin, one or two 5 grain tablets daily." His report goes on to state: "Approximately 8000 men and women adopted the regime . . . not a single case of detectable coronary or cerebral thrombosis occurred among patients who faithfully adhered to this regime during a period of eight years."[11]

Archie quickly warmed to the idea of a randomised controlled trial of low dose aspirin and he co-opted the help of a local pharmacologist, Jimmy Graham, in the Department of Therapeutics in the Welsh National School of Medicine (now the University of Wales College of Medicine). Graham became involved with us in planning the trial, and in turn he involved Ross Renton, and others in Aspro-Nicholas, a pharmaceutical firm, and they agreed to supply the aspirin and matching placebo. These were produced in capsule form to disguise the taste of the aspirin.

The first randomised control trial of aspirin

It was 1970 when the first patients were approached. In those heady days for research, formal ethical approval was unknown. Nevertheless, like most researchers of the time, Archie sought peer comment widely, and was very sensitive to any suggestion that any project of his might be unethical. He was equally concerned about the scientific standards set in his unit. On this latter, he is perhaps best remembered by his staff for the remarkable standards he set in response rates in surveys and follow up studies. Within his unit we devised the index "Cochrane units" a response rate of 91% having one Cochrane, 95%, five Cochranes, and so on. Negative Cochranes were unthinkable. We knew that Archie would find a response rate below 90% totally unacceptable and we would be sent back to do better! The standards Archie expected were especially demanding in randomised controlled trials and he was one of the first to produce evidence that participants lost to follow up are different from participants who remain in a study, and are therefore a most likely source of important bias.

The method in this first trial was that male patients were identified immediately after discharge from one of a number of local hospitals, having been diagnosed as having had a myocardial infarct. The general practitioner (GP) of the patient was contacted, and the suitability of the man for the trial agreed. The patient was then visited in his own home, the trial explained, and his cooperation sought. A copy of the randomisation code was kept by Peter Sweetnam, the statistician in the Unit, and the code was broken only if a physician or GP required to know what his or her patient was receiving.

The dose of aspirin which was used in this trial had been long debated. Inhibition of platelet aggregation was judged to be the effect of aspirin of relevance to infarction and laboratory evidence from the studies by O'Brien and others, strongly indicated that a single tablet (then 5 grains or 330 mg) daily would be more than adequate.

Moreover a small dose was attractive because undesirable side effects would be less likely to occur. On the other hand, colleagues other than clotologists considered a single tablet inadequate. They recommended multiple daily doses, and all the trials which were set up later reflected the persuasiveness of clinical opinion, rather than evidence, and larger doses were generally used.

Amongst colleagues the trial received general support—and not a little amusement. In the field, however, the reception was rather different. Several aspects came under attack, not least the dose of aspirin, which some physicians dismissed as "homeopathic". On the other hand, aspirin was under a cloud because of its irritant effect on the gastric mucosa at high doses. For these and other reasons not a few physicians were reluctant to allow the inclusion of their patients in the trial, though only one physician refused to collaborate. Many patients were also reluctant to become involved. The idea that aspirin might actually be beneficial was quite novel to them, and seemed even bizarre, or contrived, to some. At the end of the explanation about the trial an occasional patient would ask: "Come off it, Doc, what do these capsules really contain?"

When the trial had been running for about a year, a most dramatic series of events took place. On a Saturday morning early in 1972, one of us received a telephone call from a pharmacologist in Boston, Herschel Jick. Jick was director of the Boston Drug Surveillance Scheme and working with him at that time was Martin Vessey of Oxford. Vessey knew something of the unit's work at that time.

In a study by Jick and his colleagues, patients admitted to a number of hospitals in and around Boston had been interviewed and asked about the drugs they had taken in the week prior to admission to hospital. These data were later linked with the diagnosis on discharge, the main idea being to identify previously unsuspected harmful effects of drugs. In one of their analyses the group had come up with evidence that patients discharged after myocardial infarction had a marked deficiency in aspirin taking prior to admission to hospital. The risk ratio for aspirin taking was around 0.3 compared with all other patients, after elimination of those who had had conditions with a possible positive relationship to aspirin.[12]

This evidence put us in a most serious dilemma. Clearly there were two possible explanations for the association. Either, aspirin could be harmful, leading to the death of patients before they could be interviewed, or aspirin could be protective, and the taking of aspirin could reduce the chance of admission to hospital and discharge with a diagnosis of myocardial infarction. Both these had most important implications for our trial. If the first had been true, then the sooner our trial was stopped the better. If the second was true, we would have to consider expediting our trial by expanding it rapidly.

Archie has described our dilemma in his autobiography: *One man's medicine.*[13] He and I remembered the details of the situation somewhat differently—but he was a much better story teller than I! Certainly wide and intensive discussions took place. Again, Archie's reluctance to compromise a research study became clear and with considerable reluctance he agreed that the code of our trial should be broken. In those early days of the randomised controlled trial the idea of an independent monitoring group had not arisen and so we had to take the decision ourselves, and as director of the unit the decision had to be Archie's. Of course the numbers in the trial at that stage were small, and so we expected nothing conclusive from the results, unless—and the thought did occur to us—all, or most of the 18 deaths that had occurred up to that point had been in men on aspirin! Of course, it was not so. Eleven patients on placebo and six who had been on aspirin had died. We were reassured sufficiently to continue with the trial, and were encouraged sufficiently to expand it.

A number of important meetings followed as we persuaded other groups to set up similar trials. The most prestigious meeting at which our evidence was presented was in Boston, and was organised by the United States National Institutes of Health. Some of the people attending were names I knew well and had long held in awe. I remember little of the discussions but both my children and I well remember an event which immediately followed my return from Boston. My children were small at that time, far too young to have understood the reason for my excitement. My wife and I therefore took them to an expensive restaurant and told them to select one of the most expensive items on the menu. We told them that something wonderful had happened which they would not understand, but that when they were older they would remember this occasion and we would explain. They remember it all to this day!

Of course, as is often the case, our excitement proved to have been somewhat over the top! When the trial had run its course the results were analysed and published. The difference in total mortality between aspirin and placebo was not significant at conventional levels of significance but suggested a 24% reduction in all cause deaths in the men given aspirin. The trial had been set up to test aspirin's effect on total mortality, so we did not report the fact that had we added 10 and 15 non-fatal infarctions, the difference between aspirin and placebo would have been significant (a 24% reduction, 95% confidence interval = 5.3 to 42.4%). Although the index total coronary incidence came to be used freely by later trial participants, Archie always regarded it as representing special pleading. If an intervention reduces ischaemic heart disease mortality, then a reduction will be seen in all cause death—and the identification of death requires no special skill and is open to no diagnostic bias.

Our report was published in the *BMJ*,[1] together with a paper by Jick *et al* on their observational data.[12] Both were under a subheading: "For debate". At the time we felt somewhat miffed by this last, but in view of the later recognition of the need for overviews of evidence from a number of trials we would now judge the caution of the editor to have been most commendable.

Further randomised control trials of aspirin

The publication of our first aspirin trial had two very obvious effects. Firstly, there was a growth in laboratory and other work on platelets, evidenced by an enormous and rapid increase in the number of published reports on platelet function in the literature. Publication of the trial also brought the unit a number of friends with an interest in platelets, including Serge Renaud of INSERM, who, together with John O'Brien, has made an enormous and continuing contribution to the work of the unit. Indeed, the collaboration with these men led later to the Unit including a range of tests of platelet function within the Caerphilly Collaborative Prospective Study of Heart Disease and Stroke.[14–16]

The other effect of publication of our first trial was the setting up of randomised controlled trials by other research groups. The first of these was based on a residue of patients who had been involved in the Coronary Drug Prevention Studies (CDP) in the United States.[17] We ourselves set up two further trials.[18,19] One of these was closely similar to the first, other than that patients were identified and admitted while still in hospital after the myocardial infarct, and the dose of aspirin was increased to 300 mg three times a day. We were persuaded on this last by several very eminent physicians—and we have regretted the change ever since!

While this second MRC trial was in progress, Archie and I decided to mount a trial in which aspirin would be given very early in infarction, in the hope that the thrombotic process might be arrested and perhaps even reversed, with a consequent reduction in mortality. In addition to the current laboratory and other evidence, we were encouraged by reports of benefit from aspirin in amaurosis fugax. This is a condition of temporary partial blindness in which a platelet aggregate plugs a retinal vessel. Relief is almost instantaneous on taking aspirin and the restoration of blood flow can occasionally be watched through an ophthalmoscope.[20] Animal work on the prevention of myocardial damage after ligation of a coronary vessel by Folts *et al*[21] and postmortem studies by Haerem *et al*[22] were also crucial in our thinking. These latter authors had reported the finding of platelet emboli in the coronary microcirculation of patients whose deaths had been sudden. Our hope was that aspirin might disperse such emboli.

Archie and I requested a list of members from the Royal College of General Practitioners. The College collaborated willingly and generously.

Six thousand GPs were written to and 2500 agreed to cooperate in our proposed trial. Archie loved simplicity and the strategy to be followed in this trial was simplicity itself. Each co-operating GP was sent six sealed envelopes. Each contained two capsules (300 mg aspirin or placebo), which we had sealed in foil, and a numbered, prepaid record form. The GP was instructed to give the two capsules to any patient to whom he had been called and who was experiencing chest pain or other symptoms which he or she judged likely to be due to a myocardial infarct. A few clinical details were then to be entered on the record form, including blood pressure to give possible evidence on the severity of the attack, and the form returned to us. One month after reception of these, the GP was written to and the survival or death of the patient ascertained. We did not ask that aspirin be continued after that first dose, lest this might influence a decision about admission to a coronary care unit. We were also highly optimistic about the possible effect of aspirin in this situation.

Over two thousand patients were entered into the trial. The mortality at 28 days after infarction, and at lesser intervals was homogeneous in the two groups, placebo and aspirin (difference equivalent to a reduction in deaths of 5.2%; 95% CI = −9 to 19.4%).

This study was reported, and it carries a number of lessons. Later overviews of all the available evidence have indicated unequivocally that aspirin is beneficial after infarction and yield no evidence suggestive of a difference in aspirin whether this is given early after infarction, or later.[23] Why our trial was not more conclusive remains a mystery. The effect of aspirin on platelet function is prolonged and so the single dose should have covered the period of highest risk of death.[24] One uncertainty relates to the possibility that many of the patients might have vomited the aspirin. We doubt this, but unfortunately we did not make appropriate inquiries. The main message is, however, that conclusions should never be based on a single trial. It is certainly interesting to think that had that trial been the first, we certainly would not have proceeded with work on aspirin and its reporting could well have deterred others from setting up appropriate trials.

In any case, any disappointment we might have felt from the somewhat lukewarm reception our report had with the *BMJ* was balanced by the encouragement we received from others. In particular we valued a comment from Sir Richard Doll who said to us: "Well, gentlemen, the evidence may not be certain, but it is more convincing than that for most of the other drugs in the *British Pharmacopoeia*."

The development of "overviews"

Archie believed that the most important single development in medical research had been the introduction of the randomised controlled trial. I believe that had he lived to see more recent developments, he would have judged that the development of the "overview" or "meta-analysis" is a development of equal importance. The aspirin trials played a significant part in this further development.

Within a relatively short time after the publication of the first MRC trial, five other trials were reported. The results of none of these achieved statistical significance at conventional levels. Archie and I, however, found the consistency of the results of the six trials most impressive and we believed that they were virtually conclusive in support of aspirin. However, two developments in the wider scene alarmed us. One was a claim which was being made by a group that had conducted a small trial of aspirin in patients who had presented with unstable angina.[25] The results of this trial achieved statistical significance at conventional levels and this led the authors to claim that aspirin was of value *only* in unstable angina, and not in infarction. The other development at that time which alarmed us was a suggestion based on results from the Aspirin and Myocardial Infarction Study (AMIS),[26] that benefit from aspirin might be present in male patients, but there seemed to be no suggestion of any effect in females. The particular subgroup analysis behind this statement was based on exceedingly small numbers, but journalists did not understand such limitations and sexist headlines appeared in some of the papers at that time.

These conclusions seemed to Archie and me to be so flagrantly untenable, and the results which had been reported from the six trials similar to our own seemed to us to be so supportive of a beneficial effect of aspirin, that we conducted our own, somewhat primitive, overview of all the evidence available at that time from trials of aspirin in the secondary prevention of death.

The following box is taken from a slide that Archie and I prepared and showed at many meetings in the United Kingdom, in Berlin, Seoul, New Orleans, and elsewhere in the very early 1980s.

Trial	Number of patients	Reduction in all-cause mortality by aspirin (%)
MRC I (1974)	1239	26 NS
CDP (1976)	1529	30 NS
MRC II (1976)	1725	30 NS
German (1978)	626	18 NS
AMIS (1980)	4524	10 NS
PARIS (1980)	1216	18 NS

All six trials: 10 859 patients
Weighted overall effect of aspirin: 23% reduction, P<0.0001

Archie was immensely gratified when, around this time, Richard Peto took up the matter of aspirin and presented a considerably more elegant overview of these six trials to the first meeting of the Society for Clinical Trials in Philadelphia.[27] After this, Peto and his colleagues began to conduct a series of overviews that have become monumental in medical research.[28] As a result of all this work, aspirin is now a drug, the uses of which are probably the most conclusively established in the whole modern pharmacopoeia.

The most recent overview, based on 145 randomised controlled trials, which yielded 10 943 vascular events in 96 316 patients, shows that aspirin reduces all cause mortality by about 20–25%, and re-infarction by about 25–30%. Furthermore, as Archie had always predicted, there is no evidence of any difference in the effect of aspirin in the reduction of thrombotic events whatever the clinical event, and whatever the type of patient. Thus the effect is homogeneous in unstable angina, post-myocardial infarction, post-stroke, and transient ischaemic attack, post-CABG, post-PCTA, post-valve replacement, and in peripheral vascular disease. Nor is there any significant heterogeneity in the effect in males or females, diabetic or non-diabetic, hypertensive or non-hypertensive, or older or younger people.[28]

One other aspect of the reporting of the results of trials was insisted on by Peter Sweetnam, the senior unit statistician who analysed the data from all our trials. It was, and still is, conventional to report the results of randomised controlled trials in terms of the observed reduction in mortality, either in crude percentage terms, or as a reduction in risk of an event, or reduced odds of an event. Thus aspirin given after myocardial infarction reduced mortality by about 25%. Although this is true, it focuses solely on the patients who die and takes no account of those who survive to the end of the trial. As Sweetnam pointed out, it is far more meaningful to state the effect of aspirin in terms of an increase in survival, and typically this raises the survival of post-infarction patients by about 2%, from about 88% to just over 90%. Such a statistic gives a far more comprehensive impression to the clinicians who care for myocardial infarction, patient by patient. These two views, the epidemiological and the clinical, are valid, but were often referred to by Archie as the clinical view and the truth!

The Cochrane Collaboration

This all leads naturally to the Cochrane Collaboration.[29] If the introduction of the randomised controlled trial was one of the most important developments in medical research, and the use of overviews another, then the setting up of the Cochrane Collaboration is yet another. Indeed, although the Cochrane Collaboration is clearly dependent upon the earlier two developments, in importance it is probably second to no other development within modern medical practice and in turn this has played a crucial role in the development of evidence based clinical practice.

Again, the humble aspirin played a key role in all this, albeit somewhat indirect. One of the statements of Archie that has come to be quoted frequently was made in 1979: "It is surely a great criticism of our profession that we have not organised a critical summary, by speciality or subspeciality, adapted periodically, of all relevant randomised controlled trials."[30] Archie's involvement in the long arguments about aspirin, the lack of acceptably conclusive results from any of the early trials, our own "back of envelope" overview of the results of the first six trials, and the eventual triumph of the meticulous overviews of Peto and his colleagues, was formative in Archie's thinking, and hence this statement, which, in retrospect, was clearly monumental.

Sadly, Archie did not live to see the Cochrane Collaboration launched. But in the introduction he contributed to a report that was published after a pilot project for the Collaboration. He wrote: "... the systematic review of the randomised trials of obstetric practice that is presented in this book is a new achievement. It represents a real milestone in the history of randomised trials and in the evaluation of care, and I hope it will be widely copied by other medical specialities."[31]

In fact, despite his involvement in this promising beginning, Archie probably never fully envisaged what has developed. He would, however, have been thrilled beyond measure with what has happened and grateful to Iain Chalmers, who, with others has taken his suggestion and turned it into a worldwide collaboration. The Cochrane Collaboration is a most fitting memorial to this great man. One can only surmise, with delight, the enormous benefits likely to come from the further development of this initiative in evidence based health care.

New uses of aspirin

The aspirin story is not over. It continues to surprise. Further uses of aspirin in conditions with a thrombotic basis are perhaps not surprising, but some of its newer possible uses are certainly unexpected. Thus beneficial effects on pre-eclampsia and on retarded fetal growth, while controversial[32] have a reasonable basis in the antithrombotic effect of aspirin. Other possible uses of aspirin, however, do not seem to be related to its antiplatelet effects.

It has been observed in a number of cohort studies and case-control comparisons that aspirin intake is associated with a reduced incidence of colon cancer and mortality from this condition.[33–35] Aspirin inhibits the proliferation of colon adenocarcinoma cells in vitro and appears to arrest the cell mitotic cycle. Another effect, which opens up a vast new field for investigation, is that within certain plants, and probably in humans, aspirin promotes cellular apoptosis or cell suicide.[36]

Aspirin has effects on the eye which lead to the suggestion that it may reduce cataract formation. Aldose reductase, an enzyme which seems to play a pivotal part in cataract formation, is inhibited by aspirin[37] as is intraocular fibroblast proliferation.[38]

Dementia

Archie concluded his autobiography *One man's medicine*[13] with a quotation:

> *I can cope with my bifocals.*
> *My dentures fit me fine.*
> *I can live with my porphyria,*
> *But, my God, I miss my mind.*

In fact, Archie never lost his mind and he remained keenly interested in the work of his unit until only a very few weeks before his death in June 1988. Dementia was however a fear of his and so he would therefore have been keenly interested in yet another possible use of aspirin. This is in the reduction of cognitive decline.

Vascular dementia is probably one of the leading causes of cognitive impairment and the syndrome "multi-infarct dementia" is probably the only major cause of dementia that is likely to be preventable at present.[39] Published estimates suggest that about 25% of elderly people have multi-infarct dementia, in half of whom it is combined with other processes. The prevalence is not well established but the range of estimates in the literature of the contribution of multi-infarct lesions to the total burden of dementia varies from about 15 to 50%. Clearly aspirin is of interest in this situation and there have been calls for controlled trials.[39] There has however been only one trial of aspirin and cognitive decline reported and it was so compromised in design and in conduct that Archie would have found it totally unacceptable.[40]

Undoubtedly Archie would have been especially delighted that his successor as director of his unit has set up a randomised controlled trial of aspirin and cognitive decline in older men. Unfortunately however, the success of aspirin is now mitigating against the investigation of its further possible uses, and setting up further randomised controlled trials is proving to be difficult. There is often a "window of opportunity" for intervention trials and in the case of aspirin it would seem that this window is closing. An ever increasing proportion of older people seem to be taking aspirin, and many of these probably take it somewhat intermittently and haphazardly. While some take it on the recommendation of their GP, many decide themselves to take it because a friend has had a myocardial infarction or stroke, or they read in a magazine about the likely benefits. Data from the Caerphilly Cohort Study[41] indicate that almost 30% of the oldest men are taking aspirin regularly. Add to these the men who are unacceptable in a randomised trial such as those who have had a recent myocardial infarction or stroke, and those who are sensitive or intolerant of aspirin, and only about 50% of the men seen in the Caerphilly Cohort Study were available for the current MRC randomised controlled trial of aspirin and cognitive decline.

Conclusion

The aspirin story, like the memory of Archie, will never die. One of the first drugs to be used by humans (Hippocrates, 400 BC), the first drug to be synthesised (by Bayer in 1897), and the drug that is reckoned to be the foundation of the modern pharmaceutical industry, aspirin may have more benefits yet to be identified, quantified, and exploited in clinical practice. In the same way, Archie, specialist in tuberculosis, pioneer of field epidemiology, international expert on pneumoconiosis, random reflector on the health services, stimulator of the concept of the overview, key figure behind the Cochrane Collaboration, and contributor to the concept of evidence based medicine—Archie Cochrane lives on in the work of those he encouraged.

1 Elwood PC, Cochrane AL, Burr ML, *et al.* A randomised controlled trial of acetyl salicylic acid in the secondary prevention of mortality from myocardial infarction. *BMJ* 1974, **1**: 436–40
2 Mather HG, Morgan DC, Pearson NG, *et al.* Myocardial infarction: a comparison between home and hospital care for patients. *BMJ* 1976;**2**:925–9.
3 Palmer JW. Smoking, caning and delinquency in a secondary modern school. *British Journal of Preventive and Social Medicine* 1965;**19**:18.
4 *Holy bible.* Daniel 1, 8–16.
5 Cochrane AL. Sickness in Salonica: my first, worst, and most successful clinical trial. *BMJ* 1984;**289**:1726–7.
6 O'Brien JR. An in-vivo trial of an anti-adhesive drug. *Thrombosis et Diathesis Haemorrhagica* 1963;**9**:120–25.
7 O'Brien JR. Aspirin and platelet aggregation. *Lancet* 1968;**203**:779–83.
8 O'Brien JR. Two in-vivo studies comparing high and low aspirin dosage. *Lancet* 1971; i: 399–400.
9 Zucker MB, Peterson J. Inhibition of adenosine diphosphate induced secondary aggregation and other platelet functions by acetylsalicylate acid ingestion. *Proc Soc Exp Biol Med* 1968;**127**:547–51.
10 Weiss HJ, Aledort LM. Impaired platelet/connective tissue reaction in man after aspirin ingestion. *Lancet* 1967;ii:495–7.
11 Craven LL. Prevention of coronary thrombosis and acetylsalicylic acid. *Mississippi Valley Medical Journal* 1956;**78**:213–215.
12 Boston Collaborative Drug Surveillance Group. Regular aspirin intake and acute myocardial infarction. *BMJ* 1974;**1**:440–3.
13 Cochrane AL, Blythe M. *One man's medicine: an autobiography of Professor Archie Cochrane.* London: British Medical Journal Memoir Club, 1989.

14 Elwood PC, Renaud S, Sharp DS, *et al.* Ischaemic heart disease and platelet aggregation. The Caerphilly Collaborative Heart Disease Study. *Circulation* 1991;**83**:38–44.
15 Elwood PC, Beswick AD, Sharp DS, *et al.* Whole blood impedance platelet aggregometry and ischaemic heart disease. The Caerphilly Collaborative Heart Disease Study. *Arteriosclerosis* 1990;**10**:1032–6.
16 Renaud SC, Beswick AD, Fehily AM, *et al.* Alcohol and platelet aggregation. The Caerphilly Prospective Heart Disease Study. *Am J Clin Nutr* 1992;**55**:1012–7.
17 Coronary Drug Project Research Group. Aspirin in coronary heart disease. *Journal of Chronic Disease* 1976; **29**:625–42.
18 Elwood PC, Sweetnam PM. Aspirin and secondary mortality after myocardial infarction. *Lancet* 1979;ii:1313–5.
19 Elwood PC, Williams WO. A randomised controlled trial of aspirin in the prevention of early mortality in myocardial infarction. *Journal of the Royal College of General Practitioners* 1979;**29**:413–6.
20 Weller M, Leokottler B, Berg PA, *et al.* Effective suppression of crescendo amaurosis fugax associated with antiphospholipid antibodies by low-dose aspirin. *Neuro-ophthalmology* 1991;**11**:195–7.
21 Folts JD, Crowell Jr, EB, Rowe GG. Platelet aggregation in partially obstructed vessels and its elimination with aspirin. *Circulation* 1976;**54**:365–9.
22 Haerem JW. Platelet aggregates and mural micro-thrombin in the early stages of acute fatal coronary disease. *Thromb Res* 1974;**5**:243.
23 Deeks J, Watt I, Freemantle N, Aspirin and acute myocardial infarction: Clarifying the message. *Br J Gen Prac* 1995;395–6.
24 O'Brien JR, Finch W, Clark E. A comparison of an effect of different anti-inflammatory drugs on human platelets. *J Clin Pathol* 1970;**23**:522–5.
25 Lewis HD, Davis JW, Archibald DG, *et al.* Protective effects of aspirin against acute myocardial infarction and death in men with unstable angina. Results of a Veterans' Administration cooperative study. *N Engl J Med* 1983;**309**:396–403.
26 Aspirin Myocardial Infarction Study Research Group. A randomised controlled trial of aspirin in persons recovered from myocardial infarction. *JAMA* 1980;**243**:661–9.
27 Editorial. Aspirin after myocardial infarction. *Lancet* 1980;**1**:1172–3.
28 Antiplatelet Trialists. Collaborative overview of randomised trials of antiplatelet therapy—I: prevention of death, myocardial infarction, and stroke by prolonged antiplatelet therapy in various categories of patients. *BMJ* 1994;**308**:81–106.
29 Sheldon T, Chalmers I. The United Kingdom Cochrane Centre and the NHS Centre for reviews and dissemination: retrospective roles within the information system strategy of the NHS programme, coordination and principles underlying collaboration. *Health Econ* 1994;**3**:201–3
30 Statement by AL Cochrane in: *Scarce resources in health care.* Office of Health Economics. London: HMSO, 1979.
31 Cochrane AL. Foreword in Chalmers I, Enkin M. Keirse MJNC, eds. *Effective care in pregnancy and childbirth.* Oxford: Oxford University Press, 1989. Quoted in Chalmers I. What would Archie have said? *Lancet* 1995;**346**:1300.
32 CLASP (Collaborative Low-dose Aspirin Study in Pregnancy) Collaborative Group: a randomised trial of low-dose aspirin for the prevention and treatment of pre-eclampsia among 9364 pregnant women. *Lancet* 1994;**343**:619–29.
33 Thun MJ, Namboodiri MM, Heath CW Jr. Aspirin use and reduced risk of fatal colon cancer. *N Engl J Med* 1991;**325**:1593–6.
34 Greenberg ER, Baron JA, Freeman DH Jr, *et al.* Reduced risk of large-bowel adenomas among aspirin users. The Polyp Prevention Study Group. *J Natl Cancer Inst* 1993;**85**: 912–16.
35 Giovannucci E, Egan KM, Hunter DJ, *et al.* Aspirin and the risk of colorectal cancer in women. *N Engl J Med* 1995;**333**:655–7.
36 Shiff SJ, Koutsos MI, Qiao L, Rigas B. Nonsteroidal antiinflammatory drugs inhibit the proliferation of colon adenocarcinoma cells: effects of cell cycle and apoptosis. *Experimental Cell Research* 1996;**222**:179–88.

37 Gupta SK, Joshi S. Relationship between aldose reductase inhibiting activity and anti cataract action of various non-steroidal anti-inflammatory drugs. In: Sasaki K, Hockwin O, eds. *Distribution of cataracts in the population and influencing factors*. Developments in Ophthalmology. Basel: Karger, 1991;**21**:151–6.
38 Kahler CM, Kieselbach GF, Reinisch N, Troger J, Gottinger W, Wiedermann CJ. Fibroblast growth-promoting activity in proliferative vitreoretinopathy: antagonism by acetylsalicylic acid. *Eur J Pharmacol* 1994;**262**:261–9.
39 Haskinsky V. Preventable senility: a call for action against the vascular dementias. *Lancet* 1992;**340**:645–7.
40 Myer JS, Rogers RL, McClintic K, Mortel KF, Lotfi J. Randomised clinical trial of daily aspirin therapy in multi-infarct dementia. A pilot study. *J Am Geriatr Soc* 1989;**37**:549–55.
41 Caerphilly and Speedwell collaborative heart disease studies. The Caerphilly and Speedwell Collaborative Group. *J Epidemiol Community Health* 1984;**38**:259–62.

6: Social work: beyond control?

GERALDINE MACDONALD

Introduction

In *Effectiveness and efficiency*, Archie Cochrane expressed the hope that Seebohm's recommendation for the creation of large, generic social services departments, realised in the early 1970s, would augment the professional status of social workers and social administrators. He had two worries, though. The first centred on the likely scope of the new profession. In much the same way that the traditional view of medicine suggested there was "a bottle . . . a pill, an operation, or a holiday to cure every ailment", he was concerned that the appointment of a social worker would be seen as the answer to every social need "whether or not there is any evidence that the social worker can alter the natural history of the social problem".[1] His concerns in this regard were prescient, with the role and responsibilities of local authority social services departments growing considerably during the 1970s. It is on Cochrane's second, inextricably related worry that this chapter will focus. Cochrane was concerned about the attitude of the profession towards evaluation, which he noted was generally antagonistic, viewing the task as essentially a moral rather than a technical endeavour. He cites Paul Halmos:

> "The certainty of value is not rooted in empirically verified results; it is rather the assurance derived from an unanalysable moral imperative."[2]

Not only was Cochrane right to be concerned, but social work's ambivalence towards evaluation persists, if somewhat tempered in recent years by a belated sense of political threat. Its antipathy towards randomised controlled trials, however, remains white hot. Anyone who acknowledges randomised controlled trials as the benchmark of rigorous evaluative research and tries to persuade social work practitioners, managers, researchers, or funders of their crucial role in the evaluation of social interventions will know what it is like to be a voice calling in the wilderness, markedly less popular than John the Baptist, and with a keen eye for Herod family look alikes.

The reasons why randomised controlled trials are considered to be the gold standard in evaluative research are well rehearsed elsewhere[3,4] and probably taken for granted by many medical readers. This is not so within social work, where controlled trials in general, and randomised controlled trials in particular, are regarded with great suspicion.

Salad days

This present day antipathy towards randomised controlled trials is somewhat surprising given that social work can boast involvement in large randomised controlled trials from as early as the mid-1930s. These prize fights (for example, social work *versus* delinquency) were undertaken in a spirit of unprecedented optimism that social work's principal modus operandi, social casework (a combination of relationship based counselling, advocacy, and practical assistance), could make a real difference in the erstwhile trajectories of personal and social problems. This confidence in the effectiveness of the intervention was matched by a view of the "scientific method" (controlled trials) as a valid and ethically robust means of scrutinising the effects of people's good intentions:

> "There are value-assumptions, and ethical consequences, in every step the social scientist takes ... and his own research and writing, whether he likes it or not, are bound to reflect (these). It was during the tragic experiences of the second world war that most social scientists began to think clearly about this issue. The Youth Study, however, some years previous to the war had accepted the logical marriage of science and ethics. It assumed that to prevent delinquency and to foster spiritual growth were worthy ends. But it knew that starting with such assumptions the tools of science (even awkwardly applied at the beginning) might be counted on to hasten the achievements of these goals, or might (as has happened) demand that the goals be better defined. In the long run, social science working hand in hand with ethics can help mankind evolve a clearer, sounder, and more viable statement of its own moral objectives."[5]

The Youth Study in question was the Cambridge-Somerville Youth Study, a randomised controlled trial of delinquency prevention, initiated in 1936 by Richard Cabot. Then as now, delinquency was a topical subject, defeating both understanding and successful management. There was already a body of evidence suggesting that reformatories did not reform, and that precious little else seemed to make much difference once criminality was established.[6] Cabot, familiar with this material, had developed the view that delinquency could be prevented by securing for those at risk a friendly, understanding and supportive relationship with an adult, outside the family, who would provide them with an "ego-ideal" Cabot was aware, however, that this was "merely a hunch—a hypothesis needing verification".[5] Therefore he considered it ethically incumbent on him to test this in the most rigorous way available, and he subsequently designed, funded, and initiated a randomised controlled trial of the effectiveness of long term counselling for boys identified at risk of delinquency. The staff of the study were not restricted to those with social work qualifications, but the person specification, so to speak, was in this mould. Thus, the study sought "men and women of good character, intelligence, and tact, who had had professional experience in dealing with people . . . A social worker, no matter how well trained, was not to be preferred to a warm, outgoing person who had that vital spark so essential in human relationships, but who had not had the benefit of formal social work education". Precursors of Margaret Thatcher's "streetwise granny" perhaps.

Views of the ethics of randomised controlled trials appear to have undergone a transformation since Cabot's day, with those who argue for their relevance decidedly *not* seen as being on the side of the angels. This chapter takes as its starting point that randomised controlled trials constitute the "gold standard" of evaluative research and does not rehearse these particular arguments here. It reviews some possible reasons for the apparent change in attitudes towards randomised controlled trials in particular and scientific methodology in general (sometimes referred to as empiricism); provides some evidence of contemporary challenges faced by those who would see randomised controlled trials assume a more certain and authoritative position (all other methodological issues being equal) within outcome research; and offers some technical and ethical reasons why funders, policy makers, and practitioners concerned with social interventions should take more seriously than they do the issues of validity that randomised controlled trials are designed to tackle.

Shooting the messenger

Despite the rather dated language of the Cambridge-Somerville Youth Study, the idea that delinquency has (at least some of) its roots in early childhood and socialisation, that a confiding relationship which provides an opportunity for insight and a role model to support change, and that it is possible to identify those at risk of delinquency, remain common currency today. Although an American study, conducted in two towns in Massachusetts, nothing about it compromised its relevance to the United Kingdom, except perhaps the amount and duration of contact time between workers and young people, which was luxurious by present day standards. Further, between 1936 and 1972, 16 other large scale controlled trials were conducted, predominantly but by no means exclusively focused on delinquency, 11 of which were randomised.

Why then did this enthusiasm for the controlled trial run so dramatically into the sand? Festinger provides one possible explanatory mechanism—namely, dissonance reduction.[7] The results of these early trials were hard to take. Generally, those in receipt of the independent variable (for example, counselling) fared no better than those whose lives were marred by its absence. Worse, in some studies, including the Cambridge-Somerville Youth Study, the data indicated deterioration effects.[8,9] The ministrations of professional helpers, it seems, can be deleterious to health and welfare. The poor showing of the profession's efficacy in these studies led those whose practice mirrored that under scrutiny to conclude that it must be the methodology that was at fault, rather than the tools of their trade.

Another reason was possibly the means whereby the results of these studies were disclosed to the troops. Typically, the abreaction of the social work profession was triggered not by the publication of these studies (the existence of which is *still* unknown to most students and qualified workers) but by the publication of a narrative review by Fischer in 1973. Fischer's conclusion was as follows:

> "The available controlled research strongly suggests that at present, lack of evidence of the effectiveness of professional casework is the rule rather than the exception. A technical research corollary to this conclusion and a comment frequently appearing in the social work literature, is that we also lack good scientific proof of ineffectiveness. This assertion, however, taken alone, would appear to be rather insubstantial grounds on which to support a profession."[10]

The news was not quite what had been expected. Fischer's review elicited a series of articles and letters from the righteously indignant who wrote to complain that scientific methodology was much too blunt an instrument with which to poke about in the necessarily mysterious dynamics of what passes between would be helper and might be helped. The antipathy towards scientific methodology remains virulent,[11,12] despite improvements in patterns of findings.[13,14]

The reasons marshalled in opposition to scientific methodology, in which the randomised controlled trial elicits most opprobrium, fall into three categories: *philosophical* (positivism, and therefore trials, are wrong headed), *ethical* (neither trials, nor positivist approaches, are compatible with the ethical principles underpinning social work), and *technical* (trials are simply not practicable ways of evaluating the effects of social work). The philosophical objections are probably more pronounced in social work than in medicine and we begin with these.

Not the place to seek the Emperor

One objection has already been alluded to—namely, that much as one should be wiser than to look for the sacred Emperor in a poor teahouse, one should not seek to reveal the subtle mechanisms of social work's helping strategies through the blunt instruments of scientifically directed research. What in other fields are reasons *for* conducting randomised controlled trials—the difficulty of controlling for other influences on the trajectories of personal and interpersonal problems—are here miraculously transformed into the reasons for *not* doing them.

As a predominantly (though by no means exclusively or necessarily) quantitative method, the randomised controlled trial is thought bound to miss the subtle interplay of important non-specific variables. Social work's preoccupation with the "helping process" is perhaps attributable to its investment in relationship based forms of counselling. Whereas research supports the importance of process variables, such as the quality of the therapeutic relationship,[15,16] it does not permit the conclusion drawn by some that (as Fats Waller might have put it) "it ain't what you do, it's the way that you do it, that's what gets results!". This belief continues to be adhered to despite growing evidence that *what* is done matters considerably (see for example Macdonald and Sheldon 1992;[14] Gendreau 1996[17]).

The extreme version of this argument is the position that social work is an art, rather than a science, a stance which elicited from two antagonists the retort: "If social work is an art, then let it be funded by the Arts Council".[18] A dangerous jest to share in the current political climate. The problem with dismissing science as too blunt an instrument for the evaluative task in social work, is that one must eventually ask whether in fact the Emperor in question is the one with no clothes.

Another related problem that stymies the acceptance of randomised controlled trials in social work merits brief mention. Quite simply put, the theories and methods which currently enjoy the best empirical support, and those which have been most exposed to trial methodology, are those which are least popular in the field. Therefore, there has been a double incentive to dismiss a methodology which (quite consistently as it happens) has suggested that social workers, among other helpers, should be doing more of one kind of thing and less of another.

The method that continues to attract least evidential support—whether measured by an absence of randomised controlled trials or their results—is psychodynamic counselling, still a dominant force in the profession. The methods that attract most evidential support, again from the point of view of the sheer number of randomised controlled trials and their results, are those derived from theories of learning (cognitive-behavioural approaches).*

* Briefly, many patterns of behaviour, both adaptive and maladaptive are thought to be acquired as a result of various forms of learning (for example, modelling, operant, and classical conditioning). Therapeutically, this offers the possibility that some behaviours can be unlearned if, for example, the contingencies governing them can be altered. In recent years the definition of behaviour and learning has been extended to include cognition and cognitive processes, although these remain subject to controversy. Compared with most other interventions, the hallmark of behavioural interventions is that one doesn't learn to swim by attending a seminar on swimming. Modelling, behaviour rehearsal and reinforcement of performance are key strategies in behavioural approaches.

The flavour of the disjuncture within the profession is illustrated in the following editorial comment in a National Society for the Prevention of Cruelty to Children (NSPCC) training resource for child protection advisers, which contained within it a review of studies of effectiveness in the field:

> "Suppose, for example, we adopt a very strict criterion and consider only those methods which have been tested using the protocols of experimental research. We will quickly discover that they are very few in number and restricted almost entirely to behavioural techniques which train parents to use less abusive forms of discipline (or, more generally, make available a wider range of parenting skills)."[19]

Oh dear! In other words, there are *some* relevant, rigorously gathered, and carefully analysed studies, but the techniques that show up well are not those we would choose to use. With the exception of probation (now wrested from its social work anchorage by Government) this picture is broadly accurate. The Central Council for Education and Training in Social Work (CCETSW) omitted to mention behavioural techniques in their list of therapeutic strategies that social workers should be familiar with,[20] and there are probably only four social work courses in the United Kingdom which teach these methods to a level that would enable students to use them in their assessments and their interventions.

It is not coincidental that the theoretical foundations of behavioural approaches also enjoy greater empirical support than, for example, psychodynamic counselling or some forms of family therapy. Nor is it coincidental that those who promote evidence based practice in social work tend to accord them some status. It is puzzling, therefore, that in general a profession which purports to be concerned with people's welfare typically ignores an accumulation of promising evidence about ways of helping, across a range of problems. But it is the rather *un*mysterious, technical nature of behavioural social work—so different from Freudian counselling—that one suspects is the reason for its downright unpopularity. Discussions of the uses and abuses of cognitive-behavioural approaches[21,22] are not dissimilar to those that take place about empiricism in general, and we revert to this general issue later.

The misuse of science

More serious—because it enjoys some empirical support—is the objection that the history of quantitative methods can be shown to replicate oppressive patterns of social relationship, in the assumptions which have underpinned research questions, in the socioeconomic make-up of research teams (predominantly white, male, heterosexual) and in the uses to which research findings have been put. This has become an appropriate concern for social work, the clients of which are often from the poorest and most vulnerable groups in society, working within a political context which also conspires to maintain the status quo. The need to develop a model of research that reflects the experiences and world views of oppressed groups—for example, disabled people,[23] black people,[24] and gay and lesbian people[25]—has been persuasively argued. Less persuasive is the often linked argument that to do this it is necessary to reject scientific methodology in favour of qualitative, interpretist models of research which look to be more sympathetic to individual subjective and collective experiences.[26] By equating the masculinist, racist, or heterosexist assumptions underpinning much research with the methodology, the proverbial baby has often been thrown out with the bathwater. Oakley summarises, but does not endorse, the situation as follows:

> "Qualitative methods . . . are seen to be more suited to the exploration of individual experiences—the representation of subjectivity within academic discourse and to facilitate, (in practice if not in theory) a non-hierarchical organisation of the research process. . . . Conversely, quantitative methods . . . are cited as instituting the hegemony of the researcher over the researched, and as reducing personal experience to the anonymity of mere numbers."[27]

The call for dichotomous allegiance is, of course, an artificial construct, and one that is crippling the development of a research paradigm which is both methodologically sound and which attends to important qualitative data. Preventing further physical abuse of a child by a parent who none the less continues to despise him, may be improvement on the easy to measure continuum, but would be a rather pyrrhic victory.

Oakley's own study of the effects of social support in pregnancy[28] demonstrates how even the randomised controlled trial can be deployed in such a way as to benefit those with little power—in the case of maternity care, it offers the possibility of calling a halt to (or at least evaluating) the rise in unevaluated technology. There is nothing intrinsically incompatible in conducting scientific research from an anti-oppressive perspective. Oakley's summary of the tenets of a feminist perspective towards the process of research as: (*a*) not employing methods oppressive either to researchers or to the researched, and (*b*) "oriented towards the production of knowledge in such a form and in such a way as can be used by women themselves", offers a guide to good research generally, particularly in a field where the nature of the task is, in part, to address oppression and its consequences.

Social work has rightly been concerned to tackle forms of oppression such as racism and sexism, both within its own organisations and practice, and this needs no defence. Further, it is right to evaluate critically the philosophical and value judgements underpinning research (necessary for *all* research, not just randomised controlled trials). But beyond this, we must take care that in pursuing our own ideological goals we do not deprive those who have little voice of those methods of helping which would be most effective and most acceptable.

Randomised controlled trials are not the only fruit

At all levels in social work, from practice through to research funders, the most difficult task facing those wishing to persuade the *cognoscenti* of the value of randomised controlled trials, is the unavoidable discussion of their methodological superiority over other methods—else why would we bother? Now this is problematic in a profession which sees itself as concerned with human justice and—though one might wish to take issue with its formulation—has always held as a central principle, the uniqueness of the individual. These are laudable aspirations when applied to human beings, but comprise rather large errors of judgement when extended to theories or concepts. It is difficult to have a discussion in social work—with students, managers, workers, or research funders—without being told that randomised controlled trials are just *one* method among many, and that we must not cede them any particular primacy. For example, here are some statements taken from feedback from four UK government departments approached for funding of a research proposal aimed at establishing a register of trials pertinent to social work and the work of the personal social services.*

> "... we have concerns that the emphasis in the proposal on controlled trials is too strong given the body of available scientific work on PSS and the likely paucity of randomised controlled trials of social work interventions. ... In general we have chosen to move forward with an approach which looks at research literature on particular issues, covers several aspects of each issue not only effectiveness, and includes all relevant and valid scientific designs.
>
> [X is] still concerned at the overwhelming emphasis under 'experimental designs' on randomised controlled trials. These are not the only experimental methodologies, and, especially in the Social Care field, they feel randomised controlled trials may not be the most appropriate. They require further written confirmation that all types of methodology and protocols would be looked at fairly in the study.
>
> There was ... a view expressed by several of the people consulted that it will be important to look at a range of social service research methods in order to assess where 'softer' approaches have something to offer. There was some concern that useful 'softer' methodologies could be further downgraded if they did not involve 'controlled trials'."

---

* The Department of Health and Social Services in Northern Ireland has since funded the proposal referred to, albeit without the support of its sister departments.

Again, leaving aside the logic of whether "softer methodologies" can "involve controlled trials", it is a striking feature of such objections that they highlight precisely those reasons why many would consider such approaches essential. The irony is that during two one-day seminars organised by Barnardo's and the Social Science Research Unit (and funded by the Economic and Social Research Council) to explore the issue of methodology in welfare interventions, those opposed to randomised controlled trials—certainly most participants involved in government funded social work research—would have given an independent observer the impression that the problem was that social work's research profile was simply teeming with randomised controlled trials to the exclusion of other methods which had much to offer. In the last decade the number of trials of social work itself has fallen; those conducted are generally smaller, and less methodologically secure, than in earlier years.[14] Be assured, the social work world is not about to be overrun with randomised controlled trials, which remain a rather rare sight in the methodological fruit basket.

This is the case even if we extend our scope beyond social work to the research activities of other professionals. In the field of child abuse and neglect, for example, Fink and McCloskey[29] found only 13 studies which met what they regarded as minimum criteria of methodological rigour ("clearly defined outcomes and valid measures, explicit criteria for including and excluding participants, and random assignment to experimental and control groups") only four of which were published after 1985. Oates and Bross[30] found only 25 papers in 10 years which met minimum requirements of more than five subjects (at least 15% of whom had been physically abused), and one of randomisation, a matched control group or the use of a premeasure and postmeasure of effectiveness. None of these were concerned with routine service provision. Given the huge investment in this, and other areas of welfare provision, and given the stakes involved, we should perhaps be more worried than we appear to be at the *lack* of randomised controlled trials rather than discussing their tyrannical nature.

"Clean hands": the ethical objections

In broad brush terms, the ethical objections to the scientific paradigm in social work research, as epitomised in the reasons given for dismissing randomised controlled trials, are not dissimilar to those encountered within medicine.[31] However, they carry flavours and twists peculiar to the history of social work research, and the way it sees its role. In brief the objections are: (*a*) it is unethical randomly to allocate clients to one of two or more groups, only one of which will receive the "active ingredient"; (*b*) such trials are prohibitively costly and the resources they consume are better targeted at service provision; (*c*) research in general, and "scientific methodology" in particular, exacerbate an already extant power imbalance between researchers and researched. We have already considered the third objection in the context of randomised controlled trials, and shall return to it in the general context of an obligation to effective intervention. The other two objections merit some further comment.

The scandal of random allocation

The alleged breach of ethics incurred by randomisation presupposes two things, both erroneous.

Firstly, certainty that the intervention which is being withheld from those in the control group(s) is effective (delivers intended outcomes) and desirable (carries minimal adverse effects, is not prohibitively costly, does not infringe the wellbeing of others). In the first instance it is worth returning to the Cambridge-Somerville Youth Study for a poignant reminder of the dangers inherent in such assumptions. Some 30 years after the close of the study, J McCord traced over 500 of the men who had participated, and conducted a follow up study.[32] From their replies to a postal questionnaire McCord ascertained that those who had been in the experimental group, that is to say those who had received a range of services entailing an average of three and a half hours face to face contact with staff over a number of years, were:

- More likely to commit (at least) a second crime
- More likely to evidence signs of alcoholism
- More likely to manifest signs of serious mental illness (including manic depression and schizophrenia)
- More likely to have had at least one stress related illness; in particular, high blood pressure or heart trouble
- More likely to have occupations with lower prestige
- More likely to report their work as "not satisfying".

Although we now have a much better understanding of the part the system can play in this (including the adverse effects of providing intensive therapeutic endeavour at an early stage, as opposed to, for example, cautioning), the bottom line is that using the state of the art technology of the period (egopsychology based counselling) made little impact, even at a time when resources were noticeably less constrained than they are at present. Further, many of the men who responded to McCord asked her to pass on messages to their counsellors. These messages—unsolicited testimonials of affection and gratitude—testify to the gap between client satisfaction and tangible outcome, and the fallacy of relying on measures of process as evidence of effectiveness.

Secondly, objections to randomisation presuppose that routine service delivery embodies those ethical principles that lead it to reject randomisation—for example, fairness, equity, respect, and dignity. But consider the following.

Some years ago I was invited, with a colleague, to evaluate a promising development in the provision of group based support to families whose children were considered at risk of abuse, and whose names were on the child protection register. On learning that the borough concerned, like many at the time, had on the register about 40 families for whom there was no allocated social worker (and no other service provided), and from whom eight families would be selected for the project, we proposed a randomised controlled study rather than the before and after test they were seeking. We were told that it would be unethical to allocate clients randomly. No-one was interested in a discussion of the ways in which this could be achieved without compromising concerns about vulnerable clients. It seemed to escape notice that the personal social services are delivered daily in the context of a large scale uncontrolled trial. Organisations are, it seems, only beset with ethical qualms when asked to formalise arrangements they happily operate as long as they result from organisation constraints or chance events, and as long as we do not attempt to learn anything en route.

Cost

Randomised controlled trials of a size that would command statistical power are indeed often costly and strategically challenging to mount within the personal social services. As indicated earlier, the trend in randomised controlled trials in social work has been towards fewer, smaller, often less methodologically robust trials, which—though by no means always—beg as many questions of validity as they seek to address.[33] But objections that trials are often inadequately conceived or executed is not a reason for rejecting them in favour of other methods. Similarly, the choice of other methods on the grounds of cost seems spurious when the arguments *for* the superiority of trials is taken seriously. In other words, what is the point of spending *any* money at all, if the results are open to challenge on the grounds of internal validity? Similarly, one must question the ethics of involving people in studies that are of doubtful value.

A cool appraisal of research expenditure on the work of the personal social services shows an imbalance between large numbers of small, descriptive studies, more accurately described as informed administration, and a paucity of rigorous studies which provide secure data. It is perfectly possible—and eminently more reasonable when it comes to evaluative research—to cut the cake a different way, producing larger more substantial slices of something that will hold sufficient calorific value to be of use.

In the context of ethical disputes in social work Archie Cochrane may have had a soulmate in Frederick Seebohm, the chairman of the Committee of Inquiry whose report resulted in generic social services departments:

> "The personal social services are large scale experiments in helping those in need. It is both wasteful and irresponsible to set experiments in motion and to omit to record and analyse what happens. It makes no sense in terms of administrative efficiency, and however little intended, indicates a careless attitude towards human welfare."[34]

Unfortunately it seems that Seebohm's words went largely unheeded in the years of plenty when, as Cochrane feared, social workers seemed to be written into every piece of social legislation. It is only now, in leaner times, constrained by government edict, that a concern with the effectiveness of professional activity is resurfacing, albeit under a flag with predominantly monetary colours. But the demand for evaluation now carries other risks and problems. Firstly, political ideology poses a major threat to perceived relevance of rigorous research, such that policies are implemented despite evidence of their ineffectiveness. Case management of the mentally ill is now national policy despite the lack of evidence that except in intense forms it is effective,[35] and we are going ahead with a policy of detention of young offenders despite decades of evidence that this certainly does not work, on any outcome measure other than that when locked up these young people are off the streets. Secondly, the increasing number of provider agencies commissioning research (which many will need to do to secure future funding) will only want certain kinds of results. Demand factors are very hard to resist in non-experimental studies. Thirdly, the wholescale nature of change within the personal social services means that it will be difficult to conduct randomised controlled trials of organisational aspects of service provision. To reiterate Seebohm's view, this surely "indicates a careless attitude towards human welfare".

Why social work research should be better controlled

In social work, lack of attention to methodological issues is exacerbated by a more fundamental problem—namely, ambivalence toward empirical data in general, and frequent hostility to the suggestion that empirically based data or evidence should carry more weight than other theories or bright ideas. This is a deeper irrationality than the "blunt instruments" fallacy examined earlier. Here is Medawar's eloquent analysis of the roots of this problem:

> "We are still so deeply steeped in the tradition of which [William] Blake was one of the founders, that we find it difficult to realise that the intensity of the

conviction with which we believe a theory to be true has no bearing upon its validity except insofar as it produces a proportionately strong inducement to find out whether it is true or not. Some theories have enjoyed an unduly long lease of life because of a certain, dark visceral appeal."[36]

This chapter is (unsurprisingly) in favour of social work on the basis of "what works", not "what appeals". This emphasis has implications for the proper nature of social work research.

Put simply, it is little use funding research, however well designed, if the problems being targeted are conceptualised in ways that enjoy no empirical support or do not lend themselves to empirical verification. This is a difficult area, because assessor bias by peers can effectively exclude the evaluation of certain kinds of intervention, as well as certain kinds of research design,[37] and we should avoid introducing a further source of exclusivity. However, in distributing scarce resources, it would not be unreasonable to require researchers to demonstrate the validity of their problem formulations and the (one hopes) logical relationship they enjoy with the intervention proposed. This might see a diminution of the "anything goes" approach to knowledge, in which mutually exclusive theories, enjoying disparate degrees of empirical support, are treated equally. At present, even at Masters level, one will still find students being offered, as if choice were a matter of personal taste or preference, a range of theoretical and therapeutic options, many of which are mutually exclusive (you cannot believe both Jean Piaget's view of the development of conscience[38] and Melanie Klein's;[39] —but both often appear in the same study).*

Like other helping professions[39] we become attached to theories and ways of working, some of which we acquire as a result of early professional socialisation (it is disturbingly easy to predict students' appetites for theories on the basis of their precourse experience), some of which are chosen because they are inherently rewarding for the practitioner. Less often, they are chosen for their apparent validity or effectiveness, irrespective of personal appeal. The consequences are serious for those on the receiving end of would be helpers (whose motivation, be it noted, is not in question):

"In the constant search for 'tools' which aid the therapeutic process with abused children and adults, we have found a new medium which seems in many ways ideal for post-disclosure therapy. The medium is ice. It can be very cheaply made in large amounts, and sustains the child's interest, especially in large quantities.

---

* For Piaget, conscience developed in middle childhood, as the result of a growing awareness of the "singular other" perspective, of intentionality, and of rules as the product of consent. For Klein, conscience developed much earlier, with the realisation that the "good breast" (satisfying, comforting) and the "bad breast" (withholding) are in fact the same, thus giving rise to guilt and providing a basis for the formation of conscience. Social work, and psychotherapy, still boast plenty of Kleinians.

> If the room and the child are hot, and the child is asked to touch the ice quickly, the experience is refreshing, exciting and meets the needs of the hot child."[40]

Such "innovative" approaches rarely elicit cries of "foul" from those concerned with ethical ground rules. Yet how ethical is it to operate a programme with little rationale, no inbuilt attempt to make sure that at the very least no harm is being inflicted, against a background of knowledge which at least raises the question of the appropriateness of the strategies used.[41,42] For example, it is by no means clear that the drama therapy techniques used by these workers, which include the rolling up of ice cubes to represent the "abusing part of the perpetrator", lead to the most appropriate associations to install in the minds of sexually abused children.

Hesitation at deploying a rigorous evaluation of such "innovations" may in part be sustained by the view shared by many social workers that professional status does not rest easy with the social work role. This is seen not as a source of expert help, but of empowerment. Now empowerment may well be a useful guiding principle, and we return to this concept later, but if this emphasis is developed independently of a concern for valid knowledge about the nature of social problems (however politically uncomfortable) or the effectiveness of particular interventions (however distasteful to the professional concerned) we are in danger of operating a double standard at the expense of the least powerful groups in society. The point is eloquently summed up by Pinker:

> "If the characteristic patterns of risk and dependency confronting social workers were to spread to the majority of the population, the general public would very soon demand services of the highest quality from professional social workers of the highest calibre, and the idea of applying egalitarian principles to standards of knowledge and skill would be laughed out of court."[43]

Debates about the relevance of empiricism in the physical and social sciences[44] make little sense when considering the effectiveness of alternative strategies of intervention: how else are we to make informed decisions, but via empirically valid, identifiable differences in effect size, cost, side effects, and so on? And it is difficult for some of us to see how we can be expected to evaluate competing theories of social problems without recourse to disconfirmable claims. Empiricism does not provide an escape route from theory to "truth" as those involved in the Cambridge-Somerville Youth Study were all too aware (see above). But it does offer a way of making explicit the theoretical underpinnings of our conceptualisations, hypotheses, or assumptions about problems and solutions, and the possibility of controlling for some of these influences when seeking to test their relative usefulness. Without such self imposed checks we will not be able to develop our knowledge base in social work beyond the anecdotal and fashionable, or answer with any degree of confidence questions about "What works best with these sorts of difficulties and with these constraints?".

Is the technology transferable?

No amount of persuasion of the desirability of controlled trials in social work will compensate for insuperable technical problems, should these exist. The tone of the discussion so far has suggested that the more routine use of controlled trials is not only a good thing, but largely a matter of persuading various groups of people whose objections are largely wrong-headed. This is not the case. There are substantive problems that beset the social scientist who wishes to use controlled trials in a field such as social work, and challenges arise here that, even if encountered elsewhere, assume a sharper focus. The chapter concludes with a discussion of some of these—namely, the choice of outcome measures, isolating the "active ingredient" in compound interventions, informed consent, the impossibility of the "double blind", and other sources of bias.

Outcome measures

Social work is charged with certain tasks such as "the protection of children" and "community care". It is relatively easy to agree goals and outcome indicators within a single case, though surprisingly this is rarely done with any degree of specificity. Client and worker can agree to differ, as long as each identifies outcome measures that meet certain requirements of specificity and measurability. So, for example, in a child protection case, the worker may want to see improved child management skills on the part of the parent, the parent on the other hand, may want a better behaved child. Whereas life is easier if a parent can be persuaded of the interrelationship of the two, it is not essential to the evaluative task: both goals can be pursued. However, life is more complicated when we move from the single case to groups (for example, child abusers) and corporate or occupational tasks (for example, child protection). One of the challenges in reviewing the child abuse literature, for example, lies in finding studies which use the same definition of child abuse (let alone measures), or the same measures of successful intervention. Legal definitions have about as much specificity as "illness", and are about as useful. Decision making is therefore inherently problematic, except at the extremes, and these problems carry over into the research endeavour.

It is probable that while we can, as in medicine, hit upon solutions to problems we do not really understand (life sentences for 10 year old offenders, for example) our likely effectiveness in tackling social problems will depend to some extent on our ability to locate discrete phenomena accurately. In social interventions, this presents us with a number of matters "upstream" of the evaluative endeavour, which need to be tackled with comparable rigour. They arise from the tendency to give single category nomenclatures to multifaceted and complex phenomena such as *abuse* and *delinquency*. Here is an example from medicine. It is suggested that had doctors 50 years ago been given erythropoietin, one of biotechnology's successful drugs and an excellent treatment for many anaemias, they would have discarded it, as they did not have the right classification of anaemias to be able to pick out the patients who would respond (Biotechnology and genetics: survey. *Economist* 1995: 25 February: 15). Social work is disadvantaged insofar as the phenomena with which it is concerned have currency in common discourse. For example, abuse is used as if it is a clear, precise term across a range of situations; but it is not at all clear that sexual abuse, physical abuse, or spouse abuse are the same *kind* of thing? Nor is it the case that the term "physical abuse" has analytical utility. Such taken for granted terms belie a lack of conceptual clarity, which lead researchers and practitioners into a range of difficulties (see Macdonald and Macdonald[37] for a discussion of the problems generated by assumptions about "the family").

In part, the problem for setting occupational or problem specific goals arises from the fact that we are considering an individually interventionist social service, rather than, for example, public health, which logically and in fact, enjoys a group or societal focus. The discourse of the aims and objectives of social work in relation to social problems can lead to talk of goals which lack coherence. For example, some have argued that the primary goal of child protection work is to reduce mortality: "The most crucial issue for the child protection services is how successful or otherwise they are in their ability to prevent the deaths of children."[45]

Others have argued that such goals misperceive the logic of the task. Infrequent, often unpredictable events are not, despite their emotive value, good outcome measures, and to judge social work's success in child protection on such a basis is not rational.[46,47] Although apparently lesser goals than the prevention of homicide, the prevention of further abuse, and amelioration of misery in identified situations of risk straddle both the individual case and the "social task"; the criteria for intervention are demonstrable, the costs and benefits more accessible and existent, and the strategies for intervention and evaluation more transparent. The problem of measures which are pertinent across cases in a trial and provide sources of between group data remains, but this is surmountable. Also, as with any attempt to locate specific outcome indicators, once identified as targets, indicators become susceptible to specific optimisation irrespective of the underlying behaviour (a problem that exists in medicine once we move beyond mortality or morbidity to the discussion of, for example, quality adjusted life years (QALYs)).

At the other extreme, softer, "who could disagree?" goals are also problematic. For example, it would be a brave person who would disclaim concern with the goals of *working in partnership* or *empowerment*. But how does one assess the effectiveness of a worker, or an agency, at meeting such self professed aims? If one looks at the uses of "participation" in the broader social work literature one will find it is variously used as a way to instil confidence;[48] a device to ensure professionals do not restrict need to available services;[49,50] as a basic human need (for example, autonomy);[51] and as a device to enhance effectiveness in service delivery.[57] If one is concerned with evaluating effectiveness it is important to specify "effective in relation to what?"

Biehal[50] provides a sensitive discussion of some of the issues around client participation in relation to community care of the elderly, and some useful descriptive accounts (drawn from the Social Work in Partnership Research and Development Project) of how social workers actually comport themselves when thinking about "participation" with elderly clients. Such descriptive work is useful in understanding what people do, and in appreciating the street-level constraints on service delivery. What it does not do is address the issue of effectiveness. It is all too easy for the individual (or for aggregates of observed individuals) to find that those clients whom they have successfully engaged in participation are also those who have been most effectively helped, and then to move to regarding participation as effective. The obvious problem is that the elderly who are good at participation may well be precisely those elderly who are good at profiting from proffered help, so "participation" itself is not generating the outcome (and is therefore not the effective strategy it is claimed to be). The need for some randomised controlled trials is obvious. But whereas randomised controlled trials provide the tool to assess effectiveness, we still have to address the issues of what is "participation", what is its claimed justification and desired outcome, and what the real life constraints on delivery may be. Many social work innovations become popular precisely because they can be embraced for many motivations. It may be that we have to constrain workers to implement "thinner" versions of "participation" before we can get a lever on whether and why it might be effective.

Notice—in line with our earlier worries about social work emphases—although we have said that the need for randomised controlled trials is obvious, Biehal[50] manages to discuss participation without once considering the need for such a research strategy. More worryingly, York and Itzhaky,[53] who purport to present a research design to locate the effects of participation, and do address some of the issues of measurement, only refer to randomised controlled trials in passing, citing with apparent approval Hunt's assertion that "control groups are not relevant".[54]

Isolating the "active ingredient"

A further challenge is the identification of the "active" component in any intervention, as interventions in social work tend to be complex interactions. For example, social work is typically not providing a "single" therapeutic response to an identified psychological problem, but a battery of therapeutic, supportive, practical assistance to a range of problems, all of which shift across the lifetime of a "case". Again, the problems are not insurmountable (and do not disappear if we opt for other research models) but may well be costly in time and effort. In some interventions it is relatively easy to parcel out different aspects of a combined package to test the relative effectiveness of each. This is how, in the treatment of phobias, we have moved from systematic desensitisation (a structured package of relaxation, the construction of a hierarchy of feared situations, imagined exposure to the hierarchy, and finally in vivo exposure) to graded in vivo exposure, experimental manipulations demonstrating that the last was the "active ingredient". In other areas we again may need to be more parsimonious and restricted in our interventions to enable a future of richer, grounded, interventions.

Informed consent

Except insofar as randomisation is often dismissed as unethical, consent of any kind seems to be an under-discussed issue in social work (where trials are scarce), and within the psychological literature which informs much of social work's therapeutic endeavour, and comprises the major source of relevant controlled trials. Randomisation is often stated as a fait accompli, with no discussion of the ethical or technical difficulties around consent that may have arisen—or should have been noticed. One can hazard guesses at why this is so (it is difficult to judge from the literature, where the issue is rarely mentioned). Certainty of the *ethics* of randomisation perhaps (as delivering advancements of knowledge in situations of equipoise—idealistic, we think); the possibility that research participants in psychological experiments are often psychology graduates, or respondents to advertisements, both groups paid to participate. Indeed, one of the challenges facing researchers within psychology, is to move away from "safe and easy" problems (low level child abuse) to the severity and complexity of problems encountered daily within the personal social services.

There are some technical consent issues which present themselves specifically with regard to randomised controlled trials—what to tell people and when to tell them—and others that have more to do with protecting the welfare of research participants, particularly when they are the compulsory clients of the statutory social services. Some others, less pertinent perhaps to evaluative research, are technical research issues which masquerade as ethical dilemmas.[37]

Consent may be sought before or after randomisation; information may be collected from all participants including those who decline to participate and those who drop out, or only from those who have agreed to participate, regardless of when consent is sought. There are strong statistical arguments for collecting and analysing data on all "could be participants" (the intention to treat principle) as not to do so can distort the apparent effects of interventions. However, if people decline to participate in a study of welfare interventions, it is difficult to insist that they contribute information at a future point, even if they have provided information at the possible point of entry to a study. Which is not to say they would not be willing. The reality is that we simply do not know what potential research participants in social work would be willing to do. The dearth of randomised controlled trials in the field means this question has rarely been posed, and the lack of data extends to the question of informed consent in general. Oakley's study of the effectiveness of social support to pregnant women[27] provides evidence of a strong altruistic motivation on the part of women to participate in the study, even though some were greatly disappointed at drawing a "control straw" in the process of random allocation. It may be that working as we do with reluctant clients makes this less likely, but we do not know. The emphasis given to empowering individuals should give the profession a head start over medicine in the willingness to take this issue on board, aided perhaps by the impossibility of achieving double blind experimental conditions.

Informed consent does strain the experimental protocol. Oakley points out that the process of seeking informed consent was such that even those in the control group sometimes felt supported by being a participant, albeit not in receipt of the independent variable. She concludes that "It is probably true to say that rigorous testing of the hypothesis that social support can improve pregnancy outcome is at odds with the principle of informed consent". Informed consent in social work may similarly contaminate randomised controlled trial methodology, insofar as it alerts people to the availability of one or more different methods of helping (which they can seek elsewhere, read about, or ask for under certain statutory conditions). Informed consent, which involves a minimal description of what different methods of helping comprise, may provide some clients with sufficient insight to effect some change. Finally, there is the real problem that informed consent which leaves some people in a treatment group they are then unpersuaded of, may introduce yet another source of bias—the "lack of demand" effect. Rather than bemoaning their contamination effects, we should perhaps recognise that sometimes ethical tenets throw up technical challenges.

Whereas the medical research participant usually recognises that he or she is ill and wants effective treatment, social services clients are often those who do not accept the diagnosis and do not see the need for any kind of "treatment". The only means of engaging reluctant clients is often to negotiate a "lowest common denominator" ("I know you don't want me involved in your life, if you want to be rid of me we have to achieve. . . ."). In an already coercive situation, one must be careful not to put additional pressure on clients. Further, the close linkage of support from social workers and cooperation with them means that one must be able to assure clients that refusal to participate will not disadvantage them in other ways. The vulnerability of clients to the "process variables" of power is worryingly large, as a number of research studies have shown.[55,56] Given the high stakes at play for those who come to the attention of welfare services for statutory reasons (children at risk, the seriously mentally ill, juvenile offenders), it must be incumbent on researchers to ensure that those who give informed consent and find themselves in a control group which, at the end of the day, fares less well than the experimental group, do not find themselves having passed through a one way door in terms of consequences. In other words, if my children's welfare or family intactness depends on effective help, and this turns out to be the help available only to the experimental group, then this should be made available to me at a later point. The issue is not straightforward. Children's lives run on different time scales to those of adults. Parents who fail in one programme of help may be discouraged from trying something else. However, these problems are not generated by issues of randomisation or informed consent. These processes highlight problems that typically lie buried in daily routine, from which no-one—neither client, nor worker, nor tax-payer—has an opportunity to learn.

Dealing with bias

One especially difficult problem in social work research is that of controlling for the experimental effects—the so-called Hawthorne effects. (There is some evidence that the original "Hawthorne effect" is attributable to economic self-interest and is not in fact an exemplar of "experimental effect".) Double blind methodology is not an option within most social welfare research, and enthusiasm for the novel or the believed in becomes a serious issue. Social work is not like administration of an encapsulatable medicine in which the contents of the capsule can remain unknown to all actors. Although not unique to social work—presumably the evaluation of some surgical procedures presents similar difficulties—the fact that social interactions are the very "stuff" of much social work means that the "enthusiasm" variable is a more powerful wild card.

Working within chaos

Evaluation *is* especially challenging within social work. Problems change, sometimes daily, today's difficulties oust previous priorities. Remember Kuhn's aside about the messiness of social science:

> "A paradigm can ... insulate the [scientific] community from those socially important problems that ... cannot be stated in terms of the conceptual and instrumental tools the paradigm supplies. ... One of the reasons why normal science seems to progress so rapidly is that its practitioners concentrate on problems that only their own lack of ingenuity should keep them from solving."[57]

New information arises which brings about a modification of assessment, and a change of direction. However, it is this very complexity that makes sound evidence of what strategies are most likely to succeed with certain problems in certain circumstances so important. It is anthropologically fascinating to encounter the bewilderment expressed by other professionals when working with the challenging families that are the bread and butter of social work. For example, when they tried to implement what were essentially behavioural techniques in the chaotic families known to the National Society for the Prevention of Cruelty to Children,[58] the psychiatrist Nicol and his colleagues commented on how long it took to establish a relationship of trust with families before implementing their programmes, and how often their plans were scuppered by unforeseen events.[58] My own view is that the training received by social workers—at its best—makes them eminently unflustered by such day to day phenomena, and that we would do well to recoup the courage of our predecessors and combine our energies with those of researchers willing to tailor scientific methodology to the challenges such interventions certainly pose. We should be developing new strategies if necessary, rather than appearing to suggest that if experimental methodology is to be used then the work must be tailored to *it*.

Some final words of caution

The popular notion that social work is something that anyone *could* do, its media image, and a series of child abuse scandals (often misinterpreted; see Macdonald[45]), provides easy pickings for those in more secure, better understood, and more highly regarded occupations, such as medicine or academia. It is not my intention that the discussion of social work's failure to grasp the technical possibilities and ethical necessity of controlled trials should be used simply as a stick with which to beat an already beleaguered profession.

This is not a "special case" plea, but a cautionary note against the drawing of simplistic conclusions about an occupation which has less influence than medical personnel have over the evaluation agenda. In critical ways social work is more vulnerable to political ideology than medicine, in which the *content* of practice (if not the shape) remains largely under the control of clinical staff. It would be naive to suggest that social work is simply lagging behind medicine in embracing a more bullish approach to evaluation. At the time of writing (1996), fiscal constraints have driven social services departments to policies of working only with those in highest need. The imposition of an evaluative paradigm which ignored the bias such circumstances introduce could easily result in the erroneous conclusion that social work is not worth the treasury candle, when the more plausible interpretation of the result might be that it is social policy which should be reconsidered. It is worth considering that the medical equivalent would be an evaluation of the effectiveness of medical staff solely on the basis of their performance in circumstances in which they were only permitted to work with those beyond help, while constrained to ignore those who with some timely help could be prevented from deteriorating.

All this said, social work *is* lagging behind medicine in its appreciation of methodological issues in research; the repudiation of the importance of randomised controlled trials that appears in some quarters verges on the criminally negligent.

Although social work is not altogether without a sense of its own identity, if the basis of that identity is restricted to the ideological rather than the empirical then it will remain vulnerable; consider:

> "The scrutiny devoted to probation in recent years should be extended to the functions and effectiveness of the other areas of social work. Their training and practice should likewise be devolved to their parent services which care for children, mental health, the elderly. . . ."[57]

If social work is simply a "doing" activity, unformalisable, relying on the goodwill and moral integrity of its practitioners, then Coleman is probably right to revert to the apprenticeship model of earlier generations. But if it is an evidence-based activity, the picture changes. Universities are and can only be justified as organisations designed for the generation and dissemination of knowledge. If social work is based on knowledge then its training and development are properly university based concerns, and Coleman's argument collapses. It remains bitterly ironic that the Coleman stance on probation has been implemented. Scrutiny of the evidence of probation's effectiveness (both relative to other disposals and in some areas in its own right) should have secured its future as a research based, university trained occupation, rather than as an activity to be divorced from its academic and social work roots and opened to those deemed (on the basis of no evidence whatsoever) more suitable—namely, ex-army and police officers, who will receive on the job training; a reminder, if reminder were needed, that in the short term, outcomes in the political sphere are not determined by rational argument (any liberal believer in the efficacy of truth has to place much faith in that "short term" qualifier).

Whatever the political climate, as an interventionist discipline social work must embrace evidence-based approaches to practice if it is not to fall foul of "the peculiar repulsiveness of those who dabble their fingers self approvingly in the stuff of other people's souls".[60] If it is to do this, then the purse holders of government research funds and the Central Council for Education and Training in Social Work must radically rethink their approach to research agendas and the training curricula. At present the profession's ability to prepare, maintain, and disseminate the findings of systematic reviews of the effects of their interventions in a manner that will sustain evidence-based practice, is seriously hampered by its inability to agree on what shall count as evidence. In research terms, social work is not beyond control, although this may be more difficult to achieve than in other fields. Our lack of attention to the methodology of evaluative research leaves us in a weak position to challenge those who would see the shape and remit of the profession changed to suit prevailing ideology, but more important is the ultimate disservice to vulnerable people. If not evidence-based practice, then what?

1 Cochrane A. *Effectiveness and efficiency: random reflections on health services*. London: Nuffield Provincial Hospitals Trust, 1972:68. (Reprinted in 1989 in association with the BMJ.)
2 Halmos P. *The faith of the counsellors*. London: Constable, 1965.
3 Campbell DT, Stanley JC. *Experimental and quasi-experimental designs for research*. Chicago: Rand McNally College Publishing Company, 1980.
4 Cook TD, Campbell DT *Quasi-experimentation: design and analysis: issues for field settings*. Chicago: Rand McNally College Publishing Company, 1979.
5 Allport GW. The forward. In: Powers E, Witmer H. *An experiment in the prevention of delinquency: the Cambridge-Somerville youth study*. New York: Colombia University Press, 1951:xxix.
6 Glueck S, Gleuck E. *500 criminal careers*. Cambridge MA: Harvard University Press, 1931.
7 Festinger L. *A theory of cognitive dissonance*, Evanston IL: Row Peterson, 1957.
8 Powers E, Witmer H. *An experiment in the prevention of delinquency: the Cambridge-Somerville youth study*. New York: Colombia University Press, 1951.
9 Lehrman LJ, *et al*. Success and failure of treatment of children in child guidance clinics of the Jewish Board of Guardians. *Research Monographs No 1*, 1949.
10 Fischer J. Is casework effective: a review. *Social Work* 1973;**17**:1–5.
11 Cheetham J, Fuller R, McIvor G, Petch A. *Evaluating social work effectiveness*. Buckingham: Open University Press, 1992.
12 Fuller R. Evaluating social work effectiveness: a pragmatic approach. In: *What works?: effective social interventions in child welfare*. Report of a Conference Organised by Barnardo's and the Social Science Research Unit, Basingstoke: Barnardo's, 1996.
13 Reid W, Hanrahan P. The effectiveness of social work: recent evidence. In: Goldberg, EM, Connelly N, eds. *Evaluative research in social care*. London: Heinemann, 1980:9–20.
14 Macdonald G, Sheldon B. Contemporary studies of the effectiveness of social work. *British Journal of Social Work* 1992;**22**:615–43.

15 Orlinsky DE, Grawe K, Parks BK. Process and outcome in psychotherapy. In: Bergin AE, Garfield SL, eds. *Handbook of psychotherapy and behavior change*. New York: John Wiley and Sons, 1995:270–368.
16 Beutler LE, Machuado PPP, Neufeld SA Therapist variables In: Bergin AE, Garfield SL, eds. *Handbook of psychotherapy and behaviour change*. 4th ed. New York: John Wiley, 1994.
17 Gendreau P. Offender rehabilitation: what we know and what needs to be done. *Criminal Justice and Behavior* 1996;**23**:144–61.
18 Brewer C, Lait J. *Can social work survive*? London: Temple Smith, 1980.
19 Paley J, ed. *Child protection adviser's resource pack* London: NSPCC/DoH, 1990.
20 Central Council for Education and Training in Social Work. *Paper 30 (revised edition)*. London: CCETSW, 1995.
21 Hudson B, Macdonald G. *Cognitive-behavioural approaches in social work*. Basingstoke: Macmillan, 1997.
22 Sheldon B. Cognitive-behaviour therapy: *Research, practice and philosophy*. London: Tavistock, 1995.
23 Morris J. *Pride against prejudice. Transforming attitudes to disability*. London: The Women's Press, 1991.
24 Lorde A. *Sister outsider*. New York: Crossing Press, 1984.
25 Kitzinger J. Sexual violence and compulsory heterosexuality. In: Wilkinson S, Kitzinger C, eds. *Heterosexuality*. London: Sage, 1992:219–38.
26 Rose H. Hand, brain and heart: a feminist epistemology for the natural sciences. *Signs: Journal of Women in Culture and Society* 1983;**11**:73–90.
27 Oakley A. Who's afraid of the randomised controlled trial? Some dilemmas of the scientific method and "good" research practice. *Women and Health* 1989;**15**:25–59.
28 Oakley A, Rajan L, Grant A. Social support and pregnancy outcome. *Br J Obstet Gynaecol* 1990;**97**:155–62.
29 Fink A, McCloskey L. Moving child abuse and neglect prevention programs forward: improving program evaluations. *Child Abuse and Neglect* 1990;**14**:187–206.
30 Oates RK, Bross DC. What have we learned from treating physical abuse? *Child Abuse and Neglect* 1995;**19**:463–73.
31 Chalmers I. Scientific inquiry and authoritarianism in perinatal care and education. *Birth* 1983;**10**:151–64.
32 McCord J. A thirty-year follow-up of treatment effects. *American Psychologist* 1978;**33**: 284–9.
33 Stein J, Gambrill E. Facilitating decision-making in foster care. *Social Services Review* 1977;**51**:502–11.
34 Seebohm Report. *Report of the committee on local authority and allied personal social services*. London: HMSO, 1968. (CMND 3703.)
35 Marshall M, Gray A, Lockwood A, Green R. Case management for people with severe mental disorders. In: Adams C, Anderson J, de Jesus Mari, eds. *Schizophrenia module of the Cochrane Database of Systematic Reviews*, 1996, Issue 3.
36 Medawar P. *Pluto's Republic*. London: Methuen, 1982:17.
37 Macdonald GM, Macdonald KI. Ethical issues in social work research. In: Hugman R, Smith D, eds. *Ethical issues in social work*. London: Routledge, 1995:46–64.
38 Piaget J. *The child's construction of reality*. London: Routledge and Kegan Paul, 1958.
39 Klein M. *The psychoanalysis of children*. Rev ed. Hogarth Press/Institute of Psychoanalysis, 1975.
40 Zelickman I, Martin J. Feeling the way forward. *Community Care* 1991;16–17.
41 Hawton K. The behavioural treatment of sexual dysfunction. Symposium on sexual dysfunction. *British Journal of Psychiatry* 1982;**140**:94–101.
42 Jehu D. *Beyond sexual abuse: therapy with women who were childhood victims*. Chichester: John Wiley, 1989.
43 Pinker R. An alternative view: a note by Professor RA Pinker. In: *Social workers: their role and tasks* London: Bedford Square Press/National Institute for Social Work, 1980:257–8.
44 Heineman M. The obsolete imperative in social work research. *Social Services Review* 1981;**55**:371–97.

45 Pritchard C. Re-analysing children: homicide and undetermined death rates as an indication of improved child protection: a reply to Creighton. *British Journal of Social Work* 1993;**23**:645–52.
46 Macdonald GM. Allocating blame in social work. *British Journal of Social Work* 1990;**20**: 525–46.
47 Macdonald KI. Comparative homicide and the proper aims of social work: a sceptical note. *British Journal of Social Work* 1995;**25**:489–97.
48 Challis D. Case management and consumer choice: the Kent community care scheme. In: Clode D, Parker C, Etherington S. eds. *Towards the sensitive bureaucracy: consumers, welfare and the new pluralism*. Aldershot: Gower, 1986:91–104.
49 Sinclair I, O'Connor P, Stanforth I, Vickery A. *Bridging two worlds—social work and the elderly living alone*. Aldershot: Gower, 1988.
50 Biehal N. Participation, rights and community care, *British Journal of Social Work* 1993; **23**: 443–58.
51 Gough I, Doyal L. A theory of human needs. *Critical Social Policy* 1984:**10**;6–38.
52 Griffiths R. Does the public service serve? The consumer dimension. *Public Administration* 1988;**66**:195–204.
53 York AS, Itzhaky H. How can we measure the effects of client participation on the effectiveness of social work intervention? *British Journal of Social Work* 1991;**21**:647–62.
54 Hunt SM. Evaluating a community development project: issues of acceptability. *British Journal of Social Work* 1987;**17**:661–7.
55 Dingwall R, Eekelaan J, Murray T. *Protecting children*. Oxford: Blackwell, 1983.
56 Satyamurti C. *Occupational survival: the case of the local authority social worker*. Oxford: Blackwell, 1981.
57 Kuhn TS *The structure of scientific revolutions*. 2nd ed. Chicago: University of Chicago Press, 1970.
58 Nicol AR, Smith J, Kay B, Hall D, Barlow J, Williams B. A focused casework approach to the treatment of child abuse: a controlled comparison. *Journal of Child Psychology and Psychiatry* 1988;**29**:703–11.
59 Coleman D. *Social work or crime prevention? a better future for probation*. London: Centre for Policy Studies, 1995.
60 Wooton B. *Social science and social pathology*. London: Allen Unwin, 1959.

Part 3
Efficiency

7: Health economics: has it fulfilled its potential?

ALAN MAYNARD, TREVOR A SHELDON

Introduction

Economic analysis as applied to health care is a relatively recent activity in the United Kingdom. It was stimulated by the crisis of healthcare expenditure which coincided with a number of critical reviews of the delivery and effectiveness of healthcare interventions in the late 1960s and the early 1970s. Economics provides a dimension that was missing from most clinical epidemiological work—that of efficiency—which is still not sufficiently emphasised by the "evidence based" healthcare movement of today.

This chapter explores the circumstances in which health economics arose and the conceptions of efficiency which were put forward by Cochrane in *Effectiveness and efficiency*.[1] We examine the limited contribution which the subdiscipline of health economics has made to health services research in the United Kingdom and point to the channelling of economics resources into economic evaluation at the expense of the broader areas of the financing, organisation, and delivery of health care. The overconcentration on economic evaluation of treatments reflects the lack of interest in health services research in the United Kingdom. To make the maximum contribution to the formulation and execution of health policy, health economists should return to "basics", forge closer links with economics, and adopt a broader perspective.

Effectiveness and efficiency in its historical context

Economic and social change

The period after the second world war and until the late 1960s was one of continuously high employment with relatively mild fluctuations in gross domestic product (GDP), employment, and unemployment (never exceeding 2.4% in the United Kingdom).[2] This period was accompanied by relatively low rates of inflation and modest cyclical (stop-go) policies, and was characterised by what has been called a "Keynesian consensus" during which public expenditure and public employment increased. The cost of social services in Britain as a share of GNP rose dramatically from around 4% before the second world war to 29% in 1975.[3] In the 1960s expenditure on the NHS increased as a percentage of all social expenditure, partly fuelled by the biggest hospital building programme since the Victorian era.[4]

By the early 1970s the growth of public expenditure was seen to be unsustainable and it was thought that a crisis of funding would occur if costs continued to grow.[5] The policies of the Conservative and Labour parties were less convergent and the limited consensus began to fracture. The unchallenged rapid expansion of the welfare state in Britain and abroad came to an abrupt end in the mid 1970s[6] in the aftermath of the first oil crisis in 1973 which precipitated a sharp downturn in GDP and employment.

The ending of the postwar boom, the fracture of the Keynesian consensus, and the pressure to constrain public expenditure concentrated the thoughts of government on improving the efficiency of public services and what Thatcher later called "value for money". The "white hot technological revolution" of the Wilson Labour governments (1963–70) led both to a greater infusion of academics into government and the recognition, epitomised in the Fulton Committee report[7] on the civil service, of the need for greater quantification in public policy formation.

The increasing demands on public finances made by the development of the health service, technological change, and higher public expectations could not all be met and had to be modified in the light of the financial constraints imposed by the recession. This presented policy makers with sharper choices about how to allocate limited resources. Such choices needed to take into consideration the likely costs and benefits of alternative investments. Addressing these issues is at the very heart of economics. From the late 1960s onwards, the number of professional economists within central government increased dramatically from 25 in 1964 to 350 in 1975.[8] Both within the Department of Health (the then chief economic adviser, David Pole, was appointed in the early 1970s) and from academia (for example, Alan Williams, on secondment from York University to the Treasury, was deployed into the Department of Health to assist in the appraisal of the hospital building programme) economic argument was injected into a policy debate dominated previously by medical science and rhetoric.[9,10]

The increased expenditure on the NHS of the previous decade was mainly disbursed geographically according to historical patterns and used for services as determined by the medical profession (see below) with little analytical attention to the likely outcomes either in terms of absolute health benefits or their social distribution. Now the attention of economists, who hitherto had not been closely involved in healthcare policy issues, began to be focused on the uses of NHS expenditure in a significant way. In doing so they brought with them the analytical approaches and techniques developed in other areas such as investment appraisal, transport, and the environment.

Health care under scrutiny

The 1960s and early 1970s were also periods of social and political upheaval in which the organisation of society, distribution of political and economic power, and the mechanisms by which social relations were maintained came under sustained critique. The period was notable for the impressive concentration of intellectual re-examination and critique of health care and healthcare systems in developed countries.

Some doctors, historians, and social scientists questioned the contribution of health care in general and medicine in particular, to improving levels of health.[11–15] Illich[16] went further, drawing on the work of Cochrane among others, noting the medicalisation of society and accusing medicine of expropriating peoples' ability to deal with ill health and indeed of causing significant disease.

The unequal social distribution of health care was analysed by Cooper and Culyer[17,18] and Hart[19] among others, who showed that substantial inequality of health care remained despite over two decades of the NHS.

This period saw the coming of age of medical sociology[20,21] which, for example, critically examined the medical profession's monopoly over the definition of illness and other aspects of the role of doctors and the power they exercise.[22] The hegemony of the medical profession was also threatened by the increasing evidence of variations in clinical practice in Britain[23] and internationally[11] and that much clinical activity had not been shown to be effective. In the United States, this erosion of professional prestige and power also seen in other (most notably the legal) professions was perhaps best signified by the rise in medical malpractice litigation.

The need to evaluate health care was appreciated increasingly by researchers and policy makers aided by the Donabedian framework for approaching evaluation.[24] By the early 1970s, the idea was growing that not only did doctors have to concern themselves with the efficacy of care and its acceptability to patients[25–27] but also economic efficiency.[1,28]

Cochrane's radical critique,[1] which raised his public profile and was for many the starting point of a re-examination of the way in which health services are delivered, was therefore very much of its time. It was one of the most concise and accessible summaries of several critical currents prevalent in the late 1960s and early 1970s.

Cochrane's view of economics

Whereas Cochrane's focus was on what is now termed efficacy, his book was permeated by statements about economics. His opening polemical statement in *Effectiveness and efficiency*[1] (p 1) was "all effective treatment must be free". He defined effectiveness as "the effect of a particular medical action in altering the natural history of a particular disease" (p 2). What Cochrane defined as effectiveness, as derived from randomised controlled trials in idealised settings, is what today is termed efficacy. Cochrane recognised that he was defining effectiveness as efficacy: he used the term ambiguously because he wrote that he disliked the word efficacy!

His definition of efficiency combined the notion of effectiveness (the effect of the intervention on patient health in everyday settings) with the "optimum use of personnel and materials" (p 2). He argued (p 1) that "if we are ever going to get the 'optimum' use from our national expenditure on the NHS we must finally be able to express the results in the form of the benefit and the cost to the population of a particular type of activity, and the increased benefit that could be obtained if more money were made available".

Cochrane returned to economic issues throughout his book. He argued (p 26) that "BCG (TB vaccination) might be abandoned when it costs more to prevent a case of tuberculosis through BCG vaccination than to treat a new case of TB when it occurred". Later (p 43) he recognised the need for good cost data to inform hospital decision making and his discussion of home versus hospital confinements includes clear advocacy of the measurement of costs and outcomes: "what is needed is a series of measurements of the cost and effect of hospitalising various percentages of confinements".

The centrality of the economic component in decision making is clearly set out again towards the end of his book (p 83): "allocation of funds and facilities are almost always based on the opinion of senior consultants but, more and more, requests for additional facilities will have to be based on detailed argument with hard evidence as to the gain to be expected from the patient's angle and the cost. Few could possibly object to this".

Many in medicine continue to object, with varying degrees of explicitness, to this approach. Some advocates of evidence-based medicine explicitly argue that, at the level of the individual clinical encounter, the imperative is to identify efficacy and to try to apply such knowledge to the care of individual patients, regardless of cost issues.[29]

The economists' argument is that choices should be informed by knowledge of an intervention's benefit and cost and that the limited budget of the NHS should be targeted at those treatments which give incrementally the greatest health gain per £ spent. This is what Sackett *et al* call evidence-based purchasing which they regard as the domain of the manager and not the clinician.

Cochrane did not agree with this position.[1] He argued (p 71) "surely priority should be given to finding out which treatments are effective and then ensuring that these treatments are efficiently given to all who need them". While this statement is somewhat ambiguous it probably means identifying what is "effective" (Cochrane's term for efficacy knowledge derived from randomised controlled trials) and then the evaluation of the efficiency of these interventions (that is, their costs and effects).

He found the notion of measuring effects or outcomes in terms of broader quality of life issues "repugnant" (p 77). At one level he believed that the task was too complex, describing the eased death of a Russian prisoner of war in his arms as the product of tender loving care which was difficult to quantify. However, he recognised the inevitability of outcome measurement as a part of the unavoidable process of prioritisation which he observed was executed then (and now!) "unconsciously and inaccurately".

An influence on his reluctant conversion to broader outcome measurement was Alan Williams, the York economist. Cochrane and Williams had a very intense interaction in the early 1970s and each taught and was taught by the other. Williams convinced Cochrane of the need:

> "to quantify value judgements" and measure outcomes—that is, "if the saving of a man's life aged 20 and the restoration of normal expectation of life is rated 100, what number would be assigned to the case of a severe schizophrenic?" (p 77).

Cochrane's concern was the optimisation of output—"the division of the medical budget among all medical activities" (p 76). He recognised the need to identify, measure, and value both outcomes and costs at the margin. Thus:

> "the next stage would be to enumerate the various outputs at the present financial level of allocation of money. The outputs will vary from the prolongation of life through reduction of morbidity to home and hospital care for those who cannot look after themselves. These outputs . . . will then be costed and calculations made as to how the various outputs could be increased by, say, a 10% increase in financial allocation" (p 77).

For most of the succeeding 25 years Cochrane's economic arguments have been ignored by most clinicians. Clinicians gradually recognised the merits of rigorous evaluation of health services (particularly using randomised controlled trials) but were much slower to recognise the merits of including cost and quality of life elements in such trials. This continuing reluctance to adopt economic (cost) and generic, comprehensive, non-disease specific (quality of life) outcome measures which reflect patient valuations is, in part, a product of the continuing clinical conflict between the doctor's obligations to the individual patient to provide all effective treatment, and the social perspective, which emphasises opportunity cost. In other words, the treatment of some patients deprives other patients of care from which they can benefit.

Cochrane's early dictum that, "all effective care should be free" was implicitly transformed in his book into an alternative dictum "all cost effective care should be free". That clinicians, economists, psychologists, and others still fail to produce data to inform the provision of cost effective health care by the NHS deprives potential patients of care from which they can benefit. This inefficiency is unethical for a public service because it fails to maximise population benefit from a cash limited publicly financed budget. Perhaps the severe threats to clinical autonomy and professional practice posed by managed care in the United States and more aggressive purchasing in the United Kingdom NHS will finally convince the profession that Cochrane was right and the production of enhanced survival and good patient care at least cost ideally depend on cooperation with health service researchers in general and health economists in particular. That such convictions were expressed by Cochrane[1] and Doll[28] and subsequently ignored has generated much interprofessional conflict and the maintenance of inefficiency in the NHS, the costs of which have been detrimental to patient welfare.

The early days of health economics

A leading architect of the subdiscipline of health economics was Alan Williams. His secondment to the Treasury in the late 1960s[10] led to his advocating the use of investment appraisal techniques in the public sector and him being asked to review the hospital programme of the Ministry of Health. He sought to identify the criteria for these ambitious investments and found, unsurprisingly, that it was the principle of "Buggins' turn" constrained by a preference to replace the oldest hospitals first. There was no evidence that "old" was less cost effective than "new" but it was clear that new hospitals tended to be more physically isolated, and thus less accessible to patients, and more costly to run.

Williams sought to convince a Ministry dominated by medical practitioners that the relative benefits of old and new be identified in terms of cost and population health outcomes. He failed, and was told that "experience" was the best way of allocating hospital investments! However, as a consequence of these ministerial debates, he encountered Archie Cochrane, and was encouraged by him to develop his health outcome measurement work.

These efforts, and the development of the economic input to the Ministry's policy making, was encouraged by Dick Cohen (chief scientist 1972 to 1973) and Douglas Black (chief scientist 1973 to 1977), the latter choosing to invest government resources into a postgraduate training programme in health economics at York in 1976 and, in so doing, providing the personnel to develop the subdiscipline in the 1980s and 1990s.

Until the maturation of these York trained health economists, the subject area was dominated by researchers who converted from areas such as public finance (Williams), social policy (Culyer), and transport economics (Mooney). The intellectual issues addressed by pioneers such as these were largely related to economic evaluation. Williams (see Cuyer *et al*[30]) developed his interest in outcome measurement initially in the field of social indicators as a result of meeting Vincent Watts during his sojourn at the Treasury in the late 1960s. Watts at that time had been developing an index of crime seriousness in the Home Office and introduced Williams to his wife Rachel Rosser. The Rosser-Watts work led to the disability and distress matrix which was used subsequently by Williams, Kind, and Rosser and later by Williams[31] to "guestimate" cost quality adjusted life years (QALY) data for various interventions.

The Rosser inputs to the paper by Williams[31] are obvious but less obvious is the role of Martin Buxton and the Department's health economists. Buxton and his Brunel colleagues supplied Williams with data from their heart transplant study, an exemplary and very influential evaluation of an expensive and high profile therapeutic programme.[32] The economic advisers in the Department of Health provided Williams with technical inputs. Both they and Buxton are acknowledged by Williams but were unwilling to be coauthors for political reasons. The application of the techniques of economic evaluation led to an increasing volume of studies (see for example, the study of Piachaud and Weddell[33] working with Cochrane) and the annotated bibliography of the area by Culyer *et al.*[34]

Separately, economists addressed the issue of the geographical distribution of NHS resources. In the late 1960s an American student at Oxford published a complex analysis of the English hospital system which, inter alia, highlighted the inequalities in resources allocation: this study, which used intermediate outcome measures, stimulated Williams to focus on population health outcomes. This work, by Martin Feldstein,[35] was complemented by the work of Cooper, Culyer, and others[17,18] and led the Labour minister, Richard Crossman, to conclude that these inequalities were the most significant NHS problems of the time.

It was left to his Conservative successor, Keith Joseph, to introduce the first crude resource allocation formula for hospital funding in England. The limitations of this were exposed by economists and epidemiologists and led, subsequently, to the development of the resource allocation working party (RAWP) formula in England and similar weighted capitation formulae in Wales, Scotland, and Ulster.[36] Recently, further work has led to a new (York) formula in England.[37]

Health economics, and health economists, have proved to be an "insidious poison in the body politic". Like many pharmaceuticals which are poisons if used in the wrong dosage, a balanced input of economics is essential for the maximisation of individual and population health in a world of constrained resources. This input can be contentious—for instance, the continuous challenge by economists to decision makers to face explicitly the finite nature of resources and the inevitability of "rationing" has often antagonised clinicians because of the challenge to clinical autonomy.[38]

However, gradually antagonism is yielding to weary acquiescence in the need for explicit rationing criteria and the mobilisation of the knowledge base to direct scarce resource towards those patients who can benefit, in terms of health outcome, the most.[39] It is this which Cochrane articulated so nicely and which, regrettably, has been less than fully developed in the past 25 years.

The selective absorption of health economics into the research process

The research processes of medicine are insular and powerful, in no small part because of the level and targeting of funding by the state and the pharmaceutical industry at clinicians. Cochrane's book influenced his colleagues and led to an increased acceptance of randomised controlled trials. However, the medical professional tended to monopolise this work, in general focusing on the randomised controlled trials design, but largely ignoring costs and often adopting intermediate end points, although with some notable exceptions such as the RAND health insurance experiment.[40] For example, many studies evaluating cancer treatments adopted randomised controlled trials but rarely measured cost consequences, and used intermediate and incomplete end points such as tumour growth and survival, ignoring the measurement of the quality of survival. This was not what Cochrane advocated: he wanted measurement of efficacy, outcomes, and costs. Why was his advocacy so limited in its success?

There are no doubt many causes of the separation of economics from medicine in the decades since Cochrane. One reason is the inherent conflict between the individual ethic of doctors to do all they can for their patients and the societal ethic of economists who emphasise that a decision to treat one patient in the private sector is a decision to deny treatment to several other patients in the public sector. Medical training has generally offered only superficial consideration of these issues. Robust presentation of such issues by economists among many healthcare groups has sometimes led to economists being accused of being "doctor bashers" when their real concern has been to articulate and facilitate the bridging of the individual patient-societal divide.[41]

This rationing controversy has absorbed much of the effort of economists and, as a consequence, the development of the subdiscipline of health economics in the United Kingdom has been distorted with too much effort being put into the broad advocacy of the techniques of economics evaluation and too little emphasis being placed both on methodological quality and development and on the broader application of the economics techniques to health policy.

The techniques of economic evaluation were well established by the 1960s and early 1970s.[42–45] Williams refined these techniques to produce the first checklist of questions to be used to interrogate and appraise economic evaluations in health care (table 7.1).[46]

TABLE 7.1—*Williams' checklist for appraising economic evaluations*

1	What precisely is the question which the study was trying to answer?
2	What is the question that it has actually answered?
3	What are the assumed objectives of the activity studied?
4	By what measures are these represented?
5	How are they weighted?
6	Do they enable us to tell whether the objectives are being attained?
7	What range of options was considered?
8	What other options might there have been?
9	Were they rejected, or not considered, for good reason?
10	Would their inclusion have been likely to change the results?
11	Is anyone likely to be affected who has not been considered in the analysis?
12	If so, why are they excluded?
13	Does the notion of cost go wider or deeper than the expenditure of the agency concerned?
14	If not, is it clear that these expenditures cover all the resources used and accurately represent their value if released for other uses?
15	If so, is the line drawn so as to include all potential beneficiaries and losers, and are resources costed at their value in their best alternative use?
16	Is the differential timing of the items in the streams of benefits and costs suitably taken care of (for example, by discounting, and, if so, at what rate)?
17	Where there is uncertainty, or there are known margins of error, is it made clear how sensitive the outcome is to those elements?
18	Are the results, on balance, good enough for the job in hand?
19	Has anyone else done better?

From Williams 1974.[46]

This checklist has been developed by Williams' students and subsequently by colleagues.[47,48] It continues to be refined in part due to the continuing need to reiterate the "gospel" and convert reluctant clinical scientists to the techniques of economic evaluation. Thus, although the proliferation of such lists and guidelines on the presentation of evaluations is a useful dissemination activity, the marginal product in terms of intellectual coherence and the advance of the methods of the subdiscipline have been quite limited.

The prolonged efforts of health economists have over the years resulted in the techniques of economic evaluation being utilised in the way Cochrane advocated. The pharmaceutical industry, faced by cost containment policies which curtailed their profit growth, looked increasingly at the use of the techniques of economics evaluation, apparently to demonstrate value for money but more often as a marketing device.[49] The implementation of the fourth hurdle—that is, addition of the cost effectiveness test in addition to the safety, efficacy, and quality controls which determine the acquisition of a product licence—in Australia in 1991 was also a landmark for the development of economic evaluation.[50] The decision of the Australians to test for cost effectiveness to determine Medicare reimbursement of new drugs, meant that the industry had to invest intensely worldwide in such techniques.

Whereas coordinated technology assessment work had developed significantly in the United States from the late 1970s (when the term QALY was first used), its development in the United Kingdom, despite the work of Cochrane and Williams, was slow and unfocused. The Medical Research Council had absorbed a tranche of Department of Health research funding (the Buller monies) but failed to apply this to health services research in a way which was recognisable as health services research to researchers. By the second half of the 1980s, the Department, recognising that they had been duped, applied pressure on the MRC and persuaded them to create a Health Services Research Committee (initially with no budget!). This Committee was dominated by clinicians, initially having token statistician and economist members who gradually grew in influence as it was recognised that all clinical trials might need economic (cost) and quality of life components.

Despite this rather narrow perspective, economists have helped to shape policy discussion about allocative efficiency in the NHS. For instance, the Department of Health limited the development of the heart transplantation programme until the results of an evaluation were available. This excellent study formed a knowledge base for subsequent development of the programme and helped prevent the uncoordinated expansion of heart transplant capacity in the NHS.[32] Williams generated a generic methodology to inform investment decisions between different diagnostic and treatment programmes. Although the methods were embryonic, the cost per QALY estimates he produced focused attention on both methodological issues and the practicality of such an approach. The subsequent patterns of investment in coronary artery bypass grafts as opposed to transplants and in hip replacements are compatible with the results of this early study.[31]

These important studies demonstrated the potential power of economic techniques in the evaluation of clinical practice and their use in helping to shape policy to promote allocative efficiency. However, the early promise of economic evaluation techniques has not been adequately developed.

The theoretical and methodological base on which economic evaluation should rest has not progressed significantly despite the important consequences which such developments may have on policy. Furthermore, Udvarheyli *et al*[51] pointed out the variable quality of economic evaluations, Sheldon[52] raised questions about the use of modelling in health care evaluations, and Rigby *et al*[53] have demonstrated the poor quality of many health economic reviews. Only recently have serious attempts been made to produce recommendations on the conduct of cost effectiveness analyses to promote quality and comparability.[54]

Mugford[55] for example, recently listed a range of familiar issues in economic evaluations which remain controversial: treatment of indirect costs; discounting health gains and resource use; valuation of health benefits; choosing correct comparator; selection of appropriate research design; translation of efficacy measures of randomised control trials into estimates of effectiveness; choice of the measure of effectiveness; when is it appropriate to use cost benefit analysis, in particular, when and how can willingness to pay be used; and how to use human capital measurement and other measures for indirect costs.

The application of economic techniques in health care have been slow and restrictive. For instance, it is only in the last year that a group has been commissioned to evaluate the cost effectiveness of the liver transplantation programme. On the other hand, economists have often invested considerable energy evaluating limited alternatives which reflect more the marketing interests of pharmaceutical companies rather than what may be the optimal intervention (therapeutic or preventive). For instance, the gastrointestinal complications of alternative oral non-steroidal anti-inflammatory drugs varies considerably and their cost effectiveness has not been demonstrated to be superior to paracetamol for arthritis. Reductions in gastrointestinal bleeds and costs may be more easily achieved through a change to first line paracetamol prescribing rather than the addition of (say) supplementary therapies.[56] Unfortunately only the latter have been evaluated.[57]

There is a risk that the pecuniary interests of the pharmaceutical industry are leading to a narrowing of the focus of economic evaluations and thereby a distortion of resource allocation in the NHS. Only if economists harness their skills to the broader interest of the health service will economic evaluations necessarily promote efficiency.

The increasing importance of demonstrating cost effectiveness, particularly in the pharmaceutical area, and the use of national guidelines which link reimbursement decisions to evidence of relative cost effectiveness, ironically may have had a perverse effect on the ability of economics to contribute more broadly to important health service decisions. By absorbing a disproportionate amount of economists' time, which is scarce (and also inflating salaries), it has diverted these resources from activities which are central to the efficient provision of health care in all societies.

Health economists have won the battle to make people see the relevance of the results of economic evaluations to decision making, but in doing so they have contributed to their professional isolation from the corpus of economic analysis and in some ways reduced the ability of the NHS and universities to afford to harness these skills in their broader application to a wide range of analytical challenges.

It is no surprise therefore that clinical trials with economic and quality of life components are what many clinicians think are the sole potential contributions of economics to health services research. In fact, the role of the economist is much broader, encompassing behavioural issues such as incentives, the demand for health and health care, and the supply of labour.

The potential contribution of economics to health services research

The resistance of the clinical establishment to the use of the techniques of economic evaluation has led to health economists investing heavily in dissemination and trials, many of which are for drugs. The opportunity cost is that their expertise has not been available to tackle the many other methodological and applied areas in which the economists' "tool kit" could produce new knowledge to inform clinical and policy choices.

The areas in which economics can contribute is usefully considered according to the schema devised by Williams in the early 1980s and used in the bid to the Department of Health and Social Science Research Council to acquire initial funding for York's Centre for Health Economics (figure 7.1). It is evident from this that economists can investigate a variety of policy issues—for example.

Supply of health care

What determines providers' behaviour? How should doctors be paid? How should the hospital capital market be organised (for example, the relative balance of public and private funding)? Does the creation of hospital trusts affect behaviour? What is the effect of changing the skill mix on the delivery and outcomes of primary and secondary health care?

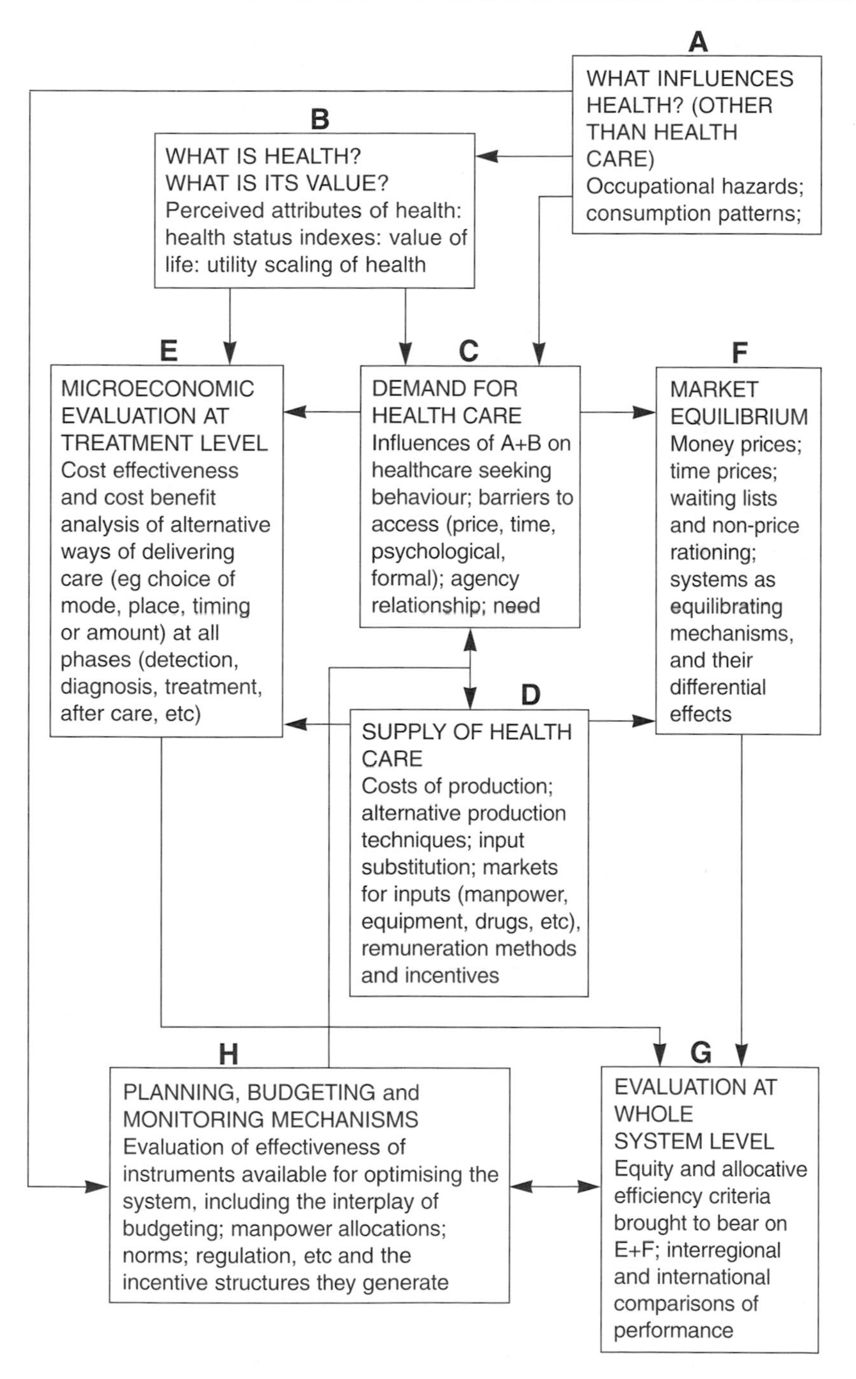

FIG 7.1—*Health economics: structure of discipline.*

Demand for health and health care

What influences the consumption of patients (for example, time costs, prices, income)? What is the impact of user charges on the consumption and distribution of drugs and dental services? What are the determinants of health related behaviour such as tobacco consumption and the use of illicit drugs?

Market equilibrium or methods of allocation

What are the effects of alternative methods of allocating health care services to competing needs (prioritisation)? It was remarkable that the first critique of the NHS internal market pricing rules came from someone who was not a health economist but a lecturer in land economy.[58] She pointed out that the NHS rule that price should equal average cost would inhibit competition (the principal aim of the reforms). In competitive markets, prices tend to vary according to the size and duration of contracts.

Equity and allocative efficiency

Whereas the NHS has emphasised the equitable allocation of resources by the development of national formulae based on epidemiological type measures of need (morbidity and mortality), little attention has been focused on ensuring equity in "health gain" which is related to ability to benefit. Economics can, therefore, make the necessary link between equity issues and efficiency but in fact little work has been done.

These and the other issues illustrated in figure 7.1 are all ones in which there is a body of economic knowledge which has not been thoroughly applied in the United Kingdom. It is remarkable how an enormous social experiment such as the internal market in the NHS, was created with all too little recourse to the knowledge base and implemented without exploitation of relevant and available techniques of appraisal. Williams[59] listed over 60 researchable questions arising from the Thatcher reforms and most of these questions remain ignored by the bulk of the health economics profession in Britain.

This behaviour reflects both the lack of a "customer" for this type of research (before and during the NHS reforms) and the lack of interest in this field by the bulk of health economists in the United Kingdom as opposed to their United States counterparts who focus more on market regulatory issues.

Although Cochrane did not allude to the topics outside economic evaluation, he was concerned with incentive issues: if you can lead the clinician horse to the waters of new knowledge, how could you make him drink? The considerable research effort on implementing the results of health research has relatively ignored the potential role of economic incentives (monetary and non-monetary).

Conclusions

Economics, through the subdiscipline of health economics, has not fulfilled its potential role in contributing to the development of health services research in the United Kingdom. This reflects both the diversion of resources and intellectual capacity into the narrow confines of the evaluation of clinical interventions, an area which has become increasingly appropriated by commercial interests. Economists in their eagerness to disseminate the importance of economic evaluation have often found themselves the hand maidens of clinical trialists. As the NHS research and development programme developed, with its insistence on the incorporation of economic analysis in health technology assessment, economists became inundated with requests to act as cost accountants on other peoples' studies. Such offers, because they represented a coming of age of economic evaluation and because they generated cash, were difficult to refuse.

The Government's research and development programme, being narrowly focused on clinical interventions, provided little or no funding for the broader elements of health services and health systems research. As a consequence there was insufficient funding of major policy initiatives such as the creation of the NHS internal market. The lack of a broad health services research perspective in the United Kingdom was noted by Cochrane in his autobiography (pp 244–6).[60]

The "blinkered" vision of health economists who ignore issues other than narrow economic evaluation and "coat tail" government, industrial, and clinical imperatives, may have rendered many incapable of applying economic analytical techniques to the broader issues of health policy. The regeneration of health economics in Britain requires a reorientation. Practitioners may need to return to basics and with it a much closer relationship with academic departments of economics. The desirability of specialisation by economists into health economics at the predoctoral level is questionable. Health economists, while seeking to colonise the clinical mind[41] (chapter 2, pp 10–29) may have lost their disciplinary head!

1 Cochrane AL. *Effectiveness and efficiency: random reflections on health services*. London: Nuffield Provincial Hospitals Trust, 1972.
2 Artis MJ, ed. *The UK economy: a manual of applied economics*. 11th ed. London: Weidenfeld and Nicolson, 1986.
3 Heald D. *Public expenditure*. Oxford: Martin Robertson, 1983.
4 Glennester H. Social policy since the second world war. In: Hills J, ed. *The state of welfare*. Oxford: Clarendon Press, 1990:11–27.

5 O'Connor J. *The fiscal crisis of the state*. New York: St Martin's Press, 1973.
6 Gough I. *The political economy of the welfare state*. London: Macmillan, 1979.
7 Fulton Report. *Committee on the civil service*. London: HMSO, 1968.
8 Colvin P. *The economic ideal in British government: calculating costs and benefits in the 1970s*. Manchester: Manchester University Press, 1985.
9 Pole JD. Programmes, priorities and budgets. *British Journal of Preventive and Social Medicine* 1974;**28**:3.
10 Williams A. *Output budgetary and the contribution of microeconomics to efficiency in government*. London: HMSO, Centre for Administrative Studies, 1967. (Occasional paper 4.)
11 Bunker JP. Surgical manpower: a comparison of operations and surgeons in the United States and in England and Wales. *N Engl J Med* 1970;**282**:135–44.
12 Fuchs VR. *Who shall live?* New York: Basic Books Inc, 1974.
13 Powles J. On the limitations of modern medicine. *Science, medicine and man* 1973;**1**:1–30.
14 McKeown T. *Medicine and modern society*. London: Allen and Unwin, 1965.
15 McKeown T. A historical appraisal of the medical task. In: McLachlan, McKeown T, eds. *Medical history and medical care*. London: Nuffield Provincial Hospitals Trust, 1971: 27–55.
16 Illich I. *Medical nemesis: the expropriation of health*. London: Calder and Boyars, 1974.
17 Cooper MH, Culyer AJ. An economic assessment of some aspects of the National Health Service. In: *Health services financing (the Jones report)*. London: British Medical Association, 1970.
18 Cooper MH, Culyer AJ. Equality in the National Health Service: intentions, performance and problems in evaluation. In: Hauser MM, ed. *The economics of medical care*. Allen and Unwin, 1972:47–57.
19 Hart JT. The inverse care law. *Lancet* 1971;i:405–12.
20 Cartwright A. *Patients and their doctors*. London: Routledge and Kegan Paul, 1967.
21 Illsley R. Promotion to observer status. *Soc Sci Med* 1975;**9**:63–7.
22 Freidson E. *Professions of medicine*. New York: Dodds Mead and Co, 1970.
23 Heasman MA, Carstairs V. Inpatient management variations in some aspects of practice in Scotland. *BMJ* 1971;i:495.
24 Donabedian A. Evaluating the quality of medical care. *Milbank Memorial Fund Quarterly* 1966;**44**:166.
25 Morris D, Ward AW, Handyside AJ. Early discharge after hernia repair. *Lancet* 1968;i: 681–5.
26 Mather HG, Pearson WG, Read KLQ, *et al*. Acute myocardial infarction: home or hospital treatment? *BMJ* 1971;**3**:334.
27 Hayes MJ, Morris GK, Hampton JR. Comparison of mobilisation after two and nine days in uncomplicated myocardial infarction. *BMJ* 1974:**3**;10.
28 Doll R. Surveillance and monitoring. *Int J Epidemiol* 1974;**3**:305–14.
29 Sackett D, Rosenberg WM, Gray JA, Haynes RB, Richardson WS. Evidence based medicine: what it is and what it isn't [editorial]. *BMJ* 1996;**312**:71–2.
30 Culyer AJ, Lavers R, Williams A. Social indicators: health. *Health Trends* 1971;**2**:31–42.
31 Williams A. Economics of coronary artery bypass grafting. *BMJ* 1985;**291**:326–9.
32 Buxton M, *et al*. *Costs and benefits of heart transplant programmes at Harefield and Papworth Hospitals*. London: Department of Health and Social Security Research Report, HMSO, 1985.
33 Piachard D, Weddell A. The economics of treating varicose veins. *Int J Epidemiol* 1972; **1**:287–94.
34 Culyer AJ, Wiseman J, Walker A. *An annotated bibliography of health economics*. London: Martin Robertson, 1977.
35 Feldstein MS. *Economic analysis of health service efficiency*. Amsterdam: North Holland, 1967.
36 Department of Health and Social Security. *Sharing resources for health in England*. Report of the Resource Allocation Working Party. London: DHSS, 1976.
37 Smith P, Sheldon TA, Carr-Hill RA, Martin S, Peacock S, Hardman G. Allocating resources to health authorities: results and policy implications of small area analysis of use of inpatient services. *BMJ* 1994;**309**:1050–4.

38 Williams A. Health economics: the end of clinical freedom. *BMJ* 1988;**297**:1183–8.
39 New B, on behalf of the Rationing Agenda Group. The rationing agenda in the NHS. *BMJ* 1996;**312**;1593–601.
40 Brook RH, Ware JE, Rogers WH, *et al.* Does free care improve adults' health results from a randomised controlled trial. *N Engl J Med* 1983;**309**:1426–1434.
41 Ashmore M, Mulkay MJ, Pinch TJ. *Health and efficiency: a sociology of health economics.* Milton Keynes: Open University Press, 1989:58–85.
42 Litchfield N, Williams AH. Cost benefit analysis: a bibliography. *Journal of the American Institute of Planning* 1960:**26**;4.
43 Mishan EJ. *Cost benefit analysis: an informal introduction.* London: Allan and Unwin, 1971.
44 Mishan EJ. *Elements of cost benefit analysis.* London: Allen and Unwin, 1972.
45 Williams A. Cost-benefit analysis: bastard science and/or insidious poison in the body politick? *Journal of Public Economics* 1972;**1**:199–255.
46 Williams A. The cost-benefit approach. *Br Med Bull* 1974;**30**:252–6.
47 Drummond MF. *Principles of economic appraisal in health care.* Oxford: Oxford University Press, 1980.
48 Drummond MF, Stoddart G, Torrance G. *Methods for economic evaluation of health care.* Oxford: Oxford University Press, 1987.
49 Evans RG. Manufacturing consensus, marketing truth: guidelines for economic evaluation. *Ann Intern Med* 1995;**123**:59–60.
50 Henry D. Economic analysis as an aid to subsidisation decisions: the development of Australia's guidelines for pharmaceuticals. *PharmacoEconomics* 1992;**1**:54–67.
51 Udvarheyli IS, Colditz GA, Rai A, Epstein AM. Cost effectiveness and cost benefit analysis in the medical literature: are methods being used correctly? *Ann Intern Med* 1992;**116**: 238–44.
52 Sheldon TA. Problems of using modelling in the economic evaluation of health care. *Health Econ* 1996;**5**:1–11.
53 Rigby K, Silagy C, Crockett A. Health economics reviews: are they compiled systematically? *Int J Technol Assess Health Care* 1996;**12**:450–9.
54 Russell LB, Gold MR, Siegel JE, Daniels N, Weinstein MC. The role of cost-effectiveness analysis in health and medicine. *JAMA* 1996;**276**:1172–7.
55 Mugford M. *How does the method of cost estimation affect the assessment of cost-effectiveness in health care* [D Phil Thesis]. Oxford: Exeter College, 1996.
56 Gabriel SE. Economic evaluation using mathematical models: the case of misoprostal prophylaxis. *J Rheumatol* 1995;**22**:1412–4.
57 Bloor K, Maynard A. Is there scope for improving the cost-effective prescribing of nonsteroidal anti-inflammatory drugs? *PharmacoEconomics* 1996;**9**:484–96.
58 Dawson D. *Costs and prices in the internal market: markets vs the NHS Management Executive guidelines.* Discussion paper. York: University of York, Centre for Health Economics; 1994.
59 Williams A. Research implications of the NHS review. In: Culyer AJ, Maynard A, Posnett JW eds. *Competition in health care: reforming the NHS.* London: Macmillan, 1990:237–52.
60 Cochrane AL, Blythe M. *One man's medicine: an autobiography of Professor Archie Cochrane.* London: British Medical Journal Memoir Club, 1989.

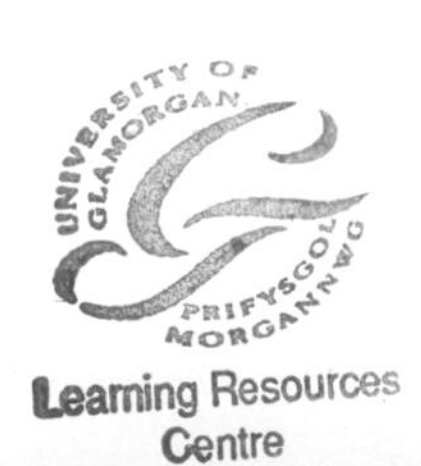

Part 4
Equity

8: Beyond effectiveness and efficiency . . . lies equality!

ALAN WILLIAMS

Introduction

Archie Cochrane's analytical thinking was guided by three key concepts: effectiveness, efficiency, and equality. It is probably his own fault that the third of these has not enjoyed the prominence of the other two. After all, he left it out of the title of his book! Moreover, in the single chapter devoted to "equality", his insistence elsewhere on the importance of *outcome* as the ultimate criterion of success seems to have weakened somewhat: the inequalities he dwells on are mostly to do with resources (structure) and utilisation (access and process).

It is worth considering the line of thinking that led Cochrane down that path. If effectiveness is about altering the natural history of a disease for the better, and efficiency is about "the optimum use of personnel and materials in achieving those results" in actual practice (minimising the sacrifices imposed on others), equality is about minimising differences between people. But differences in what? His starting point is revealing:

> "Having chosen two indices, effectiveness and efficiency, ... I soon discovered that they were only applicable to a part of the NHS. I see the NHS, rather crudely, as supplying on the one hand therapy, and on the other board and lodging and tender, loving, care. My two indices are very relevant to the former, but only to a limited extent to the latter. I needed another index with which to compare the two branches of the NHS and add a little humanity to my approach. Returning to my early enthusiasm for the idea of an NHS, I soon discovered what I wanted: equality. The difference in the medical care of the rich and the poor was sufficient to touch the hardest-hearted student in the 1930s (pp 2–3)."

He goes on to observe that:

> "I have devoted most of the space to an analysis of effectiveness and efficiency in the 'cure' section, because so much more is known about it. There has been so little work done in the 'care' section that I decided to discuss it under

'Equality'. Changes in the 'standard of living' of that side of the NHS may well produce such marked changes that the evaluation of 'care' is difficult until equality with the cure side has been achieved (p 3)."

It was a pity that Cochrane gave so much ground here. He should have pursued the line of argument that with an appropriately comprehensive and generic measure of health related quality of life it should be possible to compare both of his two sectors (cure and care) with respect to *all three* of his criteria. After all, the care sector needs to demonstrate effectiveness and efficiency too, and the cure sector needs to be concerned about equality. He harks back to this from time to time later in the book, but his early concern with equality in *provision* continues to dominate his thinking. Elsewhere he warns against thinking that more is better, but here he sees deprivation as being about differential levels of service provision, rather than being about the much more fundamental matter of differential levels of health.

Cochrane on equality

In his chapter on equality, he is rather dismissive of social class differences. In the space he does devote to them he concentrates on the utilisation rates for different services. The closest he gets to equality of outcomes are the data on the incidence of different diseases. He thinks that the only way to satisfy those who crusade for the reduction of such differences would be to produce data showing that

"... GP consultation rates, standardized by age, sex, and social class correspond exactly with incidence rates standardized in the same way (p 71)."

He accuses them of being unaware of the technical difficulties involved in making such comparisons rigorously. So he suggests instead that

"... priority should be given to finding out which treatments are effective, and then ensuring that these treatments are efficiently given to all who need them (p 71)."

But any given "disease" may have much more serious consequences for people in one occupational group compared with another (for instance the impact of a hernia on a manual worker is very different from its impact on a sedentary worker). So conducting the discussion at the level of "disease", rather than at the level of impact on health related quality of life, is a major weakness here.

Cochrane's expectation seemed to be that the use of effectiveness criteria alone would result in an equitable distribution of health, and do so more successfully than concentrating attention on utilisation, which may be of ineffective services anyway. Later I will return to this point, to take the more pessimistic view that the pursuit of effectiveness alone may not be enough, because it neglects any *explicit* consideration of distributive justice.

In his equality chapter, Cochrane concentrates his attention on differential "standards of living" in different sorts of hospital, which he regards as "the least excusable and the most easily remedied of the many inequalities in the NHS" and one to which he would give "considerable priority over social class inequality". Again attention is focused on the resources available rather than the outcomes produced with them, a deficiency which could have been remedied had he had access to reasonable quality of life measures. These would have enabled him to set outcome based standards and bring his "effectiveness" and "efficiency" concepts to bear here. He would also have been able to test his judgement that these differences are more important than the social class ones.

When he turns to variation in the quality of medical care, he goes back to outcomes as the ultimate criterion, carefully adjusted for case mix, and rejects process based policies which amount to "keeping up with the Thomases" (p 76). He is even more explicit about this when it comes to his final category of inequality, that between diseases. What he actually means by this is "between medical specialties", and he argues here that to attain an ideal distribution "which reduces to a minimum inequality between diseases" (p 76), it will be necessary to undertake "the quantification of all the various types of output" despite people's "reasonable dislike of quantifying value judgements" (p 77), and to have all such outputs costed.

Because he gives me the credit for leading him to this view (p 77), I will take this as a licence to speculate on where I might have led him "beyond effectiveness and efficiency" if I had had the opportunity to do so! It seems that he had accepted the idea that resources should be redeployed so as to equalise health gains at the margin across specialties and disease groups, and hoped that even though this might not take care of all the problems perceived by those with egalitarian views on distributive justice, at least it would go a long way to improving the situation as he saw it at the time. So where might he have gone to next?

Equality of outcome

I take the naive view that the primary purpose of health care is to improve people's health, so all healthcare activities should in principle be evaluated by measuring their impact on people's health.[1] Moreover, by "people's health" I do not mean the health of one or two people, but the overall health of the population as a whole (as that is the population served by a national health service). This stress, on the overall impact of healthcare activities on population health, is important because it puts costs in their proper perspective. As economists constantly remind people, *costs are sacrifices*, and in every budget-constrained healthcare system, the consequence of committing resources to one activity is that some other activity suffers, or, more precisely, the people who would have benefited from that other activity suffer. Thus equalising cost effectiveness at the margin will ensure that no rearrangement of resources will produce greater health benefits for the population as a whole.

But this is no guarantee that the distribution of health within the community will be "fair", in the sense that the benefits will go to the most deserving. There are many alternative conceptions of what it means to "deserve" health benefits from health care. On the negative side it might be argued that people who have knowingly contributed to their own poor health are less deserving of treatment than those who have taken good care of their health. On a different tack, it might be argued that people who are making a highly valued contribution to the general welfare of society deserve better treatment than those who are a liability to society. Yet another approach might be to say that someone on whom many other people depend is more deserving than someone on whom nobody depends. People might also feel that those who have been induced to behave in a particular way because of a promise to provide the benefits of health care should the need arise, have a prior claim over those to whom no such promises were made. The whole matter gets extremely fuzzy when these promises are not written into a specific individualised contract of insurance, but instead form part of a general understanding about what "the government" will provide if certain vaguely specified contingencies (like "getting ill") arise, as embodied in some "social contract".

There is not space here to explore all of these avenues, but I will concentrate on one equality notion which I am convinced Archie Cochrane would have found attractive—namely, that *everyone is entitled to "a fair innings"*. Initially I will interpret this very crudely to mean that there is some mean life expectancy at birth in a society which constitutes a benchmark against which age at death is informally judged. For simplicity's sake, let us suppose it to be the classic "three score years and 10". Then people might say that someone who dies at 80 had had a good run for their money, whereas someone who dies at 50 has been cut off in their prime. The former person might be said to have lived to a good age, whereas the latter person died prematurely.

As one philosopher has put it:

> "While it is always a *misfortune* to die when one wants to go on living, it is not a *tragedy* to die in old age; but it is on the other hand both a tragedy and a misfortune to be cut off prematurely."[2]

Four important characteristics of the "fair innings" concept are worth noting. First of all, it is a notion of equity that is *outcome based*, not process based or resource based. Secondly, it is about a person's *whole lifetime experience*, not about their state at any particular point in time. Thirdly, it reflects an *aversion to inequality*. Fourthly, it is *quantifiable*, and even in common parlance it has strong numerical connotations, with age at death being the usual focus.

Quality adjusted life expectancy

In my view, age at death should be no more than a first approximation, because the health related *quality* of a person's life is important as well as its length. If we consider only life expectancy and age at death, it will not be possible to reflect the view that a lifetime of poor quality health entitles people to special consideration in the current allocation of health care, even if their life expectancy is normal. The measurement of health related quality of life is now under way in several countries[3], although I shall here draw only on United Kingdom material. The data from these other countries tell a similar story about the unequal distribution of health within them, by population characteristics that are relevant to their own healthcare policies.

But when we move from life expectancy to *quality adjusted* life expectancy as the basis of a "fair innings", we need a new indicator to replace the crude unit of chronological time, the year. The obvious candidate is the QALY (quality adjusted life year), or one of its variants such as the DALY (disability adjusted life year), or any one of many other similar constructs. These indicators rate any year of life as worth less than unity if it is not a healthy year of life, with the rating getting lower the worse the health state.[4] Thus if people in a particular community generally experienced good health until they were about 50, after which it got steadily worse, and they mostly died at about age 70, a fair innings might turn out to be (say) 60 QALYs. So although the average age at death might be 70 (representing the average number of years of life actually achieved) the average number of QALYs actually achieved by the time a person dies will generally be less, and will be lower the poorer their lifetime experience of health has been. Thus we could talk about "a fair innings" in such a society as being "three score QALYs" instead of "three score years and ten". It does not trip off the tongue so lightly, but it is a much better policy benchmark!

Aversion to inequality

The "fair innings" argument embodies the notion that people are averse to inequalities in lifetime experience of health within a society. But are people equally averse to *all* such inequalities, or does the degree of aversion depend on the size of the inequality and its cause? These are empirical questions which need to be investigated, and all I will do here is indicate some general considerations which are likely to be prominent as such work progresses.

It seems natural to expect that if people are averse to inequalities in lifetime experience of health, they will be more averse to large ones than to small ones. But the exact relationship between the degree of aversion and the size of the difference is more difficult to predict. It might be a simple proportional relationship, indicating that reductions in equality are equally valued whether the reductions are from large inequalities or small ones. More plausibly it might be such that a given absolute reduction is more highly valued if it brings "outliers" closer to the norm than if it affects people who are already close to the norm. The precise quantification of this relationship is important for policy purposes, and is essential from a scientific point of view if we are to get beyond the rather vague "arm waving" stage in this crucial area of social policy, which involves many other activities besides the health service.

Whether the definition of a "fair innings" should be contingent upon the cause of the observed inequalities is a much more controversial matter. It raises the fundamental issue of what individuals are responsible for, what society in general is responsible for, and what nobody in particular can be held responsible for. In this last category I suppose most people would place inequalities due to someone's genetic endowment, which has hitherto been regarded as completely beyond their own control, and indeed largely beyond anyone's control. With current advances in molecular biology, and the imminent prospect that genetic manipulation will be possible and often advantageous, this fatalistic acceptance of genetic factors as "given" may slowly change. It will probably be the major ethical challenge to our conventional thinking about health care over the next two or three decades. Its bearing on notions of distributive justice will be dramatic if we come to consider a person's genetic endowment as being (to some extent) their own responsibility, or being (to some extent) the responsibility of society generally.

The most obvious feature stemming from our genetic endowment is whether we enter this world as male or female. This seems to be a major factor in determining our quality adjusted life expectancy. But how much of it is indeed genetically determined? Discussing this very point when calculating the global burden of disease for the World Bank, Murray observes that:

> "There appears ... to be a biological difference in survival potential between males and females. The average sex differences in life expectancy at birth in low mortality populations is 7.2 years. Not all this difference is biological: a large share is due to injury deaths among young males and higher levels of risk factors such as smoking. If we examine high income groups in low mortality populations,

the gap in life expectancy between males and females narrows considerably. . . . the ultimate gap in life expectancy at birth between the sexes is likely to approach two or three years."[5]

So not all of the differences in quality adjusted life expectancy between men and women can be ascribed simply to genetic factors and therefore regarded as not a legitimate source of social concern from a "fair innings" viewpoint. There seems to be a sizeable excess above this to be worked on in the interests of distributive justice.

The role of individual lifestyle in influencing our notions of a "fair innings" is the area of debate that is most heated at present. For instance, are smokers entitled to the same consideration as non-smokers? They face the prospect of a lower (and less healthy) life expectancy, so if we say that the same "fair innings" should apply to both, then the implication is that the non-smokers should be prepared to make sacrifices to reduce that inequality. The non-smokers are likely to argue that "contributory negligence" reduces the moral force of that obligation, and that it would be better for there to be a different "fair innings" for smokers compared with non-smokers. But this line of argument obviously has wider implications, as there are many other risks to health that people take during their lives, and none of us can be held to be completely innocent of "contributory negligence". This suggests that further argument is required to justify the singling out of particular "lifestyle" factors as grounds for setting up separate criteria within the "fair innings" framework. With smoking, a further moral difficulty arises from its addictive quality, which diminishes the role of "individual responsibility" if the habit is acquired very early in life (for instance, in someone's teens). Indeed, it might be argued that society generally bears a lot of the responsibility for not taking a tougher line on the production and distribution of tobacco products in the first place, so society should bail out those who have become the innocent victims of society's own pusillanimity.

It is interesting to note that social class differences in lifetime experience of health have been a focus of social concern in many countries for a long time, with most people expressing the view that something should be done to reduce them (or at least to stop them getting any wider). It seems that for most people differences due to social class are seen as a social rather than as an individual responsibility, and in some respects even as an act of fate for which *no-one* can be held responsible. This last point refers in particular to the "accident" of which family a person is born into, which is likely to have a dominant influence over that person's subsequent life chances, through its effects on nutrition and growth, social stimulation and interaction, education, and job prospects. All these things are caught up in the portmanteau notion of "social class", and there is no doubt that it is a major factor influencing quality adjusted life expectancy at birth. If "a fair innings" is defined for the whole society, irrespective of social class, then the professional and managerial classes will, in the interests of distributive justice, be called upon to make sacrifices in their health to help the unskilled manual workers and their families. They are unlikely to be willing to do this if they believe that the fate of these less fortunate people is due in large part to their own fecklessness, or idleness, or lack of initiative.

This brief survey of a few prominent issues in this debate should suffice to demonstrate two things: firstly that *distributive justice* is a key unresolved issue in the provision of health care; and secondly that *the reduction of inequalities in health* is a central element in it. I believe that by focusing the whole debate on the notion of a "fair innings", and on how it should be defined, and on what the quantitative trade offs are to be, we shall make more progress than by any other means open to us at present. But it involves more of the same kind of quantification that caused Cochrane such unease over his efficiency index—namely, the quantification of people's *values*.

Quantification

On the whole, debates about equity are not cast in quantitative terms. The type of argument I presented above is fairly typical. The reader is offered a problem to be resolved, and arguments that are often adduced on each side, but at the end of the day the matter is left undecided. This is because ethical principles are "essentially contestable", by which is meant that "there are competing conceptions of justice, all of which have respectable arguments in their favour"[6] Most commentators observe that such principles inevitably conflict with each other, and none "trumps" the others, so that no principle is absolute. In the presence of such unanimity about the *relativity* of ethical values, it is the more surprising that there has been almost no attempt to establish empirical trade offs.

If the nature and implications of particular positions are to be clarified in a policy relevant way, this discussion has to move on to seek quantification of what are otherwise merely vaguely appealing but ambiguous slogans (for example, that access should be determined by need, without "access" or "need" being defined in an operationally meaningful manner, and without any attempt being made to estimate the costs, in terms of other benefits foregone). Only with some quantification will it be possible to devise rules that can be applied in a consistent manner with a reasonable chance of checking on performance holding people accountable. At present, although reassurance is often offered that equity considerations have been taken into account, there is no way of establishing what bearing, if any, those principles actually had upon the outcomes. Judging by the persistence of health inequalities, and the almost universal agreement that they are deplorable, it is tempting to conclude that the rhetoric is not matched by any real commitment to do anything effective. Quantification thus has potential for clarification, for performance measurement, for accountability, and for policy analysis and reappraisal. The quest for greater quantification of equity considerations seems worth pursuing on those grounds alone, despite the hostility it is likely to engender from those who mistakenly equate quantification with lack of humanity.[7]

Some illustrative United Kingdom data

The actual United Kingdom data on health related quality of life that I shall use are from a survey representative of the adult population living in their own homes, conducted by the Research Group on the Measurement and Valuation of Health at the University of York, in collaboration with Social and Community Planning and Research in London.[8] They are based on self reported health states by men[9] at each age, using the EuroQol EQ-5D descriptive system (box), valued by a set of weights derived from the whole population by time-trade methods.[10] It is clear from these data (figure 8.1) that men in social classes 4 and 5 have noticeably worse health than their contemporaries in social classes 1 and 2, especially once they are past the age of 40 years. When these data are combined with the differences in male survival rates by social class,[11] we find that the quality adjusted life expectancy at birth of males in social classes 1 and 2 is nearly 66 QALYs, but for males in social classes 4 and 5 it is only about 57 QALYs.[12] To achieve the mean value of about 61.5 QALYs (a "fair innings" as seen by a pure egalitarian) they would need to live to be 65 and 71 years old respectively, a feat achieved by about 76% of males in social classes 1 and 2, but by only 46% of males in social classes 4 and 5.

But how averse are we, as a society, to this situation? To find out, we would need to ask people what they would be willing to sacrifice to eliminate that difference, if it were possible to do so.[13] Suppose they said (on average) that it would be worth sacrificing 0.5 of a QALY overall to equalise quality adjusted life expectancy. This means that instead of settling at the mean value of 61.5 (which implies that no sacrifice is necessary) society would regard equality at 61 to be equivalent (in terms of overall social welfare) to the current situation in which one group gets 57 and the other group gets 66.

This "social equivalence" is depicted in figure 8.2 in which the horizontal axis represents the quality adjusted life expectancy at birth of male members of social classes 4 and 5, and the vertical axis the quality adjusted life expectancy of social classes 1 and 2. The situation marked "actual" is where social classes 1 and 2 expect 66 QALYs and social classes 4 and 5 expect 57 QALYs. The dotted line from the origin plots all points where

Health related quality of life descriptors as presented in EUROQOL EQ-5D

By placing a tick (thus ☑) in one box in each group below, please indicate which statements best describe your own health state today.

Mobility:
I have no problems in walking about ☐
I have some problems in walking about ☐
I am confined to bed ☐

Self care:
I have no problems with self care ☐
I have some problems washing or dressing myself ☐
I am unable to wash or dress myself ☐

Usual activities
(for example, work, study, housework, family, or leisure activities):
I have no problems with performing my usual activities ☐
I have some problems with performing my usual activities ☐
I am unable to perform my usual activities ☐

Pain/discomfort:
I have no pain or discomfort ☐
I have moderate pain or discomfort ☐
I have extreme pain or discomfort ☐

Anxiety/depression:
I am not anxious or depressed ☐
I am moderately anxious or depressed ☐
I am extremely anxious or depressed ☐

the quality adjusted life expectancy of the two groups is equal. If it could be made equal without any overall sacrifice, we could be at the mean value, which I have taken[14] to be 61.5. But to test people's *strength* of preference, we must assume that some sacrifice has to be made. The supposed willingness of people on average to sacrifice 0.5 of a QALY overall, to eliminate the inequality entirely, is here represented by the point marked "equal at 61.0".

The next stage in my argument is more tricky. We now know that the "actual" situation and "equality at 61" generate the same level of social welfare. If we further assume that people would have the same aversion to inequality were the roles reversed (that is, if it were social classes 1 and 2

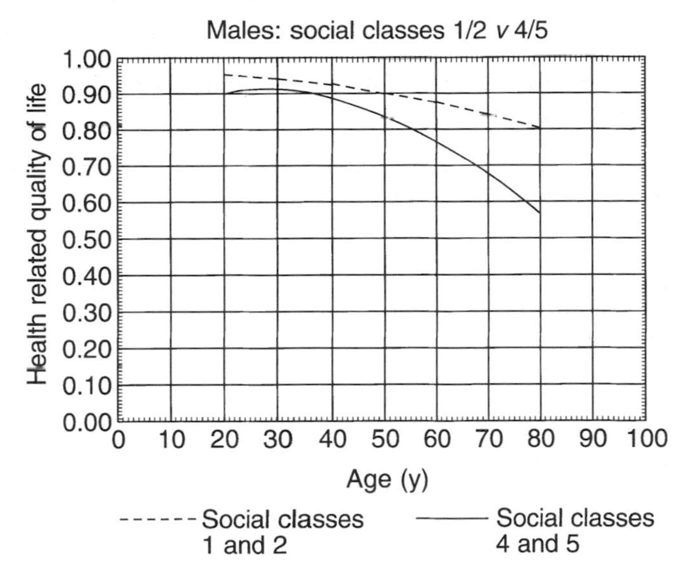

FIG 8.1—*Health related quality of life compared.*

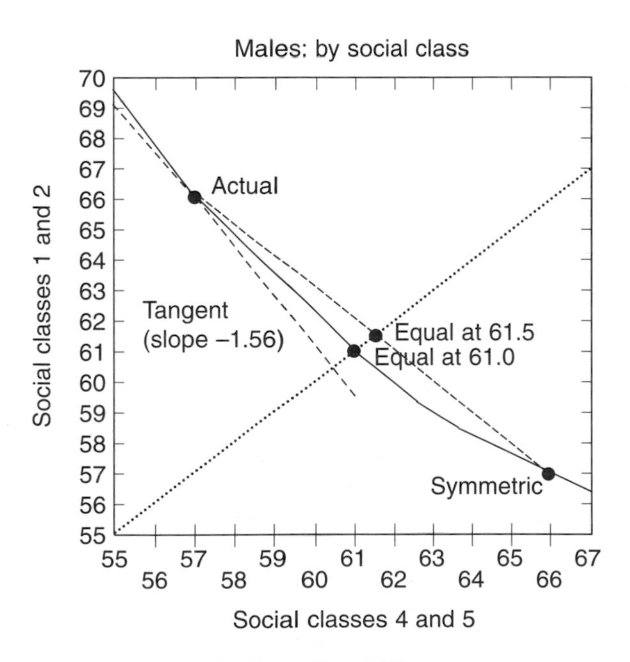

FIG 8.2—*Quality adjusted life expectancy.*

who were worse off), then the point marked "symmetric" would also generate the same level of social welfare. There is a curve drawn through these three points which is a kind of "social welfare contour" plotting all the combinations between which people would be indifferent on certain plausible assumptions (which remain to be empirically tested). One key assumption is that people's aversion to inequality increases smoothly as the size of the inequality increases. This is depicted by having the social welfare contour convex to the origin, and symmetric about the locus of points of equality (the line from the origin). This increasing marginal rate of aversion to inequality is such that, in the particular circumstances assumed here, the tangent to the social welfare contour at our actual current situation (which is plotted on the diagram) has a slope of −1.56. The meaning of this is that we would attach a 56% higher value to small improvements in the quality adjusted life expectancy of social classes 4 and 5 as we would to the same increases for social classes 1 and 2. This is the "trade off" between equality and efficiency implied by people's willingness to sacrifice 0.5 of a QALY to eliminate the difference of 9 QALYs.

It seems reasonable to suppose that if successful policies were implemented to reduce these inequalities (many of which would undoubtedly lie outside the healthcare system) then with constant overall aversion to inequality these gradients (or equity weights) would automatically decline towards 1 (their value at complete equality). The weights will obviously be higher the greater the sacrifices people are willing to make to eliminate any given inequality, and the smaller the inequality for which they are willing to make any given sacrifice. An important subject for any empirical research programme in this field will be to address in this way the issues laid out earlier. We need to know what kinds and levels of inequality people are most willing to make sacrifices to eliminate.

Beyond effectiveness and efficiency . . .

Cochrane was dismayed at the paucity of evidence that could be deployed to demonstrate scientifically the effectiveness and efficiency of most health care. Things are better than they were, but still give great cause for concern. But it would not be a wise strategy to argue that we should first of all sort out efficiency, and *then* (and only then) will we worry about equity. Firstly, we are unlikely ever to "sort out efficiency", and secondly, even if we did, we might find ourselves in such an extremely inequitable situation that there would be no way of remedying it. It is better to accept that inefficiency and inequity are both endemic in all systems, and that both have to be worked on simultaneously. For a long time I have been of the view that the best way to integrate efficiency and equity considerations in the provision of health care would be to attach equity weights to QALYs. QALYs measure benefits of health care in standard units, and equity weights allow benefit valuation to become person specific to the extent that that is policy relevant.

But there is an ever present political danger that such weights become arbitrary and capricious, and come to be used to fudge outcomes in ways that would not be acceptable if their basis were exposed to public discussion. One safeguard against this is to have some underlying (or "over arching"?) general principle enunciated, which can be confronted with evidence, so that its various implications can be explored in an open and quantitative way. The fact that it is possible to move from the general notion of a "fair innings", to specific numerical weights reflecting the marginal social value of health gains to different people, seems to me to be an important breakthrough in this respect. Perhaps it constitutes the beginning of a new crusade . . . for *evidence-based ethics*! It might also help us to develop a notion of "statistical compassion" (the ability to sympathise with the plight of the unfortunate but anonymous many) to help counteract the excesses of individual compassion (sympathy for the unfortunate but identifiable individual) which results in such severe inequity at present.

If the notion of quantitative, evidence-based, ethics is not too challenging even to contemplate, it would perhaps be a fitting tribute to Archie Cochrane to embark on such a programme of work in the 25th anniversary year of the publication of his magnum opus. It would repair a weakness in the original which he would doubtless be the first to concede, and it would help enormously to fulfil the humanitarian goals which motivated him so strongly, and which he was fearful might be undermined by the unreflective pursuit of medical virtuosity. Without implying that the old battles no longer need to be fought (for we still have a long way to go with effectiveness and efficiency), it seems to me that it is time to give equality a greater, but equally searching, share of the limelight.

Endnotes

1 This is equally true of privately provided health care, although this is not my concern here. The difference in that case is that the value of the health care is measured by the willingness and ability to pay off the patient or the insurer. This may not be closely related to the actual effectiveness of the treatment. Thus the supply of privately provided health care is not motivated by the desire to maximise the health of the population it serves, but to maximise the profitability of providing them with the health care they demand.

2 Harris J. *The value of life*. London: Routledge and Kegan Paul, 1985:94.

3 Those I know of are: Bone MR, Bebbington AC, Jagger C, Morgan K, Nicolaas G. *Health expectancy and its uses*. London: HMSO, 1995; Mathers CD. *Health expectancies in Australia 1981 and 1988*. Canberra: Australian Institute of Health: AGPS, 1991; Robine JM, Mormiche P. *L'espérance de vie sans incapacité augmenté*. INSEE première No 281, 1993; Wilkins R, Adams OB. Health expectancy in Canada, late 1970s *Am J Public Health*, 1983;**73**:1073–80. Eriksson P, Wilson R, Shannon I. "Years of healthy life." *Statistical notes* No 7 (April), National Center for Health Statistics, US Department of Health and Human Services, 1995;1–14.

4 Some of the simpler variants rate any departure from full health at zero, which means regarding all such impediments as equivalent to being dead. This seems to me so crude as to rule out the use of such measures in this kind of enterprise.

5 Murray CJL. Quantifying the burden of disease: the technical basis for disability—adjusted life years. In: Murray CJL, Lopez AD, eds. *Global comparative assessments in the health sector*. Geneva: World Health Organisation, 1994 and further references there cited.

6 For a more detailed account of this notion, see Chadwick R. Justice in priority-setting, In: *Rationing in action*. London: BMJ Publishing Group, 1993, which cites Gallie WB. Essentially contested concepts. *Proceedings of the Aristotelian Society* 1955–6;**56**:169–98.

7 Two very important, easily quantifiable, variables are going to be totally ignored in what follows, however, and they are (*a*) people's attitudes towards risk, and (*b*) their feeling about time preference. It is quite possible that aversion to inequality is as much motivated by risk aversion as by any sense of justice or solidarity. And if views about time preference are very different between the different groups whose health prospects I consider later, this will greatly complicate the rather simple welfare implications I am trying to draw. But things are complicated enough as it is, and it seems a better strategy not to tackle everything at once!

8 Not all of these results have yet been published, but a general account of the research programme is given in Williams A. The measurement and valuation of health: a chronicle, *Discussion paper 136*. University of York: Centre for Health Economics, June 1995. For some of the key data see Kind P, Gudex C, Dolan P, Williams A. Variations in population health status: results from the MVH National Survey, *CHE Seminar Paper: 14 March 1996*. University of York: Centre for Health Economics, 1996. We have no data from our study relating to the quality adjustments for those under the age of 18, so they have been assumed to be equal to those of the 18 year olds. We also have only very limited data for over 80s, so for them the trends already evident in the data have been extrapolated.

9 The restriction of this analysis to males is because social class attribution is more problematic for females.

10 See *Discussion Paper 136*, cited in endnote 8, for details of this tariff of weights and its derivation.

11 For these data see Bloomfield DSF, Haberman S. "Male social class mortality differences around 1981: an extension to include childhood ages" *Journal of the Institute of Actuaries* 1992; **119** III:545–59.

12 Obviously this assumes that a person remains in the same social class throughout their lives. Movement between social classes will make these differences less clearcut at individual level.

13 Some possibilities within the healthcare field have been reviewed in *Review of the research on the effectiveness of health service interventions to reduce variations in health. CRD Report 3*. University of York: NHS Centre for Reviews and Dissemination, October 1995.

14 For simplicity's sake I am here assuming that the two groups are of equal size. It raises no great issues of principle to work with more complex weighted averages instead.

9: Equitable distribution of the risks and benefits associated with medical innovations

WILLIAM SILVERMAN

> When shown the votive offerings to the gods of sailors who were saved after a shipwreck "because they made their vows," Diogenes the Cynic inquired, "Where are the portraits of those who perished in spite of their vows?"[1]

Many idealistic students enter medicine in the belief they will become "rescuers": active agents who will "save" the sick from untimely death. The mundane truth—most patients improve without treatment—comes later; and, for some rescuers, this humbling insight never arrives. All too often, an inflated view of medicine's prowess has led to action that is both unfair and harmful.

Cochrane's epiphany

Archie Cochrane learned about human resilience in the face of disease very early in his medical career,[2] when, as a "newly-minted" doctor, he was a prisoner of war in German hands for four years during the second world war. In a Salonica prisoner of war camp young Cochrane was often the only physician for approximately 20 000 underfed prisoners who were plagued by severe epidemics of infectious diseases that included typhoid, diphtheria, jaundice, and sandfly fever. He begged in vain for more doctors and medical supplies to cope with the overwhelming problems of attempting to care for the huge number of sick prisoners. As it happened, over this tumultuous period there were only four deaths in the camp; and three of these were related to gunshot wounds inflicted by the Germans. This revealing wartime experience convinced Archie of the relative unimportance of therapy, when compared with the recuperative powers of the human body. Subsequently, he campaigned vigorously to change the minds of all who failed to see the need for concurrent controls in the evaluation of medical innovations. Furthermore, he recognised that the postwar British invention of the randomised clinical trial provided a timely and eminently practical tool for dealing with the inevitable uncertainties about all proposed treatments.

The British streptomycin trial

Events surrounding the introduction of streptomycin for the treatment of tuberculosis provided one of the earliest and most convincing demonstrations of the urgent need for, and the inherent fairness of, randomised control methodology in the clinical assessment of most new medical interventions.[3] Streptomycin, discovered in the United States in 1946, was shown to be more effective than any previous chemotherapeutic agent in experimentally induced tuberculous infections in guinea pigs. Several exploratory clinical trials of the new agent conducted in the United States were encouraging, but the results were not convincing. The Streptomycin in Tuberculosis Trials Committee in Britain, appointed by the MRC recognised that the natural course of the pulmonary form of tuberculosis was highly variable and outcomes were unpredictable. In the past, evidence of improvement after the use of proposed agents in a number of case series had not been persuasive; the encouraging claims all failed, in the end, to fulfil their early promise. For example, over a period of 15 years there were persistent reports of benefit with gold compounds, but efficacy was never proved. Critics became convinced that only a parallel series using concurrent controls could provide the definitive proof needed for any proposed treatment. In 1944, for instance, before the arrival of streptomycin, two American experts wrote:[4] "Pairs of patients who had as nearly comparable disease as possible were selected and the toss of a coin decided which member of each pair was to receive treatment with the drug. The remaining one is considered the control." But, as Armitage observed recently,[3] despite the past tense used in the first of these sentences there was no evidence that this admirable design was ever applied in a United States study of treatment for tuberculosis; and "curiously, the same authors' (later) paper on streptomycin was based entirely on an uncontrolled series."

Austin Bradford Hill (later Sir Austin Bradford Hill, a leading participant in the historic events surrounding the first release of streptomycin in the United Kingdom for clinical study in 1946) recalled many years later[5] that Britain was able to purchase only a small supply of the new drug because the country had virtually exhausted its supply of dollars in the second world war. As a result, Hill remembered, the committee was confronted immediately with a daunting question concerning fairness: how can this small amount of a possibly curative agent for a very serious disorder be dispensed equitably? It was decided that most of the meagre supply should be made available for the treatment of miliary and meningeal tuberculosis—two forms of the infection known to be uniformly and rapidly fatal. Here there was no need for concurrent controls: any discernible improvement in a case series that departed from the expected steady downhill course could be ascribed, with confidence, to streptomycin. On the other hand, the variable natural history of pulmonary tuberculosis presented a more difficult challenge to the researchers.

Bradford Hill argued that it would be immoral *not* to conduct a rigorously planned investigation with the small amount of streptomycin remaining (enough to treat only 50 patients). The committee agreed and decided to compare bed rest (the accepted standard treatment at the time for newly acquired, uncomplicated pulmonary tuberculosis) with and without the new drug.[6] Notably, a decision was also made to use a formal scheme of randomisation to allot the treatments for eligible patients (defined as young persons—15–30 years of age—with acute progressive bilateral disease unsuitable for collapse therapy). The assignment for each patient ("S" for streptomycin plus bed rest or "C" for bed rest alone) was masked in sealed and sequentially numbered envelopes; the order of assignment was prepared in advance from random sampling numbers by Bradford Hill. The random allocation strategy and masking were chosen in this pioneering clinical trial to guard against the possibility of selection bias that might influence a decision to enrol if the clinicians knew the order of assignment in advance. (Armitage notes[3] that Hill advocated randomisation more on the grounds of common sense rather than statistical theory.) Although the intrinsic fairness of the approach was not mentioned when the streptomycin trial was reported, in retrospect (given all the fractious debate about randomisation in clinical trials since that time), the importance of the feature of equity in the (then) unusual plan needs special emphasis.

Equity and uncertainty

In choosing randomisation as a mechanism for allotting treatments under test, the planners of the streptomycin trial turned to one of the most venerable and impartial techniques ever devised for making difficult decisions under conditions of uncertainty. An appeal to the will of the gods as revealed by the machinations of chance is perhaps the oldest rite used by humankind when the need arises to make extremely difficult choices and there is paralysing uncertainty.[7] Throughout millennia, the mechanical means of divination have included pebbles, nuts, barley-corn, bones, twigs, yarrow stalks (I Ching), polished sticks, cards, coins, and dice. The list could go on, but the principle is always the same: "chance" is seen to be the action of some unseen non-human power that makes a die fall in a certain way, or an odd and not an even number of pebbles "jump" out of a buffalo horn, or causes a particular man to draw a specific lot. The process—termed *sortilege*—was, and remains to this day, an eclectic solution to the problem of doubt. As I have argued elsewhere,[8] random selection has been widely acknowledged as an eminently practical and equitable adjudicating engine: it always provides an unequivocal and unbiased decision. And sortilege is looked upon as entirely ethical; many have little difficulty in accepting the "luck of the draw" in a wide variety of risk filled imponderable situations that keep turning up in life. But some critics have had difficulty in accepting the time honoured reasoning when it is extended to random allotments in medical treatment trials.

I have suggested that the ambivalence stems from confusion about "knowing" in medicine. The dilemma has come to the fore as the profession has attempted to move away from the tradition of authoritative declarations. Impersonal rules of evidence are slowly replacing the domineering voices of respected leaders; and it is in this transitional period that the outcry is heard against formal "contests" to choose between proposed treatments. I suspect that physicians (rather than patients) object most to the use of an approach in which trusted experts, who are expected to know everything, must admit to a crucial lack of knowledge. As Zelen has pointed out;[9] some physicians believe that the doctor-patient relationship is compromised when they must inform patients about choosing treatment by what is, in essence, a toss of a coin. He put his finger on the crux of the matter when he said, "Even though, in truth, there may be no scientific evidence favouring any one treatment, physicians may find it difficult to tell patients that they do not know which treatment is best." Confession stirs up unwelcome interest in an incisive question: How does the doctor *know* which treatment is best?

The famous streptomycin trial built a firm base for a claim to know. It demonstrated the clear superiority of the new drug (at the end of six months there were four deaths among 55 patients who received streptomycin plus bed rest versus 14 fatalities among 52 patients who were treated by bed rest alone). The clinical experiment also underlined the importance of concurrent controls in revealing the limitations of the victory. For instance, clinical improvement was seen in 17 of 52 patients treated by bed rest alone. Important problems with the new drug were also disclosed: the emergence of streptomycin resistant strains of the tubercle bacilli did blunt the response to treatment in 10 of 55 patients, and toxic effects of the new drug on vestibular function were encountered in 36 of 55 patients. It was clear that the long search for the ideal drug to treat tuberculosis was not yet over.

Limiting risk

The streptomycin trial provided ample validation of Bradford Hill's arguments about the power of experimental study design.[10] There was striking contrast between the clear and quickly obtained results of the parallel comparison, and the previous trials of gold treatment (without concurrent controls) over a period of 15 years. Although the focus when planning the trial was to devise a fair way to distribute the predicted benefits of the very small supply of streptomycin, it soon became clear that randomisation was also a very effective way to reduce the total number of patients exposed to the risk of unpredicted side effects of the drug. The importance of this hedging strategy became increasingly apparent later, at the time of recurrent treatment disasters. Although the calamities could not have been prevented completely, in each instance the overall number of patients damaged by the untested intervention could have been reduced substantially by the early use of randomised control trial methodology.

For example, in one of the most tragic episodes in modern medical history, a seemingly minor change in the care of premature infants resulted in the blinding of about 10 000 babies between 1942 to 1954.[11] The 12 year epidemic of retinopathy of prematurity (originally called retrolental fibroplasia) was curbed only after a multicentre randomised trial demonstrated that the liberal use of supplemental oxygen had been the culprit. In hindsight, it is easy to see that the number of children blinded could have been markedly reduced if the original claim for the benefits of liberal oxygen had been tested before the new programme was adopted widely. But this vital lesson was ignored time after time in the introduction of new treatments. The script for potential disaster was outlined in one ordered pattern of action: an exciting new treatment proposal—enthusiastic acceptance—belated recognition of the possibility of disastrous complications—rigorous evaluation, if it took place at all, long after the untested intervention was already in wide use.

Twenty five years after the oxygen-blindness lesson, the dangerous scenario was re-enacted in a search for new drugs to suppress cardiac arrhythmias: the delay in carrying out a randomised control trial brought about what Moore labelled "America's worst drug disaster."[12] Over an eight year period beginning in 1978, flecainide and similar antiarrhythmia drugs (designated as class I agents) were administered to hundreds of thousands of asymptomatic patients with premature ventricular contractions based on the unproved assumption that this prophylactic regimen would reduce the risk of sudden cardiac death. During this very large experiment without controls, a few sceptical cardiologists began to suspect that although these drugs did suppress disturbances of cardiac rhythm, they were also capable of *inducing* lethal arrhythmias—the new agents were suspected as the cause of a worrisome number of sudden deaths. Finally, after much rancorous debate about the risk of the class I drugs, an international placebo controlled randomised trial was mounted in 1987 by the US National Heart, Lung and Blood Institutes to evaluate the effect of prophylactic use of the drugs to suppress cardiac arrhythmias in patients who had survived a heart attack. In 1989, the trial was truncated three years earlier than planned when it was found that twice as many patients receiving the active drugs (flecainide or encainide) died compared with placebo treated controls. A second trial of another promising class I agent (moricizine) also revealed more deaths in the treatment arm of the trial. The trials demonstrated, once more, the tragic consequences brought about by a delay in rigorous testing. Although there was no accurate tally of the number of the persons who died prematurely as a direct result of the widespread treatment with these untested drugs prior to the trials, the total mortality, Moore reckoned, must number in the tens of thousands.

Inequities in non-random sampling

The momentous risks of the untested intervention, in both the oxygen trial more than 40 years ago and in the cardiac arrhythmia suppression trial 25 years later, were distributed among the enrollees in the trials in the fairest way possible: impartiality was guaranteed by random allocation of compared treatments. But random *assignment* after enrolment must not be confused with an antecedent need for random *sampling* to choose trial participants. The use of random order to assign treatments for patients already enrolled does not address a prior question about justice: What is the fairest way to decide who will be chosen to participate in the comparative trial? For example, when recruitment for the cardiac arrhythmia trial was underway two thirds of eligible patients were not enrolled because many doctors were so convinced of the benefits of the drugs they refused to allow their patients to participate in what was, in essence, a lottery. But as it turned out, these eligible but not enrolled patients missed the fair chance available to those who agreed to participate in the trial: the possibility of allocation to the safe alternative (the placebo arm of the trial). Moreover, low enrolment delayed completion of the trial and, as a result, thousands of additional cardiac patients not enrolled in the study were exposed unnecessarily to the drug induced risk of sudden death. This unfortunate experience supports the view of Segelov *et al*[13] who argue that doctors must recognise that it is unethical to advise eligible patients not to enter a well planned trial. By excluding patients, doctors presume, to the possible detriment of their patients' wellbeing, to know the answer to the trial question, despite the agreed lack of proof.

Ellenberg has also charged that too little attention is paid to the inevitable selection bias in non-random methods of enrolling patients in clinical studies.[14] Only a random sample drawn from the entire pool of candidates (ensuring that every eligible patient in a clearly defined population has an equal chance of being selected) can satisfy the most stringent epidemiological requirement for representativeness, and, accordingly, the ethical demand for fairness. In time of war, for example, a national lottery is used to decide who, among all eligible young persons, shall risk their lives in battle—here random sampling is accepted as a fair and democratic solution to the problem of extremely difficult choices. But there have been no calls for a mandatory lottery to ensure fairness in selecting participants for medicine's ongoing war against disease. (The philosopher Hans Jonas rejected[15] conscription by lot as threatening and Utopian.) None the less, we need to recognise the consequences of fighting medical battles with volunteers—when only those who are willing to provide written informed consent are enrolled. Twenty five years ago, when Archie Cochrane wrote the commentary we honour in this volume, he made no mention of the volunteer issue in randomised controlled trials. In those innocent (paternalistic) days, participating doctors were expected to enrol all their eligible patients. Since that time, selection by informed consent has become an obligatory feature of clinical trials.

Maldistribution of risk and benefit

Because volunteerism honours the principle of respect for personal autonomy, self selection is widely accepted as the only ethical solution to the dilemma of who shall serve. But this interpretation of fairness, which is based on the rights of individuals, is in conflict with another principle; that of social equity. For the fairest possible distribution of risks and benefits, the canon of distributive justice decrees that every eligible patient must be required, figuratively, "to draw a lot." It is interesting that a United States commission advised that participants in research projects should be chosen so that the burdens are distributed "justly"—that is to say among all segments of society.[16] But the recommendation is silent about how this "just" standard can be achieved without a lottery.

I have argued[17] that we should be ready to question anything done in the recruitment of patients for clinical studies that exaggerates social inequalities. An interesting example of sorting by social class occurred in 1954 when public health departments in the United States conducted the famous field trial of the Salk poliomyelitis vaccine (involving almost 2 million school children).[18] A systematic difference was found between the baseline characteristics of families who volunteered their children for participation and of other families who refused to give permission: the volunteer families were better educated and more affluent than the non-participants. In addition to the clear evidence of vaccine effectiveness (the rate of poliomyelitis was lowest in the children allotted to the vaccine group), there was an interesting "volunteer effect." The highest rate of poliomyelitis was found, consistently, in children in the control group (those *allotted* to receive no vaccine); an intermediate rate was observed in children of families who refused to volunteer (those who *chose* to receive no vaccine).

In the vaccine episode, each family made their decision in the privacy of their own home, and then sent the permission form to school. They had no face to face exchange with the strangers conducting the vaccine trial. Sorting by social class may be quite different when a family must make a decision in an unfamiliar setting (the hospital) and when they find themselves confronted by strangers in positions of authority (the team of physicians and other healthcare personnel). Is it possible that the social filter effect of informed consent acts differently under the latter conditions? Does it now "select" for refusal those in the upper social classes, the least captive in society, those most likely to be fully informed? Among the consenters, are there disproportionate numbers enrolled who do not understand, who are too frightened to refuse, who are socially disadvantaged? The answer to these questions is, "Yes, at least some of the time." For instance, an interesting disparity of the latter kind was observed in an Australian survey of parents who consented and others who refused to enrol their children in a trial of a new drug for asthma.[19] The consenting parents appeared to be more socially disadvantaged and emotionally vulnerable when compared with parents who refused to allow their children to participate.

The possibility of social inequalities between participants and non-participants has not received the attention it deserves. Descriptions of the social circumstances of the enrolled patients and those of eligible patients who refused enrolment should be included in the reports of clinical trials. And the dynamics of consent and refusal need to be explored systematically if we are to understand how to improve fairness (representativeness) in randomised trials.

What is the moral standing of eligible patients who refuse to enrol in trials? When such "trial dodgers" demand the untested treatment "off study," there is a moral obligation, I believe, to turn the request down: the request is patently unreasonable. Patients do not have the right to demand that doctors prescribe untested treatments without a hedging strategy to limit the number of their patients exposed to unknown harm. The horrendous damage caused by undisciplined use of oxygen, thalidomide, and diethylstilboestrol should serve as dire warnings of the need for concurrent controls.

Cahn's criticism[20] of those who enjoy the benefits of medical research after refusing to participate in clinical trials, is particularly harsh. He condemned this evasion of social responsibility as a blatant form of hypocrisy. "To possess the end and yet not be responsible for the means, to grasp the fruit while disavowing the tree, to escape being told the cost until someone else has paid it irrevocably," he charged, "is one of the most pervasive moral syndromes of our times."

I wish to emphasise, again, that the topic of social equity in the process of evaluating medical innovations needs more *public* discussion than it has received. For example, Jonas noted[15] that the question of who should be called upon to serve can only be made "right," if the "cause" of the study is the patient's as well as the researcher's "cause." The medical profession has an obligation to convince the community that medicine's battle against pain and suffering is a just "cause;" and that the sharing of benefits and burdens in this form of warfare is a civic duty akin to national service in a conventional war. This view of medicine, as the equivalent of armed conflict, is not new. The argument was put forward more than 50 years ago by Sigerist.[21] "The war against disease and for health," he wrote, "cannot be fought by physicians alone. It is a people's war in which the entire population must be mobilised permanently."

1 Merton RK. *The sociology of science. An episodic memoir.* Carbondale, IL: Southern Illinois University Press, 1979.
2 Cochrane AL. *Effectiveness and efficiency.* London: Nuffield Provincial Hospitals Trust, 1972.
3 Armitage P. Bradford Hill and the randomised controlled trial. *Pharmaceutical Medicine* 1992;**6**:23–27.
4 Hinshaw HC, Feldman WH. Evaluation of chemotherapeutic agents in clinical tuberculosis: a suggested procedure. *American Review of Tuberculosis* 1944;**50**:202–10.
5 Hill AB. Memories of the British streptomycin trial in tuberculosis. The first randomized clinical trial. *Control Clin Trials* 1990;**11**:77–9.
6 Medical Research Council. Streptomycin treatment of pulmonary tuberculosis: a report of the streptomycin in tuberculosis trials committee. *BMJ* 1948;**2**:769–82.
7 David FN. *Games, gods and gambling.* New York: Chas Scribner's Sons, 1962.
8 Silverman WA. Gnosis and random allotment. *Control Clin Trials* 1981;**2**:161–4.
9 Zelen M. A new design for randomized clinical trials. *N Engl J Med* 1979;**300**:1242–5.
10 Malcontent. Fumes from the spleen. *Paediatr Perinat Epidemiol* 1993;**7**:230–3.
11 Silverman WA. *Retrolental fibroplasia. A modern parable.* New York: Grune and Stratton, 1980.
12 Moore TJ. *Deadly medicine.* New York: Simon and Schuster, 1995.
13 Segelov E, Tattersall MHN, Coates AS. Redressing the balance—the ethics of *not* entering an eligible patient on a randomised clinical trial. *Ann Oncol* 1992;**3**:103–5.
14 Ellenberg JH. Cohort studies. Selection bias in observational and experimental studies. *Stat Med* 1994;**13**:557–67.
15 Jonas H. Philosophical reflections on experimenting with human subjects. *Daedalus* 1969; **219**:235–41.
16 National Commission for the Protection of Human Subjects of Biomedical and Behavioral Research. *Research involving children: report and recommendation.* Government Printing

Office, Washington, DC: US Department of Health Education and Welfare, 1977. (Publ No (OS) 770004.)
17 Silverman WA. Informed consent. In: Goldworth A, *et al*, eds. *Ethics and perinatology*. Oxford: Oxford University Press, 1995.
18 Meier P. The biggest public health experiment ever: the 1954 field trial of the Salk poliomyelitis vaccine. In: Tanur JM, *et al*, eds. *Statistics: a guide to the unknown*. San Francisco: Holden-Day, Inc, 1972.
19 Harth SC, Thong YH. Sociodemographic and motivational characteristics of parents who volunteer their children for clinical research: a controlled study. *BMJ* 1990;**300**:1372–5.
20 Cahn E. Drug experiments and the public conscience. In: Katz J. *Experiments with human beings*. New York: Russell Sage Foundation, 1972.
21 Sigerist HE. *Medicine and human welfare*. New Haven: Yale University Press, 1941.

Part 5
Evolution

10: Large-scale randomised evidence: trials and overviews*

RORY COLLINS, RICHARD PETO, RICHARD GRAY, SARAH PARISH

Introduction and summary

This chapter is intended principally for those who want to know why some types of evidence are much more reliable than others. It is concerned with treatments that might improve survival (or some other really major aspect of long term disease outcome), and its chief point is that as long as doctors start with a healthy scepticism about the many apparently striking claims that appear in the medical literature, trials do make sense. The main enemy of common sense is over-optimism: there are a few striking exceptions of treatments for serious disease that really do turn out to work extremely well, but in general most of the claims of vast improvements from new therapies turn out to be evanescent. **Hence, clinical trials need to be able to detect or to refute really reliably the more moderate differences in long term outcome that it is medically realistic to expect**. Once this common sense idea is explicitly recognised, the rest follows naturally, and it becomes fairly obvious what types of evidence can and cannot be trusted. Although this chapter may also be of some interest or encouragement to doctors who are considering participating in (or even planning) some large trial, its main intended audience is the practising clinician. For, even the most definite results from large-scale randomised evidence cannot save lives unless practising clinicians accept and apply them. The chapter does not go into a lot of statistical details: instead, it tries to communicate the spirit that underlies the increasing emphasis over the last decade or so on large-scale randomised evidence.

* Adapted from Collins R, Peto R, Gray R, Parish S. Large-scale randomised evidence: trials and overviews. In: Weatherall D, Ledingham JGG, Warrell DA, eds. *Oxford Textbook of Medicine*. Vol 1. Oxford: Oxford University Press, 1996.

Unrealistic hopes about the chances of discovering big treatment effects can be a serious obstacle not only to appropriate patient care but also to good clinical research. For, such hopes may misleadingly suggest to some research workers or funding agencies that small, or even non-randomised, studies may suffice. In contrast, realistically moderate expectations of what treatment might achieve (or, if one treatment is to be compared with another, realistically moderate expectations of how large any difference between those treatments is likely to be) should, in contrast, tend to foster the design of studies that aim to discriminate reliably between (*a*) differences in outcome that are realistically **moderate but still worthwhile**, and (*b*) differences in outcome that are **too small to be of any material importance**.[1] Studies with this particular aim must guarantee strict control of bias (which, in general, requires proper randomisation and appropriate statistical analysis, with no unduly "data dependent" emphasis on specific parts of the overall evidence), and must guarantee strict control of the play of chance (which, in general, requires large numbers rather than a lot of detail). The conclusion is obvious: moderate biases and moderate random errors must **both** be avoided if moderate benefits are to be assessed or refuted reliably. This leads to the need for large numbers of properly randomised patients, which in turn leads both to large simple randomised trials (or "mega-trials") and to large systematic overviews (or "meta-analyses") of related randomised trials.[2]

Non-randomised evidence, unduly small randomised trials, or unduly small overviews of trials are all much inferior as sources of evidence about current patient management or as foundations for future research strategies. For they cannot discriminate reliably between moderate (but worthwhile) differences and negligible differences in outcome, and the mistaken clinical conclusions that they engender could well result in the worldwide undertreatment, overtreatment, or other mismanagement of millions of future patients. In contrast, hundreds of thousands of premature deaths a year could be avoided by seeking appropriately large-scale randomised evidence about various widely practicable treatments for the common causes of death, and by disseminating such evidence appropriately. Likewise, appropriately large-scale randomised evidence could substantially improve the management of many important, but non-fatal, medical problems.

The value of large-scale randomised evidence is illustrated in this chapter by the trials of fibrinolytic therapy for acute myocardial infarction, of antiplatelet therapy for a wide range of vascular conditions, of hormonal therapy for early breast cancer, and of drug therapy for lowering blood pressure. In these examples proof of benefit that could not have been achieved either by small-scale randomised evidence or by non-randomised evidence has led to widespread changes in practice that are now preventing tens of thousands of premature deaths each year.

Moderate (but worthwhile) effects on major outcomes are generally more plausible than large effects

Some treatments do have large, and hence obvious, effects on survival—for example, it is clear without randomised trials that prompt treatment of diabetic coma or cardiac arrest saves lives (and, indeed, the plaque at the entrance to our own hospital records the first clinical use of penicillin). But, perhaps in part due to these striking successes, in the past few decades the hopes of large treatment effects on mortality and major morbidity in other serious diseases have been unrealistically high. Of course, treatments do quite commonly have large effects on various less fundamental measures: for example, drugs readily reduce blood pressure, blood lipids and blood glucose; many tumours or leukaemias can be shrunk temporarily by radiotherapy or chemotherapy; in acute myocardial infarction, lidocaine can prevent many arrhythmias and streptokinase can dissolve most coronary thrombi; and in early HIV infection, antiretroviral drugs substantially reduce viraemia. But, although all of these effects are large, any effects on mortality are much more modest—indeed there is still dispute as to whether any net improvement in survival is provided by the routine use of radiotherapy for common cancers, lidocaine for acute myocardial infarction, or AZT for early HIV infection.

In general, if substantial uncertainty remains about the efficacy of a practicable treatment, its effects on major end points are probably either negligibly small, or only moderate, rather than large. Indirect support for this rather pessimistic conclusion comes from many sources, including (*a*) the previous few decades of disappointingly slow progress in the curative treatment of the common chronic diseases of middle age; (*b*) the heterogeneity of each single disease, as evidenced by the unpredictability of survival duration even when apparently similar patients are compared with each other; (*c*) the variety of different mechanisms in certain diseases that can lead to death, only one of which may be appreciably influenced by any one particular therapy; (*d*) the modest effects often suggested by systematic overviews (or "meta-analyses"; see later) of various therapies; and, in certain special cases, (*e*) observational epidemiological studies of the strength of the relationship between some disease and the factor that the treatment will modify (for example, blood pressure, blood cholesterol or blood glucose: see later).

Having accepted that, with many currently available interventions, only **moderate** reductions in mortality are plausible, how worthwhile might such effects be, if they could be detected reliably? To some clinicians, reducing the risk of early death in patients with myocardial infarction from 10 per 100 patients down to 9 or 8 per 100 patients treated may not seem particularly worthwhile—and, indeed, if such a reduction was only transient, or involved an extremely expensive or toxic treatment, this might well be an appropriate view. Worldwide, however, several million patients a year reach medical attention with a diagnosis of acute myocardial infarction, and if just one million were to be given a simple, non-toxic, widely practicable treatment that reduced the risk of early death from 10% down to 9% or 8% (that is, a 10% or 20% proportional reduction) then this would avoid 10 000 or 20 000 deaths. (Nowadays, for example, about half a million patients a year receive fibrinolytic therapy for acute myocardial infarction, avoiding about 10 000 early deaths, and large trials have shown that this difference in early mortality persists for several years afterwards.) Such absolute gains are substantial—and might, indeed, considerably exceed the numbers of lives that could be saved by a much more effective treatment for a much less common disease.

Reliable detection or refutation of moderate differences requires avoidance of BOTH moderate biases and moderate random errors

If realistically moderate differences in outcome are to be reliably detected or reliably refuted, then the errors in comparative assessments of the effects of treatment need to be much smaller than the difference between a moderate but worthwhile effect on the one hand, and, on the other, an effect that is too small to be of any material importance. This in turn implies that moderate biases cannot be tolerated, and that moderate random errors cannot be tolerated. The only way to guarantee very small random errors is to study really large numbers, and this can be achieved in two main ways: make individual studies large, and combine information from as many relevant studies as possible in systematic overviews (table 10.1). But, it is not much use having very small random errors if there may well be moderate biases, so even the large sizes of some non-randomised analyses of computerised hospital records cannot guarantee medically reliable comparisons between the effects of different treatments.

Avoiding moderate biases

Proper randomisation avoids systematic differences between the types of patient in different treatment groups

The fundamental reason for randomisation is to make possible the avoidance of moderate biases by ensuring that each type of patient can be expected to have been allocated in similar proportions to the different treatment

TABLE 10.1—*Requirements for reliable assessment of moderate effects: negligible biases and small random errors*

Negligible biases (that is, guaranteed avoidance of moderate biases)

- Proper randomisation
  (non-randomised methods might suffer moderate biases)
- Analysis by allocated treatment
  (including all randomised patients: "intention to treat" analysis)
- Chief emphasis on overall results
  (no unduly data-dependent emphasis on particular subgroups)
- Systematic overview of all relevant randomised trials
  (no unduly data-dependent emphasis on particular studies)

Small random errors (that is, guaranteed avoidance of moderate random errors)

- Large numbers in any new trials
  (to be really large, trials should be "streamlined")
- Systematic overviews of all relevant randomised trials
  (which yields the largest possible total numbers)

strategies that are to be compared, so that only random differences should affect the final comparisons of outcome. Non-randomised methods, by contrast, cannot in general guarantee that the types of patient given the study treatment do not differ systematically in any important ways from the types of patient given other treatment(s) with which the study treatment is to be compared. For example, moderate biases might arise if the study treatment was novel and doctors were afraid to use it for the most seriously ill patients—or, conversely, if they were more ready to try it out on those who were desperately ill. There may also be other ways in which the severity of the condition differentially affects the likelihood of being assigned to different treatments by the doctor's choice (or by any other non-random procedure).

It might at first sight appear that by collecting enough information about various prognostic features it would be possible to make some mathematical adjustments that would correct for any such differences between the types of patients who, in a non-randomised study, actually get given the different treatments that are to be compared. The hope is that such methods (which are sometimes called "outcomes analyses") might achieve comparability between those entering the different treatment groups, but in general they cannot be guaranteed to do so. For, some important prognostic factors may be unrecorded, while some other prognostic features may be difficult to assess exactly, and hence difficult to adjust for properly. There are two reasons for this difficulty. Firstly, it is often not realised that, even if there are no systematic differences between one treatment group and another in the accuracy with which prognostic factors are recorded, purely random errors in assessing prognostic factors can introduce systematic biases into the statistically adjusted comparison between treatments in a non-randomised study. Secondly, in a non-randomised comparison the care with which prognostic factors are recorded may differ between one treatment group and another. Doctors studying a novel treatment may investigate their patients particularly carefully, and, perhaps surprisingly, this extra accuracy can introduce a moderate bias. For example, an unusually careful search of the axilla among women with early breast cancer will sometimes result in the discovery of tiny deposits of cancer cells that would normally have been overlooked, and hence some women who would have been classified as "Stage I" will be reclassified as "Stage II". The prognosis of these "down-staged" women is worse than that of those who remain as Stage I, but better than that of those already classified as Stage II by less intensive investigation. Paradoxically, therefore, such down-staging not only improves the average prognosis of "Stage I" breast cancer but also improves the average prognosis of "Stage II" breast cancer, biasing any non-randomised comparison with other women with Stage I or Stage II disease for whom the staging was less careful.

The machinery of a properly randomised trial: no foreknowledge of treatment allocation, no bias in patient management, unbiased outcome assessment, and no post-randomisation exclusions

No foreknowledge of what the next treatment will be

In a properly randomised trial, the decision to enter a patient is made irreversibly, in ignorance of which of the trial treatments that patient will be allocated. The treatment allocation is made after trial entry has been decided upon. (The purpose of this sequence is to ensure that foreknowledge of what the next treatment is going to be cannot affect the decision to enter the patient: if it did, then those allocated one treatment might differ systematically from those allocated another.) Ideally, any major prognostic features should also be irreversibly recorded before the treatment is revealed, especially if these are to be used in any analyses of treatment. For, if the recorded value of some prognostic factor might be affected by knowledge of the trial treatment allocation, then treatment comparisons within subgroups that are defined by that factor might be moderately biased. In particular, treatment comparisons just among "responders" or just among "non-responders" can be extremely misleading, unless the response is assessed before treatment allocation.

No bias in patient management or in outcome assessment

An additional difficulty, both in randomised and in non-randomised comparisons of various treatments, is that there might be systematic differences in the use of other treatments (including general supportive care), or in the assessment of major outcomes. A non-randomised comparison, especially if it merely involves retrospective review of medical records, may well suffer uncorrectably from moderate biases due to such systematic differences in ancillary care or assessment. In the context of a randomised comparison, however, it is generally possible to devise ways to keep any such biases small. For example, placebo tablets may be given to control-allocated patients and certain subjective assessments may be "blinded" (although this is less important in studies assessing mortality).

"Intention to treat" analyses with no post-randomisation exclusions

Even in a properly randomised trial, unnecessary biases could be introduced by inappropriate statistical analysis. One of the most important sources of bias in the analysis is undue concentration on just one part of the evidence (that is, on "data-derived subgroup analyses": see below) instead of on the totality of the evidence. Another bias, which is easily avoided, is caused by post-randomisation exclusion of patients, especially if the type (and prognosis) of those excluded from one treatment group differs from that of those excluded from another. The fundamental statistical analysis of a trial should, therefore, generally compare all those originally allocated one treatment (even though some of them may not have actually received it) with all those allocated the other treatment (that is, it should be an "intention to treat" analysis). Additional analyses can also be reported: for example, in describing the frequency of some very specific side effect it may be preferable to describe its incidence only among those who actually received the treatment. (This is because strictly randomised comparisons may not be needed to assess extreme **relative** risks.) But, in assessing the overall outcome, such "on treatment" analyses can be misleading, and "intention to treat" analyses are generally a more trustworthy guide as to whether there is any real difference between the trial treatments in their effects on outcome. (For further discussion, see Peto *et al.*[3])

Problems produced by unduly data-dependent emphasis on particular results

The treatment that is appropriate for one patient may be inappropriate for another. Ideally, therefore, what is wanted is not only an answer to the question "Is this treatment helpful on average for a wide range of patients?", but also an answer to the question "For which recognisable categories of patient is this treatment helpful?". This ideal is, however, difficult to attain directly because the direct use of clinical trial results in particular subgroups of patients is surprisingly unreliable. Even if the real sizes of the effects of treatment in specific subgroups are importantly different, standard subgroup analyses are so statistically insensitive that they may well fail to demonstrate these differences. Conversely, even if there is a highly significant "interaction" (that is, an apparent difference between the **sizes** of the therapeutic effects in different subgroups) and the results seem to suggest that treatment works in some subgroups but not in others (thereby giving the appearance of a "qualitative interaction"), this may still not be good evidence for subgroup-specific treatment preferences.

Questions about such "interactions" between patient characteristics and the effects of treatment are easy to ask, but surprisingly difficult to answer reliably. Apparent interactions can often be produced just by the play of chance and, in particular subgroups, can mimic or obscure some of the moderate treatment effects that might realistically be expected. To demonstrate this, a subgroup analysis was performed based on the astrological birth signs of patients randomised in the very large ISIS-2 trial of the treatment of acute myocardial infarction.[4] Overall in this trial, the one month survival advantage produced by aspirin was particularly clearly demonstrated (804 vascular deaths among 8587 patients allocated aspirin versus 1016 among 8600 allocated control; 23% reduction; P<0.000001). But, when these aspirin analyses were subdivided by the patients' astrological "birth signs", to illustrate the unreliability of subgroup analyses, aspirin appeared totally ineffective for those born under Libra or Gemini

TABLE 10.2—*False negative mortality effect in a subgroup defined only by the astrological "birth sign": the ISIS-2 trial of aspirin among over 17 000 patients with acute myocardial infarction*

Astrological "birth sign"	No of 1 month deaths (aspirin *v* placebo)	Significance
Libra or Gemini	150 *v* 147	NS
All other signs	654 *v* 869	2P<0.000001
Any birth sign*	804 *v* 1016 (9.4%) (11.8%)	2P<0.000001

* Appropriate overall analysis for assessing the true effect in all subgroups.

(table 10.2). It would obviously be unwise to conclude from such a result that patients born under the sign of Libra or Gemini should not be given this particular treatment. Yet, similar conclusions based on "exploratory" data-derived subgroup analyses that, from a purely statistical viewpoint, are no more reliable than these are often reported and believed, with inappropriate effects on practice.

There are three main remedies for this unavoidable conflict between the reliable subgroup specific conclusions that doctors want and the unreliable findings that direct subgroup analyses can usually offer. But, the extent to which these remedies are helpful in particular instances is one on which informed judgements differ.

Firstly, where there are good **a priori** reasons for anticipating that the effect of treatment might be different in different circumstances then a limited number of subgroup analyses may be **pre**-specified in the study protocol, along with a prediction of the direction of such proposed interactions. (For example, it was expected that the benefits of fibrinolytic therapy for acute myocardial infarction would be greater the earlier patients were treated, and so some studies pre-specified analyses subdivided by time from onset of symptoms to treatment: see later.) These pre-specified subgroup-specific analyses are then to be taken much more seriously than other subgroup analyses.

The second approach is to emphasise chiefly the overall results of a trial (or, better still, of all such trials) for particular outcomes as a guide—or at least a context for speculation—as to the qualitative results in various specific subgroups of patients, and to give less weight to the actual results in each separate subgroup. This is clearly the right way to interpret the findings in table 10.2, but it is also likely in many other circumstances to provide the best assessment of whether one treatment is better than the other in particular subgroups. Of course, the extrapolation needs to be done in a medically sensible way. For example, if one treatment has substantial side effects then it may be inappropriate for low risk patients. (In this case, the side effects in a particular subgroup and the proportional benefit in that subgroup should be estimated separately, but the estimation for both might be more reliable if based on an appropriate extrapolation from the overall results rather than on the results in that one subgroup alone.)

The third approach is to be influenced, in discussing the likely effects on mortality in specific subgroups, not only by the mortality analyses in these subgroups but also by the analyses of recurrence-free survival or some other major "surrogate" outcome. For, if the overall results are similar but much more highly significant for recurrence-free survival than for mortality, subgroup analyses with respect to the former may be more stable and may provide a better guide as to whether there are any big differences between subgroups in the effects of treatment (particularly if such subgroup analyses were specified before results were available).

Avoiding moderate random errors

The need for large-scale randomisation

To distinguish reliably between the two alternatives either that there is no worthwhile difference in survival, or that treatment confers a moderate, but worthwhile, benefit (for example, 10 or 20% fewer deaths), not only must systematic errors be guaranteed to be small (see above) compared with such a moderate risk reduction, but so too must any of the purely random errors that are produced just by chance. Random errors can be reliably avoided only by studying large enough numbers of patients. It is not, however, sufficiently widely appreciated just how large clinical trials really need to be, in order to detect moderate differences reliably. This can be illustrated by a hypothetical trial that is actually quite inadequate—even though by previous standards it is moderately large—in which a 20% reduction in mortality (from 10% down to 8%) is supposed to be detected among 2000 heart attack patients (1000 treated and 1000 controls). In this case, one might predict finding about 100 deaths (10%) in the control group and 80 (8%) in the treated group. Even if exactly this difference were to be observed, however, it would not be conventionally significant (P value = 0.1; indicating that even if there is no real difference between the effects of the trial treatments, it would still be relatively easy for a result at least as extreme as this to arise by chance alone). Although the play of chance might well increase the difference enough to make it conventionally significant (for example to 110 deaths *v* 70 deaths; P<0.001), it might equally well dilute, obliterate (for example, to 90 deaths *v* 90 deaths), or even reverse it. The situation in real life is often even worse, as the average trial size may be only a few hundred patients, rather than the several thousand that would ideally be needed.

Mega-trials: how to randomise large numbers

One of the chief techniques for obtaining appropriately large-scale randomised evidence is to make trials extremely simple, and then to invite hundreds of hospitals to collaborate. The first of these large simple trials (or "mega-trials") were the ISIS and GISSI studies[4,5] in heart attack treatment, and a few other mega-trials have now been undertaken. But, in terms of medically significant findings, what has been achieved so far is only a fraction of what could quite readily be achieved by the wholehearted pursuit of such research strategies. Any obstacle to simplicity is an obstacle to large size, so it is worth making enormous efforts at the design stage to simplify and streamline the process of entering, treating, and assessing patients. Many trials would be of much greater scientific value if they collected 10 times less data, both at entry and during follow up, on 10 times more patients. It is particularly necessary to simplify the entry of patients, for if this is not done then rapid recruitment may be difficult. The current fashions for unduly complicated eligibility criteria, overly detailed "informed" consent, excessive "quality of life" assessments, extensive auditing of data, and measurements of the economic costs of treatment are often inappropriate.[1,6]

Inappropriate inclusion of cost and "quality of life" indices

Eventually, the cost effectiveness of various treatments needs to be assessed, but that does not necessarily imply that costs should be assessed in the same studies in which effectiveness is to be assessed, especially if attempts to assess costs seriously damage attempts to assess the effects on mortality and major morbidity sufficiently reliably. Moreover, what really matters is the cost of a treatment in routine practice, not its cost when given in the particular circumstances of a randomised trial.

Likewise, of course, any important ways in which treatments affect the quality of life need to be understood, but again that does not necessarily imply that "quality of life" indices should be assessed in the same trials that assess the main effects of treatment. For, although 20 000 patients may be required for reliable assessment of the effects of treatment on mortality and major morbidity, only a few hundred are likely to be needed for sufficiently reliable assessment of the effects of treatment on various proposed quality of life measures (or on costs of treatment). It may be possible to incorporate such assessments within a large mortality study as small substudies. But, this may be difficult in practice, and there are many instances where what should be a large simple trial of clinical efficacy should not be jeopardised by the measurement of such factors. Moreover, the effects of a treatment on quality of life in a trial when both the doctors and the patients are uncertain about any clinical benefits of the treatment may differ substantially from its effects on quality of life after the treatment has been shown to improve survival. Hence, it may be better to assess these other outcome measures only after having determined whether the treatment has any worthwhile effects on mortality and major morbidity, and if (as is often the case) it does not then any costs and adverse effects on quality of life may be largely irrelevant.

Simplification of entry procedures for trials: the "uncertainty principle"

For ethical reasons, patients cannot have their treatment chosen at random if either they or their doctor are already reasonably certain what treatment to prefer. Hence, randomisation can be offered only if both doctor and patient feel substantially uncertain as to which of the trial treatments is best. The question then arises: of those patients about whose treatment there is such uncertainty, which categories should be offered randomisation? The obvious answer is all of them, welcoming the heterogeneity that this will produce. (For example, either the treatment of choice will turn out to be the same for men and women, in which case the trial might as well include both, or it will be different, in which case it is particularly important to study both sexes.) **In large trials, homogeneity of patients is generally a defect, while heterogeneity is generally a strength**. Consider, for example, the trials of fibrinolytic therapy for acute myocardial infarction: some trials had restrictive entry criteria that allowed inclusion of only those patients who presented 0–6 hours after pain onset, so those trials contributed almost nothing to the key question of how late such treatment can still be useful. In contrast, trials with wider, more heterogeneous entry criteria that included some patients with longer delays between pain onset and randomisation assessed this question prospectively, and were able to show that fibrinolytic therapy can have definite protective effects when given not only 0–6 but also 7–12 hours after pain onset (see below[7]).

This approach of randomising a wide range of patients in whom there is substantial uncertainty as to which treatment option is best was used in the MRC's European Carotid Surgery Trial (ECST), which compared a policy of immediate carotid endarterectomy versus a policy of "watchful waiting" in patients with partial carotid artery stenosis and a recent minor stroke in the part of the brain supplied by that carotid artery.[8] If a patient was prepared at least to consider surgery then the neurologist and surgeon responsible for that individual patient's care considered in their own way whatever medical, personal, or other factors seemed to them to be relevant (figure 10.1), including, of course, the patient's own preferences and values:

(*a*) If they were then **reasonably certain**, for any reasons, that they **did wish** to recommend immediate surgery for that particular individual, then the patient was **ineligible** and was not part of the ECST;
(*b*) conversely, if they were **reasonably certain**, for any reason, that they **did not wish** to recommend immediate surgery, then that patient was likewise **ineligible**;
(*c*) if, but only if, they were **substantially uncertain** what to recommend, then that individual patient was automatically **eligible** for randomisation between immediate versus no immediate surgery (with all patients receiving

---

FIG 10.1—*(opposite) Example of the "uncertainty principle" for trial entry: the chief eligibility criterion for the European Carotid Surgery Trial (ECST) was that the doctors and patient should be substantially uncertain whether to risk immediate or deferred surgery. (Partly because this criterion was appropriately flexible, ECST became the largest ever trial of vascular surgery.)*

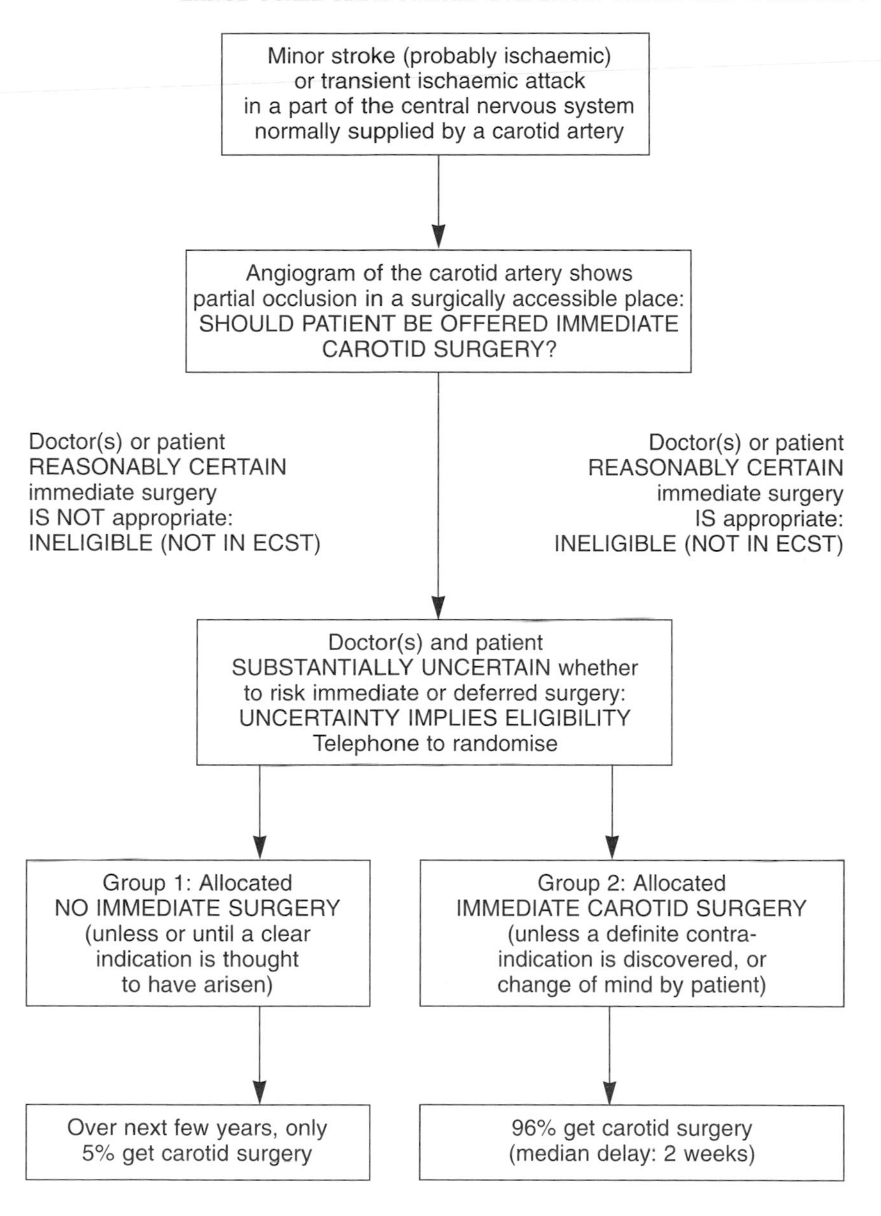
Minor stroke (probably ischaemic)
or transient ischaemic attack
in a part of the central nervous system
normally supplied by a carotid artery
Angiogram of the carotid artery shows
partial occlusion in a surgically accessible place:
SHOULD PATIENT BE OFFERED IMMEDIATE
CAROTID SURGERY?
Doctor(s) or patient
REASONABLY CERTAIN
immediate surgery
IS NOT appropriate:
INELIGIBLE (NOT IN ECST)
Doctor(s) or patient
REASONABLY CERTAIN
immediate surgery
IS appropriate:
INELIGIBLE (NOT IN ECST)
Doctor(s) and patient
SUBSTANTIALLY UNCERTAIN whether
to risk immediate or deferred surgery:
UNCERTAINTY IMPLIES ELIGIBILITY
Telephone to randomise
Group 1: Allocated
NO IMMEDIATE SURGERY
(unless or until a clear
indication is thought
to have arisen)
Group 2: Allocated
IMMEDIATE CAROTID SURGERY
(unless a definite contra-
indication is discovered, or
change of mind by patient)
Over next few years, only
5% get carotid surgery
96% get carotid surgery
(median delay: 2 weeks)
Statistical comparisons
of various outcomes over several years:
100% of Group 1 v 100% of Group 2
("INTENTION TO TREAT" ANALYSES)

whatever their doctors judged to be the best available medical care—which generally included advice to stop smoking, treatment of any hypertension, and the use of aspirin as an antithrombotic drug).

There were substantial differences between individual doctors in the types of patients they were uncertain about (in terms of the severity of carotid stenosis, as well as in various other characteristics). This guaranteed that no category—mild, moderate, or severe stenosis—would be wholly excluded, and hence that the trial would yield at least some direct evidence in each. As a result of the wide and simple entry criteria adopted by ECST, 3000 patients were randomised and the study was therefore able to provide some clear answers about who needed carotid endarterectomy. For patients with only mild (0–29%) carotid artery stenosis on their pre-randomisation angiogram there was little risk of ipsilateral ischaemic stroke, even in the absence of surgery, so any benefits of surgery over the next few years were small and outweighed by its early risks. Conversely, for patients with severe (70–99%) stenosis, the risks of surgery were significantly outweighed by its later benefits over the next few years. For both of these categories the trial stopped early, but for the intermediate category of patients with moderate (30–69%) stenosis, the balance of surgical risk and eventual benefit remained uncertain, so recruitment into the study continued, with entry still governed by the "uncertainty principle" as before.

The "uncertainty principle" meets simultaneously the requirements of ethicality, heterogeneity, simplicity, and maximal trial size. It states that the fundamental eligibility criterion is that both patient and doctor should be substantially uncertain about the appropriateness for this particular patient of each of the trial treatments. With such uncertainty as the fundamental principle of eligibility, informed consent can also be simplified. For the degree of "informed consent" that is humanly appropriate in a randomised comparison of different treatments that is governed by the "uncertainty principle" should probably not differ greatly from that which is humanly appropriate in routine practice outside of trials where treatment is being chosen haphazardly—or, to put it another way, "double standards" between trial and non-trial situations are not appropriate. The haphazard nature of many non-randomised treatment choices is reflected in the wide variations in practice between and within countries (and, even when practice is similar it may be similarly wrong: for example, before the ISIS-2 results became available (see later), almost all doctors around the world were not using fibrinolytic therapy for acute myocardial infarction). Provided that trials are governed by the "uncertainty principle", there is an approximate parallelism between good science and good ethics. Indeed, in such circumstances, excessively detailed consent procedures (which can be distressing and inhumane, and so would not be considered appropriate in routine practice) would not be either scientifically or ethically appropriate (for further discussion, see Collins *et al*[6]).

This "uncertainty principle" is just one of many ways to simplify trials, and thereby help them to avoid becoming enmeshed in a mass of wholly unnecessary traditional complexity. If randomised trials can be greatly simplified, as has already been achieved in a few major diseases, and thereby made vastly larger, then they will play an appropriately central role in the development of rational criteria for the planning of health care throughout the world.

Minimising BOTH bias and random error: systematic overviews ("meta-analyses") of randomised trials

Archie Cochrane was one of the first people to emphasise the need to bring together, by specialty, the results from all relevant randomised trials,[9] and the Cochrane Collaboration is now attempting to do this systematically.[10] For, when several trials have all addressed much the same therapeutic question, then the traditional procedure of choosing only a few of them for emphasis and fame may be a source of serious bias, since chance fluctuations for or against treatment may affect which trials become famous. To avoid this, it is appropriate to base inference chiefly on a systematic overview (or "meta-analysis") of all the results from all the trials that have addressed a particular type of question (or on an unbiased subset of such trials), and not on some potentially biased subset of the trials.[2,11] Such overviews will also minimise random errors in the assessment of treatment, as, in general, far more patients are involved in an overview than in any individual trial that contributes to it.

The separate trials may well be heterogeneous in their entry criteria, their treatment schedules, their follow up procedures, their methods of treating relapse, etc. At one extreme each trial might, in view of this heterogeneity, be considered in virtual isolation from all others, whereas at the opposite extreme all might be considered together. Both of these extreme views have some merit, and the pursuit of each by different people may prove more illuminating than too definite an insistence on any one particular approach. The heterogeneity of the different trials, however, merely argues for careful interpretation of any overviews of different trial results, rather than arguing against any such overviews. For, whatever the difficulties of interpretation of overviews may be, without systematic overviews moderate biases and random errors that may obscure any moderate treatment effects (or, conversely, may imply effects where none exists) cannot reliably be avoided.

Which overviews are trustworthy?

Over the past decade or two, a large (and rapidly increasing) number of meta-analyses of randomised trial results have been reported, not all of which are trustworthy. The two fundamental questions are how carefully the overview has been done, and how large it is. The simplest approach is merely to have collected and tabulated the published data from whatever randomised trial reports can be found easily in the literature, and sometimes this may suffice. At the opposite extreme, extensive efforts may have been made by those organising the overview to locate every potentially relevant randomised trial, to collaborate closely with the trialists to seek individual data on each patient ever randomised into those trials, and then (after extensive checks and corrections of such data) to produce, in collaboration with those trialists, agreed analyses and publications. The results of some of the largest such collaborations will be described later: the Antiplatelet Trialists' (APT) Collaborative Group,[12] the Fibrinolytic Trialists' (FTT) Collaborative Group,[7] and the Early Breast Cancer Trialists' Collaborative Group (EBCTCG).[13] Collaboration of the original trialists in the overview process, with collection of individual patient data, can help to avoid or minimise the biases that could be produced by missing trials (for example, due to the greater likelihood of extremely good, or extremely bad, results being particularly widely known about and published), by inappropriate post-randomisation withdrawals or by failure to allocate treatment properly at random. If randomisation was done properly in the first place, then post-randomisation withdrawals can often be followed up and restored to the study for an appropriate "intention to treat" analysis. Knowledge of the exact methods of treatment allocation (backed up by checks on whether the main prognostic factors recorded are non-randomly distributed between the treatment groups in a particular trial) may help to identify trials that were not, in fact, properly randomised, and that should therefore be excluded from an overview of randomised trials. Overviews based on individual patient data may also provide more information about treatment effects than the more usual overviews of grouped data, for they allow more detailed analyses—indeed, if they are really large then they may actually yield statistically reliable subgroup analyses of the effects of treatment in particular types of patient.

Conversely, however, even a perfectly conducted overview may not be large enough to be reliable. An overview that brings together complete data from all the trials that have ever been done of a certain treatment but still (because the trials were all small) includes a total of only 100 deaths will have random errors that are no smaller than those for a single trial with 100 deaths among such patients. Small-scale evidence, whether from an overview or from one trial, is often unreliable, and will often be found in retrospect to have yielded wrong answers. What is needed is large-scale randomised evidence; it does not matter much whether that evidence comes from a properly conducted overview or a properly conducted trial. The practical medical value of such evidence will now be illustrated by a few recent examples.

Some examples of important results in the treatment of vascular and of neoplastic disease that could have been reliably established only by large-scale randomised evidence

Definite result from a single very large trial: benefit from medium-dose aspirin for patients with suspected acute myocardial infarction (and benefits among other groups of patients indicated by overviews of trials)

In the ISIS-2 trial, half of 17 000 patients with suspected acute myocardial infarction were allocated aspirin tablets (162 mg/day for one month, which virtually completely inhibits cyclo-oxygenase-dependent platelet inhibition), and half were allocated placebo (dummy) tablets.[4] Before 1988, when the ISIS-2 results were published, aspirin was not routinely used in acute myocardial infarction, and no other major trial had (or has subsequently) assessed aspirin in suspected acute myocardial infarction. But, the effects of one month of aspirin were so definite in ISIS-2 (804/8587 vascular deaths among those allocated aspirin *v* 1016/8600 among those not) that even the lower 99% confidence limit would have represented a worthwhile benefit from so simple and inexpensive a treatment (figure 10.2).

As a result, worldwide treatment patterns changed sharply when the ISIS-2 results emerged, and aspirin is now routinely used in many different countries for the majority of emergency hospital admissions with suspected acute myocardial infarction. In the United Kingdom, for example, two British Heart Foundation surveys found cardiologists reporting that routine aspirin use in acute coronary care had increased from under 10% in 1987 to over 90% in 1989.[14] Worldwide, the annual number of patients with suspected myocardial infarction who would nowadays be given such treatment must be well over a million a year, suggesting that in this clinical context alone aspirin is already preventing tens of thousands of premature deaths each year. But, if the ISIS-2 trial had been 10 times smaller (1700 instead of 17 000 patients) then exactly the same proportional reduction in mortality as shown in figure 10.2 would not have been conventionally significant, and therefore would have been much less likely to influence medical practice—indeed, the result might by chance have appeared exactly

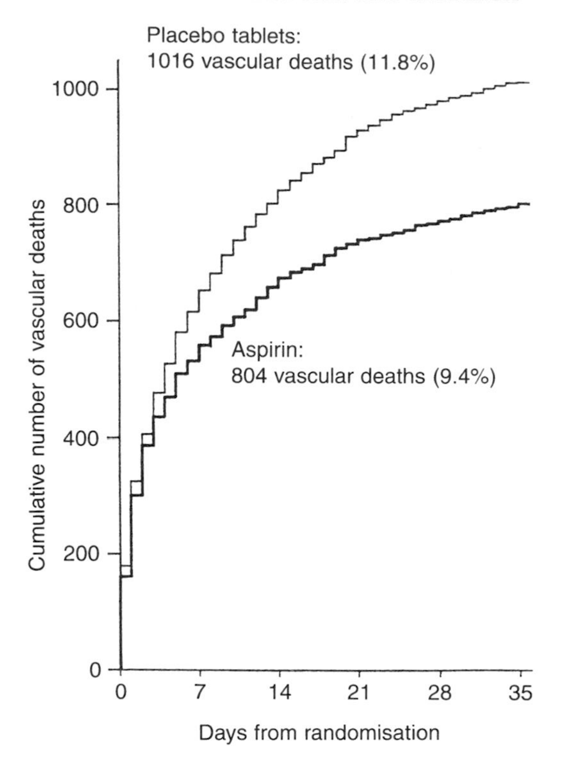

FIG 10.2—*Effect of administration of aspirin for one month on 35 day mortality in the ISIS-2 trial among over 17 000 patients with acute myocardial infarction. (Absolute survival advantage: 24 (SD 5) lives saved per 1000 allocated aspirin; 2P<0.00001.) (From* ISIS–2.[4] *© by The Lancet Ltd 1988, with permission.)*

flat, greatly damaging future research on aspirin in this context. Likewise, if the ISIS-2 trial had been non-randomised then it might well have got the wrong answer (because in a non-randomised study doctors might tend to give active treatment to patients who were particularly ill, or who were in various other ways somewhat different from those not given active treatment). And, even if a non-randomised study did happen to get an unbiasedly correct answer it would be impossible to be sure that it had actually done so, and hence again a non-randomised study might have had much less influence on medical practice than did ISIS-2.

In the ISIS-2 trial aspirin significantly reduced the one month mortality, but it also significantly reduced the number of non-fatal strokes and of non-fatal reinfarctions that were recorded in hospital. Combining all these three outcomes into "vascular events" (stroke, death, or reinfarction), 13% of those allocated aspirin and 17% of those who were not, were known to have suffered a vascular event in the month after randomisation (table 10.3:

an absolute difference of 40 events per 1000 treated—or, perhaps more relevantly, of 40 000 per million).[12] The randomised trials of aspirin, or of other antiplatelet regimens, in other types of high risk patients (for example, a few years of aspirin for those who have survived a myocardial infarction or stroke) have not been as large as ISIS-2, and so, taken separately, most have yielded false negative results. But, when the results from many such trials are combined, statistically definite reductions in "vascular events" are seen (table 10.3). Because such treatments do not seem to increase non-vascular mortality, all cause mortality is also significantly reduced.

TABLE 10.3—*Summary of overall results in trials of aspirin (or other antiplatelet drugs)* for the prevention of vascular events: the Antiplatelet Trialists' Collaboration, involving a total of about 100 000 randomised patients in over 100 trials*

Type of patient studied	Average scheduled treatment duration (and approximate numbers of patients randomised)	Proportions who suffered a non-fatal stroke, non-fatal heart attack, or vascular death during the trials		
		Anti-platelet	Control	Events avoided in these trials
High risk:				
Suspected acute heart attack	1 month (20 000)	10%	14%	40 per 1000 (2P<0.00001)
Previous history of heart attack	2 years (20 000)	13%	17%	40 per 1000 (2P<0.00001)
Previous history of stroke or TIA	3 years (10 000)	18%	22%	40 per 1000 (2P<0.00001)
Other vascular disease†	1 year (20 000)	7%	9%	20 per 1000 (2P<0.00001)
Low risk:				
Primary prevention in low-risk people	5 years (30 000)	4.4%	4.8%	4 per 1000 (2P>0.05)

* The most widely tested regimen was medium dose aspirin, involving an average daily dose of 75–325 mg, and no other antiplatelet regimen appeared to be significantly more or less effective than this at preventing such vascular events. (For comparison, in the United Kingdom or United States, a children's aspirin tablet contains about 75–80 mg of aspirin, while an adult tablet includes 300–325 mg.) Pharmacological evidence suggests that after the first few days all daily doses of aspirin in the range 75–325 mg are likely to be approximately equivalent in their effects on platelets and on the vascular endothelium. Hence, to limit any gastric discomfort with long term use, a daily dose at the lower end of this range might be slightly preferable, such as 75, 80, or 100 mg (depending on what is conveniently available). But, in acute emergencies such as suspected myocardial infarction or unstable angina, at least the initial dose should perhaps be at the upper end of the range, such as 250, 300, or 325 mg, so as to achieve a virtually complete antiplatelet effect within less than one hour (which could then be maintained by a lower daily dose).
† For example, angina, peripheral vascular disease, arterial surgery, angioplasty.

In principle these findings could, if appropriately widely exploited, prevent about 100 000 premature vascular deaths a year in developed countries alone, and there are probably at least as many vascular deaths in less developed as in developed countries. So, with realistically achievable levels of use of "medium dose" aspirin (75–325 mg/day) for the secondary prevention of vascular disease, it might well be possible in practice to ensure that aspirin is used in enough high risk patients to prevent, or substantially delay, at least 100 000 vascular deaths a year worldwide, and such use of aspirin would, in addition, prevent a comparable number of non-fatal strokes or heart attacks. (Medium dose aspirin was the least expensive and most widely tested antiplatelet regimen: it is of proven efficacy, and on review of all the antiplatelet trials no other antiplatelet regimen has been shown to be of greater efficacy in preventing vascular events: see notes to table 10.3.) This large-scale randomised evidence about medium dose aspirin is now changing worldwide clinical practice in ways that will, at low cost, prevent much death and disability in high risk patients. But, small trials, small overviews, or non-randomised studies (however large) could not possibly have provided appropriately reliable evidence about such **moderate** risk reductions.

Definite result from a very large overview of trials: benefit from "adjuvant" therapy with tamoxifen for patients with "early" breast cancer (and possible benefit suggested with ovarian ablation in younger women)

By definition, in "early" breast cancer all detectable deposits of disease are limited to the breast and the locoregional lymph nodes, and can be removed surgically. But, experience shows that undetectably small deposits may remain elsewhere that eventually, perhaps after a delay of several years, cause clinical recurrence at a distant site, which is then usually followed by death from the disease. These micrometastatic deposits may have been stimulated by the body's own hormones during the years before recurrence became detectable. So, among women who have had the detectable deposits of breast cancer removed by surgery (or by surgery with radiotherapy) there have been many trials of "adjuvant" treatments that either reduce the production of endogenous oestrogens (for example, various forms of ovarian ablation), or that block the access of those oestrogens to the tumour cells (for example, tamoxifen, which blocks the oestrogen receptor protein in some breast cancer cells).

Taken separately, most of these adjuvant trials have been too small to provide reliable evidence about long term survival.[13] But, if the results of all of them are combined then some very definite differences in 10 year survival do emerge (figure 10.3). Among women with Stage II disease who were less than 50 years old (and, therefore, generally premenopausal or perimenopausal), ovarian ablation appears to produce about a 10% absolute difference in 10 year survival (for example, 50% *v* 40%). This finding is

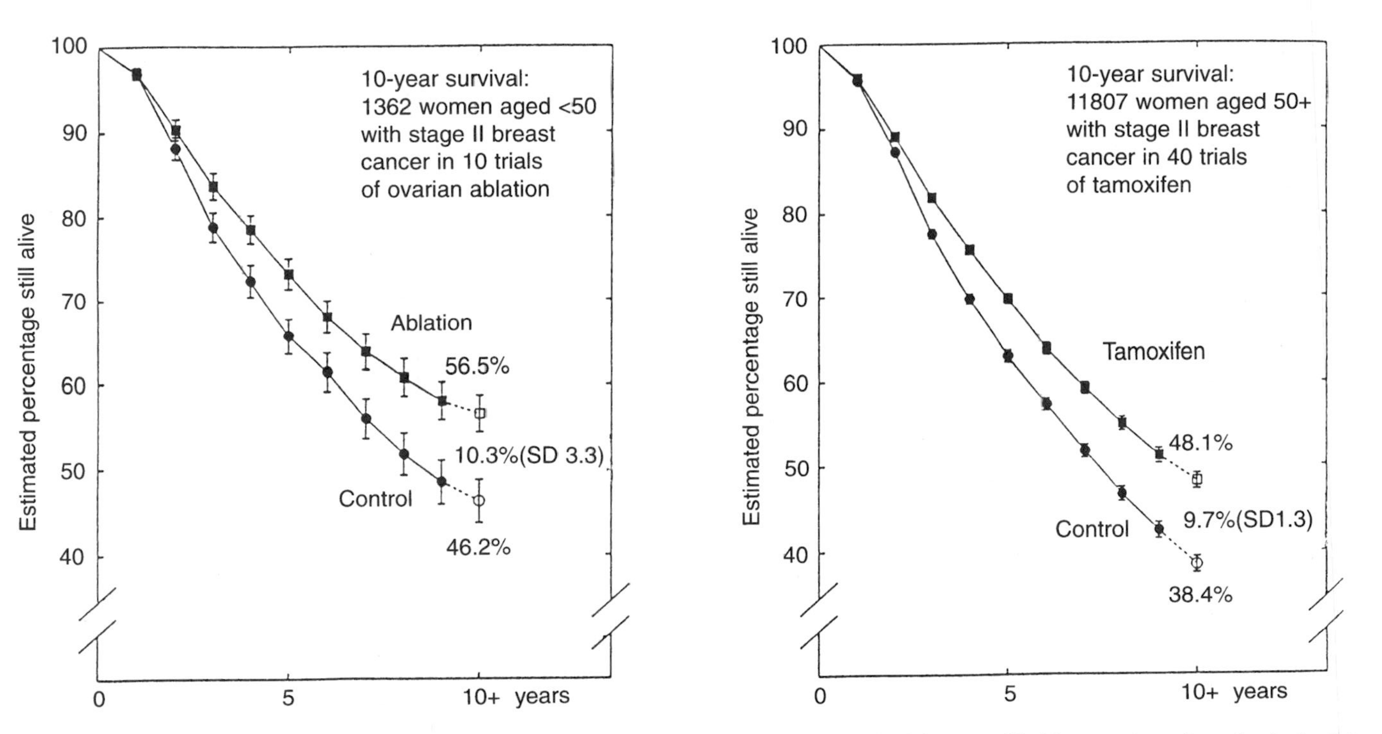

FIG 10.3—*Effects of hormonal adjuvant treatments for early breast cancer on 10-year survival in a worldwide overview of randomised trials. (From Early Breast Cancer Trialists' Collaborative Group.*[13]*)*

based on the analysis of only a few hundred deaths so it is still not as reliable as might ideally be wished, and, because substantial uncertainty remains, much larger trials are now in progress. Among older Stage II women, ovarian ablation is unlikely to be of much relevance (as most of the endogenous oestrogen at older ages comes from sources other than the ovaries) but, in aggregate, the randomised trials among such women have shown very definitely that a few years of tamoxifen likewise produces about a 10% absolute difference in 10 year survival. A smaller, but still highly significant, reduction in mortality by tamoxifen is also seen among the 10 000 randomised women with Stage I disease. Taken separately, however, 37 of the 42 tamoxifen trials were too small to have yielded statistically reliable evidence on their own (2P>0.01)—and, the five other trials were significant only because, by chance, they had results that were too good to be true.

These tamoxifen overview results have already changed clinical practice substantially, and have redirected research towards large randomised trials of the effects of different durations of tamoxifen: Should tamoxifen in asymptomatic women continue for two years, for five years, or indefinitely? Large randomised studies of the primary prevention of breast cancer among high risk women by tamoxifen are only just beginning, but they have been encouraged by the results from the tamoxifen trials overview in 30 000 patients with established cancer (Stage II or Stage I) in one breast, among whom there has been a highly significant reduction of one third in the likelihood of development of contralateral breast cancer but a small absolute increase in endometrial cancer. Again, this degree of trustworthy detail would not have been attained without large-scale randomised evidence.

Promising overview of small trials confirmed by large trial: benefit from fibrinolytic therapy as emergency treatment for a wide range of patients with acute myocardial infarction

Fibrinolytic drugs that dissolve thrombus that may be blocking a coronary artery, thereby causing an acute myocardial infarction, were introduced into clinical research in the late 1950s. But, the trials of fibrinolytic drugs in the 1960s and 1970s were too small to be statistically reliable (none involved even 1000 patients). So, by the early 1980s the haemorrhagic side effects were obvious, the benefits had not been convincingly demonstrated, and these agents were generally considered to be dangerous, ineffective, and hence not appropriate for routine coronary care. Overviews published in the mid-1980s of those previous small trials (involving a total of only about 6000 patients in two dozen trials) indicated a statistically definite benefit, but were not really believed by cardiologists—and so, again, such treatments were still not widely used. The situation has been saved by two large randomised trials, ISIS-2 and GISSI-1, both of which involved more than 10 000 patients[4,5] (and by their aggregation with the seven other randomised trials that involved more than 1000 patients; see below). In ISIS-2, not only were patients randomly allocated to receive aspirin or placebo tablets (as described before; figure 10.2), but they were also separately allocated to receive intravenous streptokinase (1.5 million units infused over about 60 minutes) or a placebo infusion. In this "factorial" design (which allows the separate assessment of more than one treatment without any material loss in the statistical reliability of each comparison), one quarter of patients were allocated aspirin alone, one quarter were allocated streptokinase alone, one quarter were allocated both streptokinase and aspirin, and one quarter were allocated neither (that is, placebo tablets and placebo infusion). Streptokinase, like aspirin, produced a highly significant reduction in mortality (and the combination of streptokinase and aspirin was highly significantly better than either aspirin or streptokinase alone; figure 10.4).

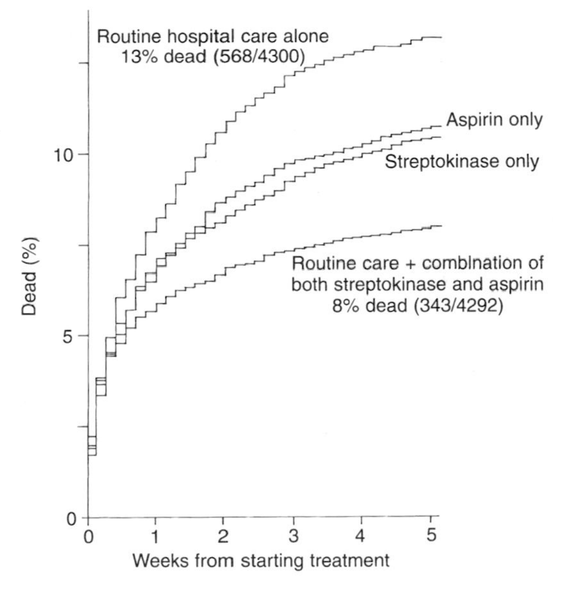

FIG 10.4—*Effects of one hour streptokinase infusion (and of one month of aspirin) on 35 day mortality in ISIS-2 among 17 187 patients with acute myocardial infarction who would not normally have received streptokinase or aspirin, divided at random into four similar groups to receive aspirin only, streptokinase only, both, or neither. (Any doctor who believed that a particular patient should be given either treatment gave it, and did not include that patient in ISIS-2.) (From ISIS-2.*[4] *© by The Lancet Ltd 1988, with permission.)*

It might appear, from figure 10.4, that there was no need for any more randomised evidence about fibrinolytic therapy, but this ignores the potential hazards of such treatment and the heterogeneity of patients. Taken separately, even ISIS-2, the largest of these trials, was not big enough for statistically reliable subgroup analyses, but when the nine largest trials were all taken together they included a total of about 60 000 patients, half of whom were randomly allocated fibrinolytic drugs. Those entering a coronary care unit with a diagnosis of suspected or definite acute myocardial infarction range from patients who are already in cardiogenic shock, with low blood pressure and a fast pulse (half of whom will die rapidly) to those who have merely got a history of chest pain and no very definite changes on their ECG (of whom "only" a small percentage will die before discharge). Fibrinolytic therapy often causes a frightening blood pressure drop: should it be used in patients who are already dangerously hypotensive? It occasionally causes serious strokes: should it be used in patients who are elderly or hypertensive, and therefore already have an above average risk of stroke (or who have only slight changes on their ECG, and therefore have only a low risk of cardiac death)? Finally, if the coronary artery has been occluded for long enough, then the heart muscle that it supplies will have been irreversibly destroyed: how late after the heart attack starts is fibrinolytic treatment still worth risking—three hours? six hours? 12 hours? 24 hours?

These questions needed to be answered reliably before appropriate and generally accepted indications for, and against, such an immediately hazardous but potentially effective therapy could be devised. To address them, all fibrinolytic therapy trialists have collaborated in a systematic overview of the randomised evidence.[7] On review of the 60 000 patients randomised between fibrinolytic therapy and control in trials of more than 1000 patients, some of the therapeutic questions were relatively easy to answer satisfactorily. For example, it seemed that most of those whose ECG was still fairly normal (or showed some other pattern that indicated only a **low** risk of death) might as well be left untreated, leaving open the option of starting fibrinolytic treatment urgently if their ECG changes suddenly for the worse in the following few hours. Conversely, among those who already had "high risk" ECG changes when they were randomised, the absolute benefit of immediate fibrinolytic therapy was, if anything, slightly greater than is indicated by figure 10.4—and age, sex, blood pressure, heart rate, diabetes, and previous history of myocardial infarction could not identify reliably any group that would not, on average, have their chances of survival appreciably increased by treatment.

The longer that fibrinolytic treatment for such patients was delayed, however, the less benefit it seemed to produce. Among those whose ECG showed definite ST-segment elevation (ST↑) or bundle branch block (BBB), the benefit was greatest (about 30 lives saved per 1000) among those randomised 0–6 hours after the onset of pain (figure 10.5). But, the mortality reduction was still substantial and significant (about 20 per 1000,

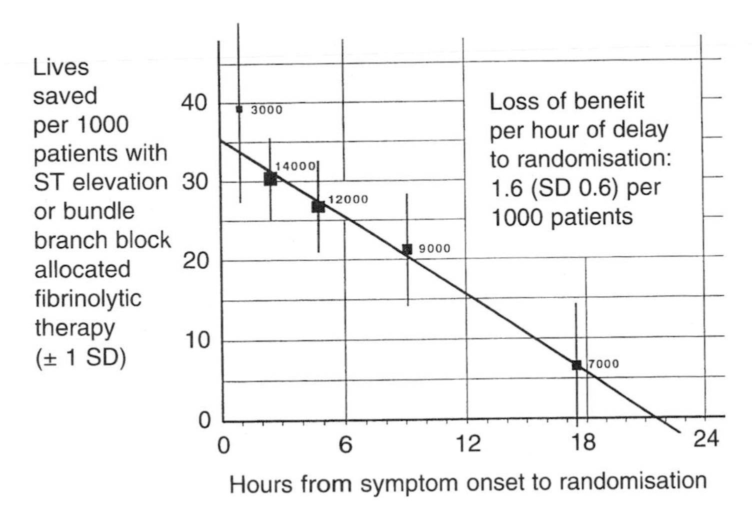

FIG 10.5—*Benefit versus delay (0–1, 2–3, 4–6, 7–12, or 13–24 hours) in the nine largest randomised trials of fibrinolytic therapy versus control in patients with acute myocardial infarction. One month mortality results for 45 000 patients with ST elevation or bundle branch block when randomised, showing the definite net benefit even for the 9000 randomised 7–12 hours after the onset of pain. (From Fibrinolytic Therapy Trialists' Collaborative group.*[7]*© by The Lancet Ltd 1994, with permission.)*

2P<0.003) when such patients were randomised 7–12 hours after pain onset. Indeed, if they were randomised 13–18 hours after pain onset there still appeared to be some net reduction in mortality (about 10 per 1000, but not statistically definite). The regression line in figure 10.5 reinforces, in a more reliable way, these separate subgroup analyses. Yet, before these large trials, it was forcefully, but mistakenly, argued that such treatments could not possibly be of any worthwhile benefit if given more than a few hours after the onset of symptoms.

Such detailed inferences are difficult enough with large-scale, properly randomised evidence, and would be impossible without it; because of their unknowable biases (see above), non-randomised database analyses are simply not a viable alternative to large-scale randomised evidence. Nor would randomisation of "only" several thousand patients have been sufficient. Indeed, in several important respects what is still needed is more, rather than less, randomised evidence about the effects of fibrinolytic therapy in various particular types of patient. Firstly, it is still not clear whether patients who do have definite ECG changes such as ST↑ or BBB but who present 12–18, or even 18–24, hours after pain onset should be treated: more randomised evidence is still needed (figure 10.5). Secondly, for one particular poor prognosis ECG category (ST depression) the one month mortality results still appear unpromising even when all currently available trials are combined (15% dead among those allocated fibrinolytic drugs *v* 14% among controls, but based on only 4000 patients). Analogy with the results in other high risk categories suggests that this result for patients with ST depression may well be a false negative. Perhaps it has arisen from unduly data-dependent emphasis on what may in retrospect prove to have been a random irregularity in the results in this particular subgroup that included only a few thousand individuals. Again, more randomised evidence is needed. Nevertheless, substantial progress has been made by the past decade of mega-trials of fibrinolytic agents. Worldwide, in the mid-1990s, about half a million patients per year are given fibrinolytic therapy, avoiding about 10 000 early deaths each year.

Small trials refuted by a mega-trial: lack of significant benefit from magnesium infusion in suspected acute myocardial infarction

It had been suggested that, in patients with suspected acute myocardial infarction, an infusion of a magnesium salt might reduce early mortality. Several small trials, involving between them a total of only about 1500 patients, had addressed this question by 1990, and their aggregated results indicated a statistically significant, but implausibly large, benefit (42/754 deaths among those allocated magnesium *v* 86/740 among the controls; $2P<0.001$).[15] Some argued that such results constituted proof beyond reasonable doubt that magnesium was of sufficient value to justify widespread usage without seeking further randomised evidence, but others remained sceptical, arguing that the apparent results were far too good to be true.

Two trials, one (LIMIT-2[16]) involving 2000 patients and one (ISIS-4[15]) involving 58 000, were therefore set up to test more reliably the possible effects of magnesium. The former yielded a moderately promising result (table 10.4) indicating avoidance of about one quarter of the early deaths, but because of its small size this result was statistically compatible with a true benefit that ranged from about zero to about a halving of early mortality. The much larger ISIS-4 trial, however, yielded a completely unpromising result, so the overall evidence, based on about 60 000 randomised patients, is now non-significantly adverse.[15]

In view of the striking disparity between the apparent effects of magnesium before and after ISIS-4 had provided large-scale randomised evidence, it is of interest to recall some of the expert views that were expressed while ISIS-4 was in progress. Some felt so strongly that magnesium was already of proven benefit (and hence that further randomisation was unethical) that the data monitoring committee of ISIS-4 was lobbied to try to have the study stopped early and all future patients given magnesium. By

TABLE 10.4—*Magnesium in acute myocardial infarction: contrast between the results of the smaller and the larger randomised trials*

	Number of patients randomised	1 month mortality			
		Allocated magnesium		Allocated control	
Nine small trials	1500	42/754	(5.6%)	86/740	(11.6%)
LIMIT-2 trial	2300	90/1159	(7.8%)	118/1157	(10.2%)
ISIS-4 trial	58 000	2216/29011	(7.6%)	2103/29039	(7.2%)
All trials	62 000	2348/30924	(7.59%)	2307/30936	(7.46%)

There is highly significant heterogeneity (P<0.001) between the group of small trials, the "hypothesis generating" results of which led to the testing of magnesium in ISIS-4, and the pair of larger trials (ISIS-4 and LIMIT-2), the results of which tested that hypothesis.

contrast, the ISIS-4 steering committee was sufficiently sceptical to want large-scale randomised evidence. They believed that the available evidence was consistent with a negligible benefit, or even a small net hazard—although they all thought it more likely that at least some net benefit would be seen. Even after the LIMIT-2 result was available, they continued to hold these opinions, and thought that if there was any real benefit then this was likely to be less than LIMIT-2 had suggested (and hence very much less than the other small trials had suggested). Those who had trusted the implausibly extreme results from the previous small trials may well have been disappointed by the results of the ISIS-4 mega-trial, which now provide strong evidence that the routine use of magnesium has little or no effect on mortality in acute myocardial infarction. But, in a world where moderate benefits are much more plausible than large benefits, it will commonly happen that striking results in small-scale trials, in small-scale overviews, or in small subgroups prove evanescent. The medical assumption that both a moderate mortality difference or a zero mortality difference may be plausible, but that an extreme mortality difference is much less so, has surprisingly strong consequences for the interpretation of randomised evidence. In particular, it implies that even quite highly significant (for example, 2P = 0.001) mortality differences that are based on only relatively small numbers of deaths may provide untrustworthy evidence of the existence of any real difference.[15]

Trials in their epidemiological context: effects of lower, and of lowering, blood pressure on the risk of stroke and of coronary heart disease

The quantitative epidemiological evidence about the effects of really long-term differences in risk factors such as blood pressure or blood cholesterol can help interpret the results from trials of the effects of reducing these risk factors for only a few years. This may help not only in interpreting the previous trials but also in planning the size and duration of any future risk factor modification trials. For, the epidemiological evidence provides approximate upper limits to the risk reductions that could plausibly be expected in the trials, and may also help to identify populations that are particularly likely to benefit from risk factor modification.

For example, appropriate analyses of prospective observational epidemiological studies of diastolic blood pressure (DBP) and disease indicate that throughout the range of usual DBP in the populations studied (about 70–110 mm Hg), a lower DBP was associated with a lower risk of suffering a first stroke or episode of coronary heart disease (that is, there did not seem to be any "threshold" or "J shape": figure 10.6).[17] The steepness of this continuous relationship between blood pressure and vascular disease suggests that the eventual reductions in risk produced by practicable blood pressure reductions (for example, with antihypertensive treatment) may well be worthwhile not only among certain "hypertensive" individuals but also among certain individuals who, although considered "normotensive", are at high risk for some reason (for example, as a result of a previous stroke or myocardial infarction).

After making due allowance for the substantial and systematic extent to which the true relationship is diluted by purely random fluctuations in the baseline measurements of blood pressure (that is, the "regression dilution" bias), the prospective studies suggest that a **prolonged** difference of only 5 mm Hg in usual DBP is associated with avoidance of at least one third of the risk of stroke and at least one fifth of the risk of coronary heart disease in late middle age. But, although non-randomised prospective observational studies may, despite the possibility of confounding by other factors, be more relevant to the eventual effects of prolonged differences in blood pressure, randomised trials of blood pressure reductions that last just a few years may be more relevant to assessing the speed with which the epidemiologically expected reductions in stroke or coronary heart disease risk are produced by reducing blood pressure. By comparing the results of a systematic overview of all randomised trials of antihypertensive therapy with the observational epidemiological evidence, it may be possible to estimate the extent to which the eventual effects of a lower blood pressure on disease incidence rates can be achieved within just a few years of treatment in middle or old age. (Ideally, these age ranges should be considered separately, as the fractional avoidance of risk may well be substantially different in middle and old age.)

Over the past few decades, numerous trials of the treatment of hypertension have been conducted to determine whether blood pressure reduction in middle age reduces the risk of stroke and of coronary heart disease. However, although it was fairly rapidly accepted that the treatment

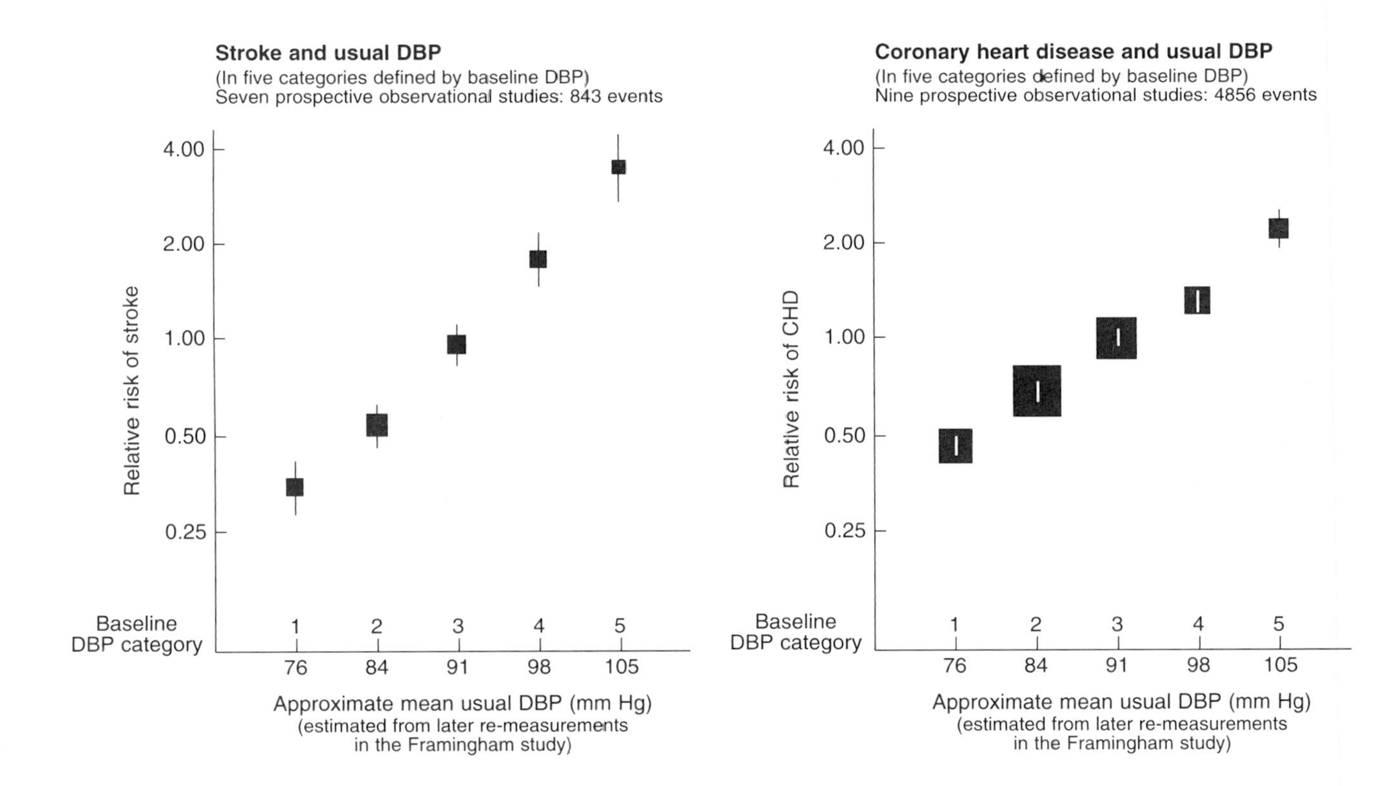

FIG 10.6—*Relative risks of stroke and of coronary heart disease for five categories of diastolic blood pressure (DBP) from the combined results of prospective observational studies. Solid squares represent the relative risks of disease in each category relative to the risk in the whole study population and 95% confidence intervals are denoted by vertical lines. (From MacMahon* et al.[17] *© by The Lancet Ltd 1990, with permission.)*

of severe hypertension could at least prevent stroke, until recently there has been controversy as to whether the treatment of even severe hypertension could also prevent coronary heart disease, and questions have also persisted about the effects on stroke of the treatment of mild to moderate hypertension. This continuing uncertainty about the benefits of lowering blood pressure may chiefly have reflected the inability of individual trials, even those with several hundred coronary heart disease events, to detect moderate coronary heart disease reductions reliably, rather than from any important heterogeneity of the real effects of treatment. The mean DBP difference between treatment and control groups in the trials was only about 5–6 mm Hg, and the epidemiological evidence suggests that a long-term difference of this magnitude is associated with only about 20–25% less coronary heart disease (and with about 35–40% less stroke). Even if such trial treatments would eventually, after many years, produce 20–25% less coronary heart disease, the effects seen within the two or three years that is available on average between randomisation and death in a five year trial might well be somewhat smaller (for example, 15%). Considered separately, however, none of the trials had recorded enough coronary heart disease events (or enough vascular deaths) for statistically reliable assessment of 15% risk reductions.

For stroke, the overview of randomised trials provides direct and highly significant evidence that most or all of the stroke avoidance associated with a prolonged difference in usual DBP appears soon after the blood pressure is lowered (figure 10.7). By contrast, the significant reduction in coronary heart disease seen in the trials (16% SD 4; 95% confidence interval 8 to 23%; 2P = 0.0001) falls somewhat short of the difference of about 20–25% suggested by the observational epidemiological evidence for a prolonged 5–6 mm Hg difference in usual DBP.[18] However, this coronary heart disease reduction is substantial and real (2P = 0.0001). Therefore, it is reasonable to hope that trials of antihypertensive regimens that can reduce blood pressure to a greater extent than the 5–6 mm Hg DBP reduction seen in these trials will demonstrate even greater reductions in stroke and coronary heart disease.

FIG 10.7—*(opposite) Reduction in the odds of stroke and of coronary heart disease in all unconfounded randomised trials of antihypertensive drug treatment (mean diastolic blood pressure differences of 5–6 mm Hg for five years). Solid squares represent the odds ratios (treatment: control) for the four larger trials and the properly stratified odds ratio for the combination of the 13 smaller trials. 95% confidence intervals are denoted by horizontal lines (for individual large trials or the combined small trials) and by diamonds (for overviews of all trials). (From Collins and Peto 1994, with permission.*[18])

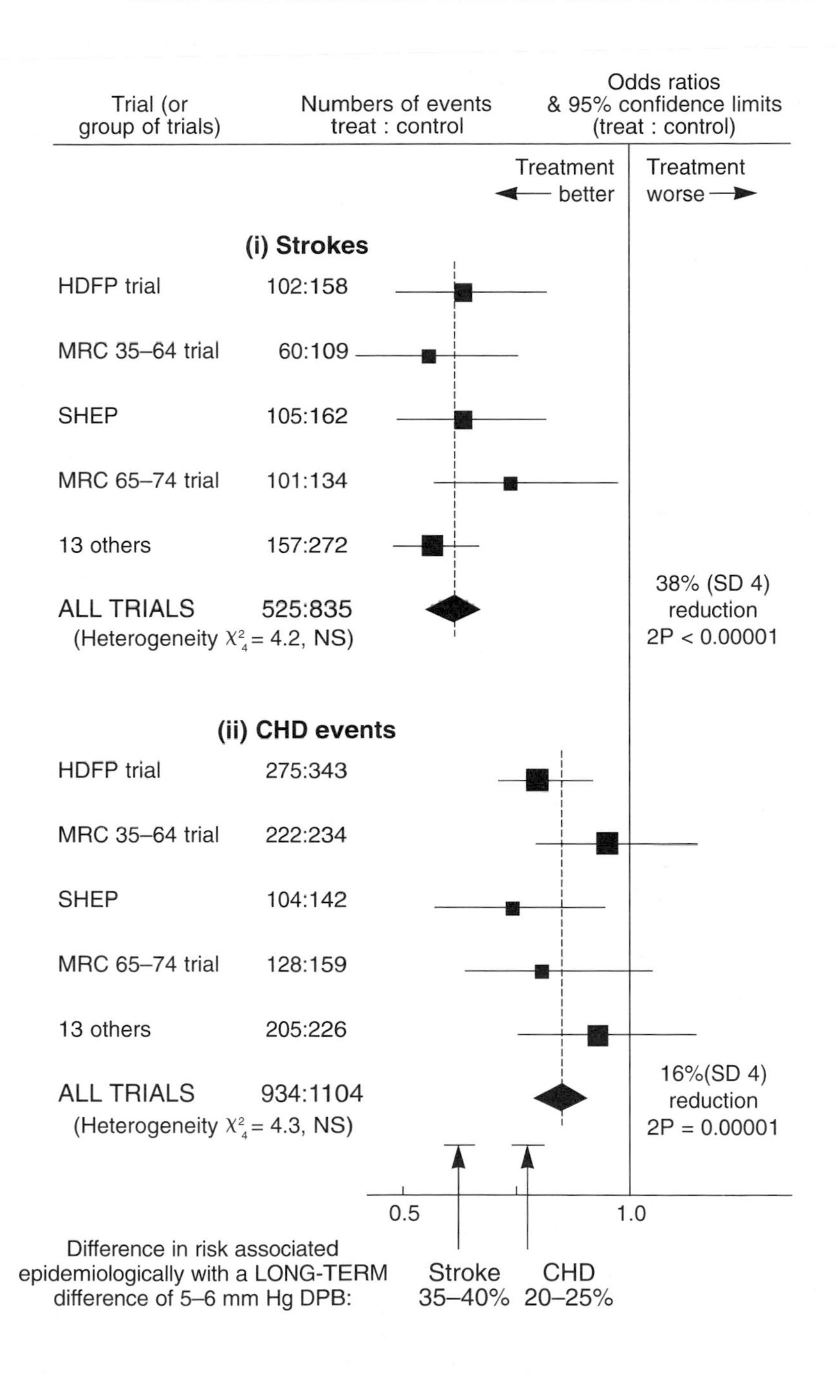
Trial (or group of trials)
Numbers of events treat : control
Odds ratios & 95% confidence limits (treat : control)
Treatment better
Treatment worse
(i) Strokes
HDFP trial 102:158
MRC 35–64 trial 60:109
SHEP 105:162
MRC 65–74 trial 101:134
13 others 157:272
ALL TRIALS 525:835
(Heterogeneity χ^2_4 = 4.2, NS)
38% (SD 4) reduction
2P < 0.00001
(ii) CHD events
HDFP trial 275:343
MRC 35–64 trial 222:234
SHEP 104:142
MRC 65–74 trial 128:159
13 others 205:226
ALL TRIALS 934:1104
(Heterogeneity χ^2_4 = 4.3, NS)
16%(SD 4) reduction
2P = 0.00001
0.5
1.0
Difference in risk associated epidemiologically with a LONG-TERM difference of 5–6 mm Hg DPB:
Stroke 35–40%
CHD 20–25%

The proportional reduction in vascular disease risk observed in the trials seemed to be similar in high risk and in low risk individuals, so that the absolute size of the reduction that is produced by treatment may be largely dependent upon the absolute risk. For high risk individuals, therefore, the absolute reduction in risk produced by antihypertensive treatment might be substantial even among those who are only moderately "hypertensive". Indeed, in view of the epidemiological evidence that there is, for stroke risk and for coronary heart disease risk, no "threshold" level of DBP within the normal range, large randomised trials might even show that blood pressure reduction is of substantial value among many "normotensive" individuals at high risk of stroke (such as those with a history of cerebral vascular disease) or of coronary heart disease (such as patients with a history of myocardial infarction, angina, peripheral vascular disease, diabetes, or chronic renal failure).

Results from large, anonymous trials are relevant to real clinical practice

A clinician is used to dealing with individual patients, and may feel that the results of large trials somehow deny the individuality of each patient. This is almost the opposite of the truth, for one of the main reasons why trials have to be large is just because patients are so different from one another. Two apparently similar patients may run entirely different clinical courses, one remaining stable and the other progressing rapidly to severe disability or early death. Consequently, it is only when really large groups of patients are compared that the proportion of truly good and bad prognosis patients in each can be relied on to be reasonably similar. One commonly hears statements such as: "If a treatment effect isn't obvious in a couple of hundred patients then it isn't worth knowing about." As the previous examples demonstrate, such statements may reveal not clinical wisdom but statistical naïvety.

It is also said that what is really wanted is not a blanket recommendation for everybody, but rather some means of identifying those few individuals who really stand to benefit from therapy. If any criteria (for example, short term response to a non-placebo controlled course of some disease modifying agent) can be proposed that are likely to discriminate between people who will and who will not benefit, then these can, of course, be recorded prospectively at entry and the eventual trial results subdivided with respect to them. There is, however, a danger in too detailed an analysis of the apparent response of small subgroups chosen for separate emphasis because of the apparently remarkable effects of treatment in those subgroups. Even if an agent brought no benefit, it would have to be acutely poisonous for it not to appear beneficial in one or two such subgroups! Conversely, if an intervention really avoids an approximately similar proportion of the risk in each category of patient, it will, by chance alone, appear not to do so in some category or other. The surprising extent to which this happens is evident from the example in table 10.2. A large, anonymous trial will at least still help answer the practical question of whether on average a policy of widespread treatment (except where clearly contraindicated) is preferable to a general policy of no immediate use of the treatment (except where clearly indicated). Moreover, without a few really large trials it is difficult to see how else many such questions could be resolved over the next few years. For example, digitalis has already been in use for over two centuries, and there is still no reliable consensus as to its net long-term effects on mortality. Trials are at least a practical way of making some solid progress, and it would be unfortunate if desire for the perfect (that is, knowledge of exactly who will benefit from treatment) were to become the enemy of the possible (that is, knowledge of the direction and approximate size of the effects of the treatment of many large categories of patient).

1 Yusuf S, Collins R, Peto R. Why do we need some large, simple randomized trials? *Stat Med* 1984;**3**:409–20.
2 Collins R, Gray R, Godwin J, Peto R. Avoidance of large biases and large random errors in the assessment of moderate treatment effects: the need for systematic overviews. *Stat Med* 1987;**6**:245–50.
3 Peto R, Pike MC, Armitage P, *et al.* Design and analysis of randomized clinical trials requiring prolonged observation of each patient. Part I: introduction and design. *Br J Cancer* 1976;**34**:585–612. Part II: analysis and examples. *Br J Cancer* 1977;**35**:1–39.
4 ISIS-2 (Second International Study of Infarct Survival) Collaborative Group. Randomised trial of intravenous streptokinase, oral aspirin, both, or neither among 17 187 cases of suspected acute myocardial infarction: ISIS-2. *Lancet* 1988;ii:349–60.
5 Gruppo Italiano per lo Studio della Streptochinasi nell'infarto miocardico (GISSI). Effectiveness of intravenous thrombolytic treatment in acute myocardial infarction. *Lancet* 1986;i:397–402.
6 Collins R, Doll R, Peto R. Ethics of clinical trials. In: Williams CJ, ed. *Introducing new treatments for cancer: practical, ethical and legal problems.* New York: John Wiley, 1992: 49–65.
7 Fibrinolytic Therapy Trialists' Collaborative Group. Indications for fibrinolytic therapy in suspected acute myocardial infarction: collaborative overview of early mortality and major morbidity results from all randomised trials of more than 1000 patients. *Lancet* 1994;**343**:311–22.
8 European Carotid Surgery Trialists' Collaborative Group. MRC European Carotid Surgery Trial: interim results for symptomatic patients with severe (70–99%) or with mild (0–29%) carotid stenosis. *Lancet* 1991;**337**:1235–43.
9 Cochrane AL. 1931–1971: a critical review, with particular reference to the medical profession. In: *Medicines for the year 2000.* London: Office of Health Economics, 1979: 1–11.
10 Chalmers I. The Cochrane Collaboration: preparing, maintaining and disseminating systematic reviews of the effects of health care. *Ann NY Acad Sci* 1994;**703**:156–63.
11 Chalmers TC, Lau J. Meta-analytic stimulus for changes in clinical trials. *Stat Methods Med Res* 1993;**2**:161–72.

12 Antiplatelet Trialists' Collaboration. Collaborative overview of randomised trials of antiplatelet therapy. I: Prevention of death, myocardial infarction, and stroke by prolonged antiplatelet therapy in various categories of patients. *BMJ* 1994;**308**:81–106.
13 Early Breast Cancer Trialists' Collaborative Group. Systemic treatment of early breast cancer by hormonal, cytotoxic, or immune therapy: 133 randomised trials involving 31,000 recurrences and 24,000 deaths among 75,000 women. *Lancet* 1992;**339**:1–15;71–85.
14 Collins R, Julian D. British Heart Foundation Surveys (1987 and 1989) of United Kingdom policies for acute myocardial infarction. *Br Heart J* 1991;**66**:250–5.
15 ISIS-4 (Fourth International Study of Infarct Survival) Collaborative Group. ISIS-4: A randomised factorial trial assessing early oral captopril, oral mononitrate, and intravenous magnesium sulphate in 58,050 patients with suspected acute myocardial infarction. *Lancet* 1995;**345**:669–85.
16 Woods KL, Fletcher S, Roffe C, Haider Y. Intravenous magnesium sulphate in suspected acute myocardial infarction: results of the second Leicester Intravenous Magnesium Intervention Trial (LIMIT-2). *Lancet* 1992;**339**:1553–8.
17 MacMahon S, Peto R, Cutler J, *et al.* Blood pressure, stroke and coronary heart disease. Part 1, prolonged differences in blood pressure: prospective observational studies corrected for the regression dilution bias. *Lancet* 1990;**335**:765–74.
18 Collins R, Peto R. Antihypertensive drug therapy: effects on stroke and coronary heart disease. In: Swales JD, ed. *Textbook of hypertension*. Oxford: Blackwell Science, 1994: 1156–64.

11: The Cochrane Collaboration

IAIN CHALMERS, DAVID SACKETT, CHRIS SILAGY

"The ward was full, so I put him in my room as he was moribund and screaming and I did not want to wake the ward. I examined him. He had obvious gross bilateral cavitation and a severe pleural rub. I thought the latter was the cause of the pain and screaming. I had no morphia, just aspirin, which had no effect. I felt desperate. I knew very little Russian then and there was no one in the ward who did. I finally instinctively sat down on the bed and took him in my arms, and the screaming stopped almost at once. He died peacefully in my arms a few hours later. It was not the pleurisy that caused the screaming, but loneliness. It was a wonderful education about the care of the dying. I was ashamed of my misdiagnosis and kept the story secret."[1]

Prelude and inauguration

This episode during Archie Cochrane's years as a prisoner of war illustrates some of the challenges which face those trying to provide effective health care. Accurate diagnosis is often important as a first step; but knowing how to provide effective help is of even greater importance. In this instance, the diagnosis—loneliness—was revealed because the care Cochrane provided had such a dramatic effect in relieving the distress of a Soviet prisoner dying from tuberculosis.

When care has such striking effects, whether these are mediated psychologically, as in this example, or through some physical, chemical, or biological medium—such as surgery, antibiotics, or blood transfusion—carefully controlled research is seldom necessary to identify whether the prescriptions and proscriptions of doctors and other health professionals are more likely to do good than harm. But as Cochrane made clear for the first time to many readers of *Effectiveness and efficiency*, carefully controlled research (using randomisation to generate unbiased comparison groups) *is* required when the effects of care are less dramatic, but nevertheless important.[2]

Cochrane had witnessed the ways in which well intentioned health professionals had been misled by uncontrolled biases in assessments of the many forms of health care which do not have dramatic effects. Uncontrolled biases in treatment comparisons have led doctors to conclude that ineffective or frankly damaging forms of care could help their patients, and sometimes that beneficial forms of care had nothing useful to offer. In the common circumstance where the differential effects of alternative forms of care are not dramatic, guidance is needed from systematically assembled, reliable research evidence. Cochrane's simple proposal in *Effectiveness and efficiency* was that such evidence is essential to inform the choices made within the health services by policy makers, practitioners, and patients.

Translating Cochrane's principle into practice, however, presents many challenges. The first of these is the lack of ready access to reliable evidence about the effects of health care. Cochrane acknowledged this obstacle in an essay he wrote seven years after his famous Rock Carling Lecture had been published. In a challenge which has now been taken up by the international collaboration named after him, he wrote:

> "It is surely a great criticism of our profession that we have not organised a critical summary, by speciality or subspeciality, adapted periodically, of all relevant randomised controlled trials."[3]

In the same essay, Cochrane also suggested that, among medical specialties, obstetrics had made least effort to seek good evidence on which to base its practices. Cochrane's jibe provided impetus to an international collaborative effort which had been established to prepare systematic reviews, using statistical synthesis (meta-analysis) when this was appropriate and possible, of all of the randomised controlled trials relevant to care during pregnancy and childbirth. In the late 1980s, substantive results of this work began to appear in journal articles, books, and in an electronic journal, in which the reviews were updated as new evidence became available and errors were identified.[4]

In 1987, the year before he died, Cochrane referred to the systematic review of controlled trials in pregnancy and childbirth as "a real milestone in the history of randomised controlled trials and in the evaluation of care," and he suggested that other specialties should copy the methods which had been used.[5] Others, too, welcomed the results of this effort to apply scientific principles to the review of research evidence across one area of health care. The systematic reviews of the effects of care in pregnancy and childbirth began to be used (by lay people as well as professionals) to inform decisions in policy and practice, for education, in quality improvement, and for helping to identify priorities for new research.[6]

The encouraging reception given to the results of this initial response to Cochrane's challenge to the health professions coincided with the inauguration of a Research and Development Programme to support the United Kingdom's National Health Service.[7] Cochrane's suggestion that the methods used to prepare and maintain reviews of controlled trials in pregnancy and childbirth should be applied more widely was taken up by the Programme, and funds were provided to establish a "Cochrane Centre", to collaborate with others, in the United Kingdom and elsewhere, to facilitate systematic reviews of randomised controlled trials across all areas of health care.[8,9]

When the Cochrane Centre was opened, in Oxford, in October 1992, those involved expressed the hope that there would be a collaborative international response to Cochrane's agenda. This idea was outlined at a meeting organised six months later by the New York Academy of Sciences.[10] By the summer of 1993, the volume of enquiries, expressions of support, and visitors received at the Centre (which, by then, had been renamed the UK Cochrane Centre) was beginning to overwhelm its small staff. Giving only two months' notice, they convened a meeting to discuss how the international collaboration required to tackle Cochrane's agenda could be organised. In October 1993—at what was to become the first in a series of annual Cochrane Colloquia—77 people from nine countries co-founded the Cochrane Collaboration—an international network of individuals committed to the preparation, maintenance, and dissemination of systematic reviews of research evidence about the effects of health care.

Evolution and consolidation

The Cochrane Collaboration has evolved rapidly in the three years since it was inaugurated at the first Colloquium (see appendix A), but its basic objectives, principles, and elements have remained the same as they were at its inception. It is an international organisation that aims to help people make well informed decisions about health by preparing, maintaining, and ensuring the accessibility of systematic reviews of the effects of healthcare interventions. The Collaboration is being built on eight values: collaboration, building on the enthusiasm of individuals, avoiding duplication, minimising bias, keeping up to date, ensuring relevance, ensuring access, and continually improving the quality of its work.

Cochrane reviews (the principal output of the Collaboration) are published electronically in successive issues of *The Cochrane Database of Systematic Reviews*. Preparation and maintenance of Cochrane reviews is the responsibility of collaborative review groups. The members of these groups—researchers, healthcare professionals, people using the health services, and others—share an interest in generating reliable, up to date evidence relevant to the prevention, treatment, and rehabilitation of particular health problems or group of problems. How can stroke and its effects be prevented and treated? What drugs should be used to prevent and treat malaria, tuberculosis, and other important infectious diseases? What strategies are effective in preventing brain and spinal cord injury and its consequences, and what rehabilitative measures can help those with residual disabilities?

Each collaborative review group (which must be international and must involve health professionals, researchers, and people using the health services) is required to prepare a plan outlining how it will contribute to the Collaboration's objectives. This plan is developed in consultation with the staff of one or more Cochrane centres (which, collectively, share responsibility for coordinating the development of the Collaboration). A collaborative review group's plan of work must be based on agreements reached at one or more exploratory meetings of those involved in the group. It defines the scope of the group and the specific topics falling within the scope. It describes who will have responsibility for planning, coordinating, and monitoring the group's work (a coordinating editor, supported by an editorial team). The plan describes how the group will identify and assemble in a specialised register as high a proportion as possible of all the studies relevant to its declared scope; and who, drawing on the studies in the register, will take responsibility for preparing and maintaining which reviews. Every group appoints an individual to organise and manage the day to day activities of the group who is based at the same place as the coordinating editor.

Members of collaborative review groups are helped to tackle these various tasks by training materials developed by the Collaboration[11] and by training workshops organised by Cochrane centres (and sometimes by the groups themselves). Whenever possible, training for people preparing and maintaining Cochrane reviews is based on the results of empirical research. Such methodological research is the focus of individuals who have come together in Cochrane methods working groups. These are tackling a wide variety of issues, ranging from statistical methods to placebo effects. Cochrane reviews may also be enhanced by input from people whose primary dimensions of interest (fields) are not individual or specific health problems, but aspects of health care, such as its setting (for example, primary health care), or a class of intervention (for example, complementary medicine), or a category of health service user (for example, older people).

To provide both an organisational and analytical framework for assembling Cochrane reviews in electronic format, software has been developed by the Collaboration. A program called Review Manager (RevMan) is used by those preparing and maintaining reviews; Module Manager (ModMan) enables the coordinating editorial team to assemble protocols and complete reviews prepared by the members of their collaborative review group, as well as information about the collaborative review group itself. This additional information includes, for example, the scope of the group's work and the strategy it is using to assemble and maintain a specialised register of relevant studies, derived both from its own searching activities and from the Cochrane central register of controlled trials (to which the group will also be contributing records). These modules of Cochrane reviews and information about the collaborative review groups, together with modules from all the other entities registered as contributors to the Collaboration (centres, fields, methods working groups, and the consumer network) are submitted at regular intervals to the Collaboration's parent database. It is from this continuously updated parent database that Cochrane reviews and information about the Cochrane Collaboration are derived for electronic publication in *The Cochrane Library*.

By the end of 1996, nearly 40 collaborative review groups had either registered or were on the way to registration as components of the Cochrane Collaboration. It seems likely that, by the fifth anniversary of the Collaboration's inauguration (October 1998), the infrastructure will be in place for preparing and maintaining systematic reviews in almost all areas of health care (see appendix A).

Potential and limitations

> "The Cochrane Collaboration is an enterprise that rivals the Human Genome Project in its potential implications for modern medicine."[12]

> "It is a fair bet that if Cochrane were alive today, he would be appalled by the use to which his name has been put."[13]

The emergence of the Cochrane Collaboration has provoked a range of reactions. Among academics, many have welcomed the Collaboration's systematic efforts to identify reliable sources of research evidence; its concern to improve the scientific quality of reviews; and its clear focus on questions of importance to people using health services. Other academics, by contrast, have disputed the Collaboration's emphasis on controlled trials,[14,15] rejected the methodologies it is adopting,[13,16,17] and raised questions about the extent to which the results of systematic reviews are likely to be applicable in the real world.[15] Among health professionals, too, there have been mixed reactions. Some have seen the Collaboration as a conscientious and concerted attempt to sift through an overwhelming volume of primary research to find studies which may be of practical importance, and to synthesise the results of those investigations which are likely to be reliable. Other health professionals see this process as an implicit rejection of the experience of individual clinicians. Some professionals, understandably, worry that systematic reviews of research evidence will be used unthinkingly by governments and others—possibly on grounds of cost—to promote or outlaw particular aspects of the care that clinicians deem either inappropriate or worthwhile for their patients; and this concern is shared by some people using the health services as well. In contrast with the differences of opinion among academics and health professionals, however, lay people who have come to learn about the Collaboration have tended to welcome it, many finding it surprising that mechanisms are not already in place for generating reliable, up to date reviews of relevant research to guide decisions and choices in the health services.

Some of the differences of opinion about the Collaboration simply reflect acceptance or rejection of the premise upon which it has been established. Those who think that the Collaboration's focus on randomised controlled trials or its commitment to systematic reviews is misguided will wish to promote alternative systems for guiding practice. These systems will need to take account of the evidence that different research designs used to assess the effects of health care,[18,19] and different methods used to review research evidence,[20] tend to yield different results. The inevitable implication is that choices will then be required about which results should be used to guide practice.

Some of the other differences of opinion about the Collaboration seem more likely to be apparent than real. Those working in the health field are relative latecomers to the science of research synthesis. This means that many of the detractors among them are unfamiliar with the body of evidence (generated largely by educational and other psychologists during the 1970s and early 1980s) identifying the biases which can compromise the validity of traditional, narrative reviews of research evidence. The science of research synthesis is still young, and insights showing how it can be pursued more effectively will continue to emerge from empirical research. Even so, it would be astonishing if there were to be any sustained complacency about the scientific quality of most of the textbooks and other narrative reviews upon which health professionals and others have had to depend in the past.[20] Signs that new standards for reviews are becoming adopted include the funding support now being provided to people preparing systematic reviews; the designation of systematic reviews ("of the Cochrane type"), published on paper or electronically, as a quality criterion for assessing academic departments[21]; and the requirement by increasing numbers of research funding agencies (for example, the British Medical Research Council) that investigators applying for support to conduct new primary research must set their application in the context of a scientifically defensible review of relevant existing evidence.

The Cochrane Collaboration's potential derives from its commitment to prepare and maintain reviews of research evidence which address questions of relevance to people using the health services; its use of transparent methods in attempts to minimise bias; and its openness to challenge. As a scientific enterprise it has at least two features which are rare if not unique.

Firstly, the protocols of Cochrane reviews (that is, information about the Collaboration's "research in progress") are routinely made available for public scrutiny and comment. Secondly, the Collaboration has established a system for incorporating new evidence in systematic reviews prospectively, and improving or correcting them when ways of doing so are identified.[22,23]

At the beginning of 1997, 199 protocols and 159 complete Cochrane reviews were available in *The Cochrane Database of Systematic Reviews*.[24] Many of the reviews provided substantial evidence of beneficial or harmful effects of healthcare interventions which are relevant to patients; and many others revealed the dearth of reliable evidence to inform choices in important aspects of health care, and thus highlighted priorities for new primary research. The relevance of the Collaboration's output for health care and health research will grow as the numbers of Cochrane reviews become counted, not in hundreds, but in thousands.

Although the Collaboration will prepare and maintain evidence of great relevance to those making choices in health care and health research, it is important that the Collaboration's limitations are clearly acknowledged—within as well as outside the organisation.

The first class of limitations relates to research evidence not currently covered by the Collaboration's objectives. It will probably take a decade or so to prepare systematic, up to date reviews of research evidence relevant to assessing the effects of all relevant elements and types of health care. The Collaboration has decided that achieving a stable state in respect of that primary objective should take precedence over any concerted attempt to broaden the organisation's objectives to cover the preparation and maintenance of systematic reviews of other research evidence relevant to decisions in health care. Examples include research relating to the accuracy and precision of diagnostic tests (including the clinical examination) and data which can help to inform patients about the prognoses of the conditions which affect them.

Whereas this first class of the Collaboration's limitations is a matter of choice, the second class of limitations is not. It relates to issues surrounding the interpretation and applicability of Cochrane reviews. The primary purpose of Cochrane reviews is to show what the data are, not to judge what the data will always mean. What the data mean will usually vary from perspective to perspective, depending on perceived needs and priorities, and the availability of resources of various kinds (figure 11.1).

One way to help ensure that Cochrane reviews cater for these different perspectives is to present their results using a variety of alternative statistics. The effects of health care can be expressed in relative or absolute terms, but people will often find the latter more helpful than the former. Measures of particular relevance to those providing care and developing policy are

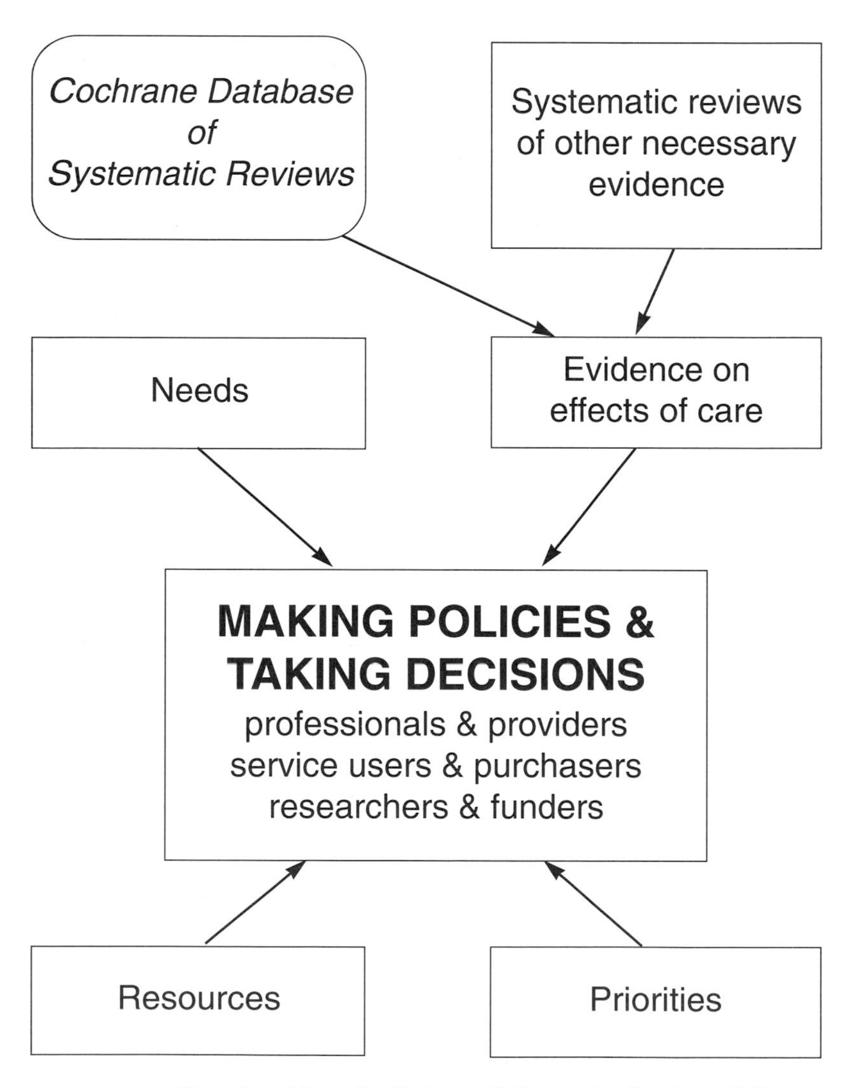

FIG 11.1—*Reproduced from the Cochrane Collaboration Brochure 1993.*

the estimated number of people who must be treated to prevent an episode of an important health problem, balanced against the number of people who, when treated, will experience, as a consequence, an additional instance of an unwanted side effect of the treatment. Measures of particular relevance from the perspective of an individual patient are the probabilities of benefiting from and being harmed by the treatment in question.

Even if Cochrane reviews have been displayed using expressions of treatment effects which are appropriate, however, it should never be assumed that the results of Cochrane reviews "speak for themselves". The authors of Cochrane reviews may well have offered their judgements about the implications of their analyses of the data for practice and future research, and their conclusions will often have been influenced by other opinions sought and offered on prepublication drafts of Cochrane reviews. But their judgements remain judgements nevertheless, and it is inevitable that they will differ from the judgements of others with different perspectives.

In making decisions about the care of individual patients, for example, the results of the reviews must be integrated with the clinician's expertise, which has been acquired through experience and practice, and the patient's expertise, which derives from their knowledge of their condition (particularly if it is a chronic or recurrent health problem), the treatments on offer, and the responsiveness or otherwise of the first to the second. If operating in synchrony, these complementary forms of expertise are reflected in more efficient diagnosis and in more thoughtful identification and compassionate use of the predicaments, rights, and preferences of individual patients in making decisions about their care.

Similar qualifications are appropriate when considering the relevance of Cochrane reviews in decisions taken in respect of whole communities.[25] The findings in a systematic review of research evidence may, very rarely, seem to have universally relevant implications. Usually, however, universal guidelines and prescriptions for the precise application of the evidence are neither wise nor workable. Local disease burdens and barriers to implementation vary widely from country to country and from place to place within countries, and local attention to these issues will help to ensure that the evidence will help those who can best benefit from it.

Relevant evidence about the effects of health care will not be applied if there are local organisational and administrative barriers. Those responsible for modifying these have to be informed and motivated to implement the enabling change. For example, more efficient overall use of limited resources is sometimes prevented because there are disincentives resulting from local budgetary arrangements and responsibilities. If applying the evidence calls for departures from tradition or other major changes in the behaviours of those who provide or receive health care, these must be identified and addressed.

The Collaboration's principle contribution to this process is through the preparation and maintenance of systematic reviews of the research evidence relevant to implementing the changes in practice through which improvements in health care must be mediated. By selecting implementation strategies which have been shown to be useful in well controlled research, people will be more likely to benefit from all of the other information prepared and maintained by those contributing to the Cochrane Collaboration.

No matter how compelling and relevant the evidence, however, it cannot be applied if people do not know about it. And although improved accessibility to *The Cochrane Database of Systematic Reviews* will always be a high priority for the Collaboration, access to the information generated through the preparation and maintenance of Cochrane reviews implies more than access to the reviews themselves. Cochrane reviews are very detailed and highly structured documents, published electronically. Neither their form nor the medium through which they are published will be acceptable to the vast majority of those whose choices in health care could be more informed by access to research knowledge. Imagination and experiment must be used to learn how key messages from systematic reviews can be distilled and disseminated. Within the United Kingdom, for example, the NHS Centre for Reviews and Dissemination in York is using a variety of formats and media for disseminating key messages from systematic reviews to professional and lay people, and evaluating the impact of some of these in controlled experiments.

Strategic alliances and the future

As an international organisation, the Cochrane Collaboration has managed to accomplish a lot in a relatively short space of time. Much of this achievement reflects the goodwill and efforts of the individuals who have contributed and continue to contribute their time and efforts to the Collaboration's activities. Their contributions take a variety of forms. They include hand-searching journals and other sources to identify relevant controlled trials; acting as reviewers or editors within collaborative review groups; supporting and encouraging colleagues involved in the Collaboration; actively developing the science which underpins the preparation of systematic reviews; stimulating interest and fostering networks within professional and community groups; and promoting the outputs of the Collaboration. Many of the contributions which have helped to establish the Collaboration have been made by individuals who have received no specific funding support, and the level of support received by others has varied widely between countries and agencies. This variation in institutional support does not alter the fact that the organisations which have provided resources for the Collaboration's activities have also contributed importantly to its success. To date, these organisations have tended to be public institutions, such as government agencies and universities; but there is considerable scope for non-profit private research funding organisations and industry to support the Collaboration's work. There is a particular role for the latter, for example, in the development of more complete registers of the controlled trials which should be considered for inclusion in Cochrane reviews.

The collaborative review groups and other registered entities within the Cochrane Collaboration (centres, fields, methods working groups, and the consumer network) elect a steering group to govern the conduct and evolution of the Collaboration. At a meeting held in August 1996, the steering group drafted a strategic plan for the development of the Collaboration (appendix B). Four goals were identified towards which the Collaboration needs to strive: (1) to ensure that high quality systematic reviews are available across a broad range of health care topics; (2) to maximise access to these systematic reviews; (3) to achieve financial sustainability; and (4) to develop an efficient and transparent organisational structure and management.

A key feature of the Collaboration's strategy is to develop appropriate alliances at local, national, and global levels. The Collaboration provides only one part, albeit an important one, of the jigsaw puzzle which needs to be completed to take full advantage of opportunities to promote health through better health care. The alliances the Collaboration must forge relate both to support of its core activities, as well as to the application of knowledge generated by its work in the wider worlds of health care and health research.

There are already many encouraging examples of the alliances that are required between the Collaboration and others. These range from links between some of the collaborative review groups and local community groups who assist in the various steps that lead to the preparation of reliable and relevant systematic reviews about the effects of health care, through to links at a national level between individual Cochrane centres and clinical guideline development programmes. At a global level, the Collaboration has begun to explore the development of strategic alliances with organisations such as the World Bank, with industry, and with international professional and consumer organisations.

The Collaboration is still very young and it is too early to try to evaluate how well it will achieve the goals which have inspired its very rapid early growth. The signs are encouraging, however. It seems probable that the continued enthusiasm and goodwill of individuals, combined with strategic alliances developed within the context of the Collaboration's eight guiding principles, will ensure that it succeeds in getting to grips with the important agenda bequeathed by Archie Cochrane.

Acknowledgements

We are grateful to Hilda Bastian, Kay Dickersin, Edward Dickinson, Monica Fischer, Jos Kleijnen, Peter Langhorne, Alan Maynard, and Beverley Shea for comments on an earlier version of this chapter; and to Joan Meyer, Tom Chalmers Jr, and Francie Chalmers for help in preparing the manuscript.

1 Cochrane AL, Blythe M. *One man's medicine: an autobiography of Professor Archie Cochrane.* London: British Medical Journal Memoir Club, 1989:82.
2 Cochrane AL. *Effectiveness and efficiency: random reflections on health services.* London: Nuffield Provincial Hospitals Trust, 1972. (Reprinted in 1989 in association with the BMJ.)
3 Cochrane AL. 1931–1971: a critical review, with particular reference to the medical profession. In: *Medicines for the year 2000.* London: Office of Health Economics, 1979: 1–11.
4 Chalmers I. Improving the quality and dissemination of reviews of clinical research. In: Lock S, ed. *The future of medical journals: in commemoration of 150 years of the British Medical Journal.* London: BMJ, 1991: 127–46.
5 Cochrane AL. Foreword. In: Chalmers I, Enkin M, Keirse MJNC, eds. *Effective care in pregnancy and childbirth.* Oxford: Oxford University Press, 1989.
6 Fox DM, Cleary PD, eds. Effective care in pregnancy and childbirth. *Milbank Q* 1993; **71**:401–533.
7 Peckham M. Research and development for the National Health Service. *Lancet* 1991; **338**:367–71.
8 Chalmers I, Dickersin K, Chalmers TC. Getting to grips with Archie Cochrane's agenda. *BMJ* 1992;**305**:786–8.
9 Editorial. Cochrane's legacy. *Lancet* 1992;**340**:1131–2.
10 Chalmers I. The Cochrane Collaboration: preparing, maintaining and disseminating systematic reviews of the effects of health care. In: Warren KS, Mosteller F, eds. *Doing more good than harm: the evaluation of health care interventions. Ann NY Acad Sci* 1993;**703**: 156–63.
11 Oxman A, Mulrow CD. *Preparing and maintaining systematic reviews.* Oxford: Handbook, Cochrane Collaboration, 1996.
12 Naylor CD. Grey zones of clinical practice: some limits to evidence-based medicine. *Lancet* 1995;**345**:840–3.
13 Shapiro S. Book review. *JAMA* 1995;**274**:667–8.
14 Hunter D. Let's hear it for R&D. *Health Service Journal* 1993;15 April: 17.
15 Black N. Why we need observational studies to evaluate the effectiveness of health care. *BMJ* 1996;**312**:1215–8.
16 Feinstein AR. Meta-analysis: statistical alchemy for the 21st century. *J Clin Epidemiol* 1995;**48**:71–9.
17 Bailar J. Quoted in: Taubes G. Looking for the evidence in medicine. *Science* 1996;**272**: 22–3.
18 Schulz KF, Chalmers I, Hayes RJ, Altman DG. Empirical evidence of bias: dimensions of methodological quality associated with estimates of treatment effects in controlled trials. *JAMA* 1995;**273**:408–12.
19 Kleijnen J, Gøtzsche P, Kunz R, Oxman A, Chalmers I. So what's so special about randomization? This volume: 93–106.
20 Antman EM, Lau J, Kupelnick B, Mosteller F, Chalmers TC. A comparison of results of meta-analyses of randomized control trials and recommendations of clinical experts. *JAMA* 1992;**268**:240–8.

21 United Kingdom Higher Education Funding Councils. *1996 research assessment exercise: criteria for assessment.* London: United Kingdom Higher Education Funding Councils, 1995. (RAE96 3/95.)
22 Chalmers I, Haynes RB. Reporting, updating, and correcting systematic reviews of the effects of health care. *BMJ* 1994;**309**:862–5.
23 Bero L, Rennie D. The Cochrane Collaboration: preparing, maintaining and disseminating systematic reviews of the effects of health care. *JAMA* 1995;**274**:1935–8.
24 The Cochrane Library. The Cochrane Collaboration, 1997, Issue 1.
25 Irwig L, Zwarenstein M, Zwi A, Chalmers I. A flow diagram to help select interventions and research for health care.

Appendix A: a chronology of the Cochrane Collaboration 1972–97

1972	*Effectiveness and efficiency: random reflections on health services* published
1974	Identification of controlled trials in perinatal medicine begins
1976	Outline plans drafted for a systematic review of controlled trials in perinatal medicine
1978	World Health Organisation and Department of Health (England) fund work at National Perinatal Epidemiology Unit, Oxford, to assemble a register of controlled trials in perinatal medicine
1985	Publication of classified bibliography of 3500 reports of controlled trials in perinatal medicine published between 1940 and 1984
	United States Public Health Service and United Kingdom Department of Health fund work to identify unpublished controlled trials in perinatal medicine and to investigate publication bias
1985–90	Preparation of systematic reviews of controlled trials in pregnancy and childbirth and the neonatal period
1989	Output of work begins with publication of: *Effective care in pregnancy and childbirth (ECPC)*, *A guide to effective care in pregnancy and childbirth (GECPC)*, and *The Oxford Database of Perinatal Trials (ODPT)*
1992	Publication of *Effective care of the newborn infant (ECNI)*
1989–92	Maintenance of systematic reviews of controlled trials of perinatal care in 6-monthly disk issues of an electronic journal, "*The Oxford Database of Perinatal Trials (ODPT)*"

February 1992	Encouraged by the reception given to the systematic reviews of care during pregnancy and childbirth, the Research and Development Programme, United Kingdom National Health Service, approves funding for a Cochrane Centre "to facilitate the preparation of systematic reviews of randomized controlled trials of health care"
October 1992	Leading articles published in the *BMJ* (Getting to grips with Archie Cochrane's agenda) and *The Lancet* (Cochrane's legacy)
	The Cochrane Centre opened in Oxford
	Pregnancy and Childbirth Group and Subfertility Group registered
November 1992	Additional funds to promote the mission of the Cochrane Centre pledged by the Nuffield Provincial Hospitals Trust and the Swedish Council on Technology Assessment in Health Care
March 1993	Neonatal Group registered
April 1993	Update Software reissues *The Oxford Database of Perinatal Trials (ODPT)* as a redesigned pilot electronic journal entitled *The Cochrane Pregnancy and Childbirth Database (CCPC)*
March 1993	Cochrane Centre renamed The UK Cochrane Centre
	Concept of the Cochrane Collaboration presented at conference organised by the New York Academy of Sciences: *Doing more good than harm*
June 1993	Development of Cochrane Collaboration *Handbook* begins with arrival of first Cochrane Visiting Fellow at the UK Cochrane Centre
August 1993	Stroke Group registered
	Canadian Cochrane Centre registered
October 1993	Formal launch of the Cochrane Collaboration at the first Cochrane Colloquium, in Oxford
	Cochrane Collaboration Steering Group nominated and appointed by participants at the first Colloquium
	Nordic Cochrane Centre and Baltimore Cochrane Center registered
	Primary Health Care Field registered
November 1993	Musculoskeletal Group registered
December 1993	Funds awarded through European Union BIOMED 1

	Programme "to identify reports of controlled trials in general health care journals in Europe"
February 1994	First meeting of Cochrane Collaboration Steering Group, Hamilton, Ontario
	Australasian Cochrane Centre registered
May 1994	Publication of Cochrane Collaboration *Handbook*
	Release of Version 1 of Review Manager (RevMan) software
	Parasitic Diseases Group registered
June 1994	Centro Cochrane Italiano registered
	Oral Health Group and Schizophrenia Group registered
July 1994	Effective Professional Practice Group registered
August 1994	Acute Respiratory Infections Group registered
October 1994	Second Colloquium, Hamilton, Ontario; first public demonstration of *The Cochrane Database of Systematic Reviews*, designed by Update Software
	Dutch Cochrane Centre registered
	Peripheral Vascular Disease Group registered
November 1994	Diabetes Group registered
	San Francisco Cochrane Center registered
December 1994	Statistical Methods Working Group registered
	Meta-analyses using Individual Patient Data Methods Working Group registered
February 1995	Software Development Group established
	Inflammatory Bowel Disease Group registered
April 1995	*The Cochrane Database of Systematic Reviews* launched in London by the Minister for Health
	San Antonio Cochrane Center registered
	Wounds Group registered
May 1995	Cochrane Collaboration registered as a Company and a Charity under English law; Executive Office established
July 1995	Airways Group registered
	Coding and Classification Methods Working Group registered
August 1995	Tobacco Addiction Group, Dementia and Cognitive Impairment Group, and Menstrual Disorders Group registered
	Screening and Diagnostic Tests Methods Working Group registered
September 1995	Cystic Fibrosis Group registered

October 1995	Third Colloquium in Oslo, Norway; third meeting of Steering Group
	Consumer Network registered
November 1995	Elections for new Steering Group
	Funds awarded to the Collaboration through the European Union's BIOMED 2 Programme for "coordinating and extending the preparation, maintenance and dissemination of systematic reviews of health care within the Cochrane Collaboration in Europe"
January 1996	Health Promotion Field registered
February 1996	Last meeting of First Steering Group and first meeting of elected Steering Group in San Francisco
	Centre Cochrane Français registered
March 1996	Hepato-Biliary Group registered
April 1996	*The Cochrane Library* launched by Update Software as a quarterly publication on CD-ROM and disk, incorporating *The Cochrane Database of Systematic Reviews*, *The Database of Abstracts of Reviews of Effectiveness*, *The Cochrane Controlled Trials Register*, and *The Cochrane Review Methodology Database*
	Physical Therapies and Rehabilitation Field and Health Care of Older People Field registered
May 1996	New England Cochrane Center registered
	Hypertension Group registered
June 1996	Movement Disorders Group, Depression, Anxiety, and Neurosis Group, and Incontinence Group registered
	Complementary Medicine Field registered
July 1996	Vaccines Field registered
August 1996	Strategic Planning Meeting in Oslo; second meeting of elected Steering Group
	Epilepsy Group and Breast Cancer Group registered
	Centro Cochrane do Brasil registered
	Placebos Methods Working Group registered
September 1996	Cochrane Collaboration and Synapse Inc sign a three year contract to make *The Cochrane Database of Systematic Reviews* available on the World Wide Web
October 1996	Fourth Colloquium in Adelaide, Australia; third meeting of elected Steering Group
	Cochrane Collaboration and Update Software sign three year contract

	Gynaecological Cancer Group registered
	South African Cochrane Centre registered
December 1996	Prostate Group registered
January 1997	Registration applications pending for Collaborative Review Groups in: Eyes and Vision; Renal Disease; Skin Disease; Pain, Palliative, and Supportive Care; Fertility Regulation; Brain and Spinal Cord Injuries; Multiple Sclerosis; Communication; and Oesophageal, Gastric, and Duodenal Disease.
	Exploratory meetings scheduled for possible Collaborative Review Groups in: Addiction; Cancers; and Behaviour Problems.
March 1997	Fourth meeting of elected Steering Group, San Francisco
October 1997	Fifth Colloquium in Amsterdam, the Netherlands, in association with the second meeting on the "Scientific Basis of Health Services"

Appendix B: Abridged version of Cochrane Collaboration Strategic Plan

Introduction

In 1979, Archie Cochrane, a British physician, criticised the medical profession for not having established a system for producing up-to-date summaries of the results of reliable research about the effects of health care. The Cochrane Collaboration was founded in 1993 to respond to Cochrane's challenge, and evolved rapidly over the subsequent three years. Building on this initial experience, the Collaboration's elected Steering Group developed a strategic plan to guide the Collaboration's evolution over the next five years. This strategic plan was accepted at the Collaboration's annual Colloquium in October 1996, and it will be modified and developed in the light of experience.

Mission Statement

The Cochrane Collaboration is an international organisation that aims to help people make well-informed decisions about health care by preparing, maintaining, and promoting the accessibility of systematic reviews of the effects of healthcare interventions.

Principles

The Cochrane Collaboration's work is based on eight key principles.

Collaboration

by internally and externally fostering good communications, open decision-making and teamwork.

Building on the enthusiasm of individuals

by involving and supporting people of different skills and backgrounds.

Avoiding duplication

by good management and co-ordination to maximise economy of effort.

Minimising bias

through a variety of approaches such as scientific rigour, ensuring broad participation, and avoiding conflicts of interest.

Keeping up to date

by a commitment to ensure that Cochrane Reviews are maintained through identification and incorporation of new evidence.

Striving for relevance

by promoting the assessment of healthcare interventions using outcomes that matter to people making choices in health care.

Promoting access

by wide dissemination of the outputs of the Collaboration, taking advantage of strategic alliances, and by promoting appropriate prices, content and media to meet the needs of users worldwide.

Ensuring quality

by being open and responsive to criticism, applying advances in methodology, and developing systems for quality improvement.

Goals and Objectives

Goal 1: To ensure high quality, up-to-date systematic reviews are available across a broad range of health care topics.

Objective 1.1: To ensure high quality in Cochrane Reviews

Objective 1.2: To ensure broad coverage of healthcare topics by Cochrane Reviews

Goal 2: To promote access to Cochrane Reviews

Objective 2.1: To ensure that Cochrane Reviews are easy to understand

Objective 2.2: To improve retrieval of information from Cochrane databases

Objective 2.3: To develop a marketing strategy for Cochrane Reviews

Goal 3: To develop an efficient, transparent organisational structure and management system for the Cochrane Collaboration

Objective 3.1: To ensure that the organisational focus of the Cochrane Collaboration supports the core function of preparing and maintaining systematic reviews

Objective 3.2: To ensure that all decision making processes within the Collaboration are transparent and explicit

Objective 3.3: To promote effective communication within the Cochrane Collaboration

Objective 3.4: To promote effective communication with those outside the Cochrane Collaboration

Goal 4: To achieve sustainability of the Cochrane Collaboration

Objective 4.1: To increase the income of the Cochrane Collaboration

Objective 4.2: To develop a three year business plan for the core activities of the Cochrane Collaboration

12: Improving the reporting of randomised controlled trials

DAVID MOHER, JESSE BERLIN

It is generally agreed that randomised controlled trials provide the most valid assessment of healthcare interventions. If such trials are to be of any value, however, the details of their conduct and results must be made available to clinicians, policy makers, researchers, and others, in such a way as to permit the reader to make informed judgements on the validity of the findings. Such informed decisions are difficult to make if knowledge of the existence of randomised controlled trials is not made publicly available—published—or if the published reports are of inferior quality. In this chapter we address these two major areas of concern.

Evaluations of medical therapies and technologies are increasingly being based on systematic reviews of the published literature. Whether or not such reviews produce a quantitative summary of the effects of treatment, scientists and policy makers assume, often implicitly, that the published literature contains either all, or at least a representative sample of the available data.[1] The selective publication of scientific findings based on the magnitude and direction of the results—termed publication bias—could lead to serious errors in the estimation (from research syntheses) of the potential benefits of interventions.

Publication bias

The existence of publication bias has been a concern for about two decades in the social science literature.[2–7] For example, Glass and colleagues[5] found systematic differences in the magnitude of effects between journal articles and dissertations in a variety of meta-analyses in psychology. Smith,[6] in summarising studies of educational innovations, found that effect sizes were considerably smaller for unpublished studies than for published studies. Coursol and Wagner[7] surveyed psychological researchers who had conducted studies of therapeutic outcome. They found that both the decision to submit an article for publication and the editorial decision to accept or reject it were associated with the results of the research, with statistically significant results favoured at each step. Specifically, they found that 82% of studies with a statistically significant outcome were submitted, compared with 43% for studies with a statistically non-significant outcome. Among articles submitted, 80% of those reporting statistically significant differences were accepted *versus* 50% of those in which no statistically significant differences were found. A consequence of these findings is that inferences based on published literature may be biased away from the null hypothesis.

The early work on publication bias led to increasing concern about its existence in the medical literature and evidence that publication bias is a problem.[8–13] In 1987, Dickersin and her colleagues showed in a survey of investigators who had co-authored reports of controlled trials that these trials were more likely to have yielded statistically significant results than trials which the same investigators had not reported.[8] Another early approach to assessing publication bias used only published literature by exploiting the relation between sample size and effect size.[9–11] The authors argued that for studies with small sample sizes to achieve significant results, those studies would have to exhibit large effect sizes. Working with a consecutive series of published reports of cancer therapy, Begg and Berlin found strong evidence of the anticipated relation between sample size and effect size.[9,10]

In some clinical fields it is possible to use a sampling frame that is unaffected by publication bias. Simes[12–13] examined studies that compared single alkylating agent therapy with combination chemotherapy in the treatment of advanced ovarian cancer. He restricted the summary to randomised controlled trials. Using several strategies, he found 20 published trials. He found an additional six studies through a database maintained by the National Cancer Institute: the Compilation of Experimental Cancer Therapy Protocol Summaries.[14] Three of the four significant trials were published but not registered, whereas all six unpublished trials yielded statistically non-significant results. When Simes performed a standard meta-analysis using only published studies, this yielded statistically significant improved survival associated with combination chemotherapy ($P=0.02$). When the analysis was restricted to the 13 of the 14 registered studies for which data were available, the observed improvement in survival was smaller, and the summary result was no longer statistically significant ($P=0.24$).

Subsequent to these studies, several empirical assessments of publication bias of a somewhat different nature were conducted.[15–18] These four studies, described in three papers, involved the identification of projects that were submitted to institutional review boards (research ethics committees) and follow up of those projects to determine whether they had obtained significant findings and whether they had been published or not.

Evidence of the existence of publication bias

The files containing all research protocols submitted to the Central Oxford Research Ethics Committee (COREC) between 1 January 1984 and 31 December 1987 provided the framework for the Oxford study of publication bias.[15] The investigators identified 720 studies approved by the COREC during the four year period. Only the studies that had been analysed were considered to have the potential for being written up and published, so tests for publication bias were restricted to the 285 studies that had been analysed, including 148 clinical trials. Data about the original studies were obtained by contacting the principal investigators or their representatives.

By May, 1990, 138 (48%) of the studies had been published. The unadjusted relation between significance of the main outcome and publication status showed strong evidence of publication bias. Sixty seven per cent of published studies had significant findings compared with only 29% of studies neither published nor presented. Only 15% (23/154) of studies with significant results remained unpublished or unpresented compared with 44% (43/97) of those with null results. The unadjusted odds ratio (OR) for publication with a significant result versus a null result was 2.96 (95% confidence interval (95% CI) 1.68–5.21), indicating a higher likelihood of publication with a significant *versus* a null result. For the 148 clinical trials alone, the association was smaller, with an unadjusted OR of 2.10 (95% CI 0.98–4.52). After adjustment for multiple other factors using logistic regression, the ORs for significant *versus* null studies were 2.32 (95% CI 1.25–4.28) for all studies and 1.59 (95% CI 0.70–3.60) for the clinical trials. In an additional subgroup analysis, the authors found that the OR for publication bias in randomised controlled trials was 0.84 (95% CI 0.34–2.09), suggesting that publication bias is less severe or absent for randomised studies. This result confirmed a similar suggestion by Berlin and colleagues.[11]

The authors also examined the association between statistical significance of a study and the likelihood of it being submitted for publication. The adjusted OR of 2.94 (95% CI: 1.43–6.01) for submission was higher than the OR of 2.32 for publication (95% CI: 1.25–4.28), suggesting that the investigators of the original studies, rather than journal editors, play a major role in publication bias.

The design of two studies at Johns Hopkins University[16] was similar to that of the Oxford study. The original studies forming the basis for this research were those appearing on the records of the two institutional review boards serving the Johns Hopkins Health Institutions and approved in or prior to 1980. The results of the Johns Hopkins studies were very similar to those of the Oxford Study.[15] At the time of the interview, 277 (81%) of the 342 studies from the Medical School had been published as had 113 (66%) of studies from the School of Hygiene and Public Health. For the medical school studies, 89% of the significant studies had been published, compared with 69% of the non-significant studies (OR=3.38; 95% CI 1.96–5.83). For the public health studies, the values were 71% and 58% respectively (OR=1.78; 95% CI 0.94–3.39).

The method for identifying eligible studies was different in an investigation of publication bias in studies funded by the National Institutes of Health than in the other two, but the strategy was similar.[17] Studies were identified from the magnetic tapes of the 1979 Inventory of Clinical Trials from the National Institutes of Health.[18] A total of 986 trials were available on the tapes, 654 funded by the National Cancer Institute (NCI) and 332 by other institutes. The NCI studies were excluded because they were thought to include a large proportion of "trials" that were not stand alone trials, but part of ongoing programmes. As in the other studies described above, principal investigators or their surrogates were contacted and interviewed about study characteristics and outcomes.

Of 332 trials listed on the tapes, 293 (83%) were eligible for the interview. Complete interviews were obtained for 217 (74%) of the trials. The 198 trials for which there was publication information form the basis of the analysis. A large proportion (184/198 or 93%) of the trials had been published. Publication was more likely for trials reporting a significant finding than for those with a non-significant finding (OR=7.04; 95% CI 1.90–26). Interestingly, publication bias appeared to be absent in multicentre trials (OR=0.84; 95% CI 0.07–9.68) but severe in single centre trials (OR=21; 95% CI 2.60–172).

Dickersin and Min[16] performed a meta-analysis of the four studies described above. Figure 12.1 summarises the results. The combined, unadjusted OR is 2.88 (95% CI: 2.13–3.89). There was little evidence of heterogeneity of the ORs across studies of publication bias.

A fifth study using this design[19] reported on 130 clinical trials using quantitative analyses with statistical tests which had originally been submitted to an Australian Institutional Ethics Committee between September 1979 and December 1988. The relative risk for publication was 3.29 (95% CI: 1.84–5.90) for statistically significant studies compared with null studies. This result is similar to the results reported by Dickersin and Min.[16]

In a study that was similar in spirit to the above, Scherer and colleagues[20] explored whether abstracts published in the field of ophthalmology in 1988 and 1989 achieved full publication status within two years after the presentation (fig 12.1B). They found that 66% (61/93) abstracts reached full publication, and that publication was, in their words, "weakly associated with significant results." In fact, the results of this study were similar to the previous studies, and the OR for the association between publication and significance was 1.72 (95% CI 0.66–4.50).

Other sources of bias

Several other potential sources of bias related to the publication process are relevant to this discussion. These include reference bias, language bias, bias that may result from financial incentives, and confirmatory bias. We shall discuss each of these, in turn.

Study references

Gøtzsche[21] examined the reference lists of published studies of trials of non-steroidal anti-inflammatory drugs in rheumatoid arthritis. He assessed whether the cited studies had found significant benefits of new therapies compared with control drugs. He found that a substantial proportion of the reference lists were not representative of all the available literature with respect to whether the new drugs showed a significant benefit over control drugs. Thus, reviews or meta-analyses that depend on reference lists for locating studies may be retrieving biased samples of the existing literature, at least in some cases.

FIG 12.1—*(opposite) (A) Meta-analysis of five studies examining the association between significant results and publication: unadjusted odds ratios and confidence intervals. JHU-Med = Johns Hopkins Medical School studies*[16]*; JHU-PH = Johns Hopkins Medical School of Hygiene and Public Health studies*[16]*; Oxford = Oxford studies*[14]*; NIH = National Institutes of Health studies.*[18]
(B) Percentages of total abstracts published over time, calculated for individual studies. Data points for individual studies were estimated in one of two ways. For some studies, values were taken directly from published linear graphs. Other studies reported percentages of published studies as bar graphs for the same and succeeding years after presentation of the abstract. For these studies, the results presented for the same year were assumed to represent the number of abstracts published by 6 months, with each succeeding year representing 6 months plus another year. (From Scherer et al.[20] *Superscripts refer to original references quoted in Scherer* et al.[20]*)*

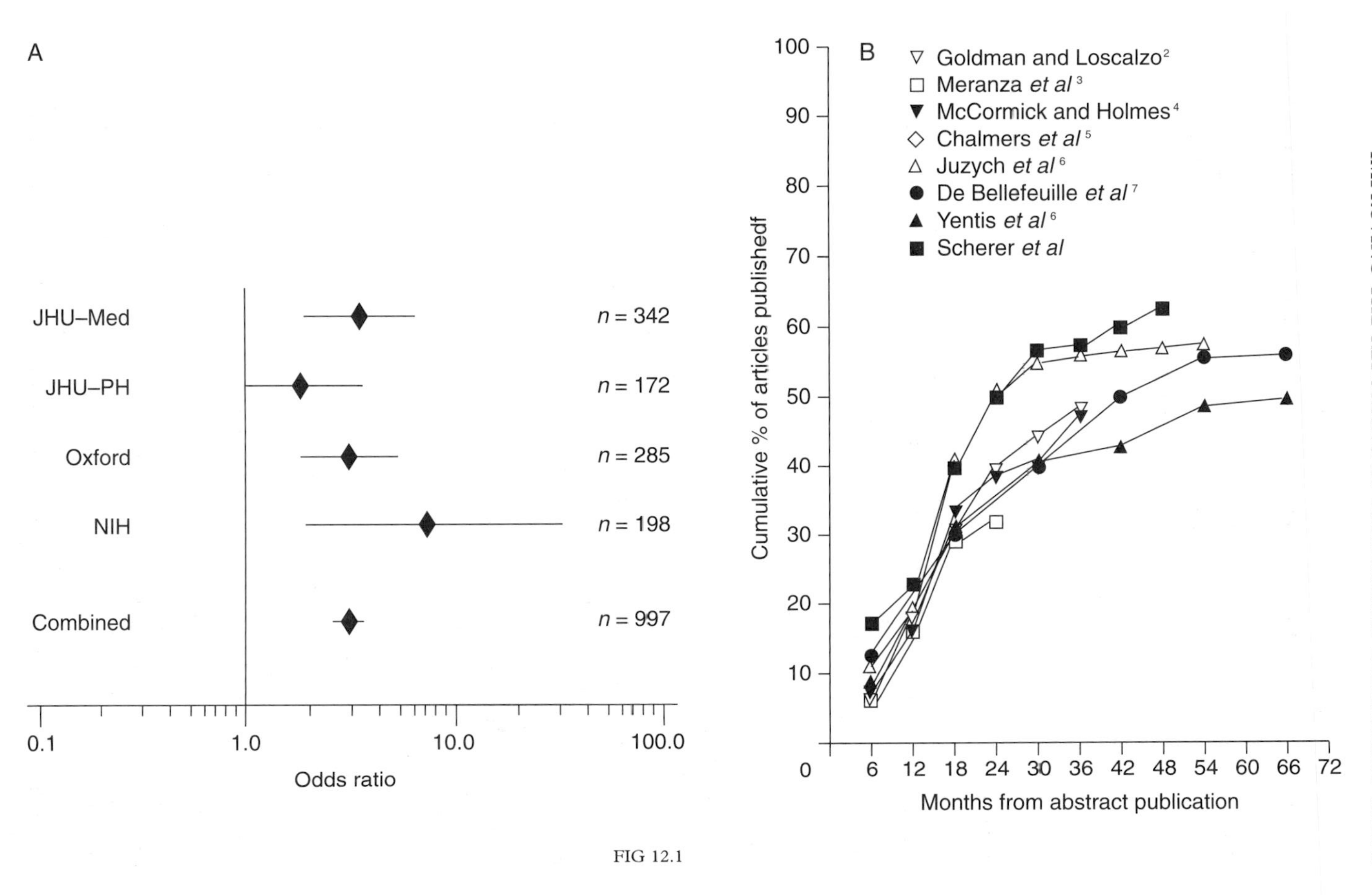
A
JHU–Med
JHU–PH
Oxford
NIH
Combined
n = 342
n = 172
n = 285
n = 198
n = 997
0.1
1.0
10.0
100.0
Odds ratio
B
Goldman and Loscalzo[2]
Meranza et al[3]
McCormick and Holmes[4]
Chalmers et al[5]
Juzych et al[6]
De Bellefeuille et al[7]
Yentis et al[6]
Scherer et al
Cumulative % of articles publishedf
0
10
20
30
40
50
60
70
80
90
100
6
12
18
24
30
36
42
48
54
60
66
72
Months from abstract publication

FIG 12.1

Language

Many meta-analyses restrict consideration to articles written in the English language.[22] Presumably this stems from a combination of lack of capacity to translate articles from other languages and, perhaps, an underlying prejudice that articles from other languages may be of inferior quality. Moher and colleagues[23] performed extensive analyses of the quality of trials reported in languages other than English, compared with those reported in English. They did not find any differences between the trials in terms of completeness and overall quality of reporting, suggesting that limiting a systematic review of trials to articles in the English language may sacrifice precision without reducing bias. However, Egger[24] has shown that, in addition to sacrificing precision, exclusion from systematic reviews of trial reports published in languages other than English risks introducing bias: German speaking authors of trials are more likely to report statistically significant results in English than in German. This echoes the findings of both Simes[12] and Easterbrook *et al*[15] that trials that have yielded statistically significant differences are more likely to be published in the more widely read journals.

Source of funding

Financial incentives can also play a part in the decision to publish or not. Davidson reviewed clinical trials published in several prestigious general medical journals during 1984.[25] He found that 89% of pharmaceutical supported studies favoured new drugs over controls, compared with only 61% of studies supported by other means. On a similar theme Cho and Bero[26] have recently reported that significantly more articles published with pharmaceutical support had outcomes favouring the drug of interest compared with those articles published without such support. Hemminki examined reports of adverse drug events in the trial reports submitted to Scandinavian drug licensing authorities.[27] She found that the proportion of subsequently published trials showing adverse effects was lower than the proportion of unpublished studies showing adverse effects. Easterbrook and colleagues[15] found that industry funded studies were significantly less likely to be published than others. Dickersin and colleagues[16] found a similar relation in unadjusted analyses, but the differences between industry funded studies and others did not persist in their multivariate analyses.

Confirmatory evidence

Mahoney[28] has described a phenomenon he terms confirmatory bias in the peer review system. He conducted a study in which he asked 75 journal reviewers to referee manuscripts describing a study with identical experimental procedures, but differing with respect to the nature and reporting of the results. He found that reviewers rated manuscripts more favourably when the results reported were statistically significant. This is consistent with the results described above from the work of Coursol and Wagner[4], who found that submitted studies were more likely to get published when statistically significant differences were reported. The studies by Easterbrook and colleagues[15] and Dickersin and colleagues[16,17] and Simes *et al*[19] suggest, by contrast, that authors are primarily, but probably not solely, responsible for publication bias. The findings by Mahoney[28] provide an explanation as to the possible reasons for authors believing that studies with no statistically significant results will not get published.

The existence of publication bias has, by now, been clearly demonstrated. Thus, the potential for obtaining biased summaries from research syntheses based solely on published studies is real and of concern. Various methods have been proposed to estimate the potential magnitude of publication bias in the context of performing a meta-analysis,[29–32] or to correct for the bias analytically.[32–34]

Avoiding publication bias

The available methods of correcting for publication bias all rely, to varying extents, on a series of assumptions about the mechanism that selects studies for publication. Because none of these quantitative approaches is entirely satisfactory, efforts should be directed at the prevention of publication bias. One way to avoid publication bias would be to obtain unpublished studies. In some cases, unpublished data can represent a large proportion of the available data. For example, in the Early Breast Cancer Trialists' Collaborative Group meta-analysis,[35] 20 of the 92 (22%) studies providing data for the meta-analysis were unpublished. It is often impractical, however, to identify unpublished studies.[36] Further, some authors have chosen not to include unpublished studies in a meta-analysis because they have not usually been peer reviewed.[37] A survey of authors of meta-analyses, meta-analysis methodologists, and editors showed that most (78%) of the meta-analysts and methodologists favoured the inclusion of unpublished material in meta-analyses under some conditions, whereas only 47% of the editors favoured the inclusion of unpublished data.[38] These authors also emphasise the potential utility of performing sensitivity analyses by summarising results both with and without unpublished data.

In the clinical trials field, there has been some movement toward the prospective registration of all initiated studies.[39–42] This would provide a sampling frame to identify studies independently of their findings, much along the lines of the Simes study described earlier.[12,13] Funding for such registries has been difficult to obtain and seems to remain an issue. A number of institutes within the National Institutes of Health support registries of studies involving humans.[41,42] The systems of ethics committees and institutional review boards in place in many countries could provide a convenient framework for such registration. In particular, Chalmers and colleagues[43] have suggested that funding agencies and ethics committees should require the registration and publication of trials that they have supported and approved. The idea of involving ethics committees in requiring registration and publication of trials has been further developed by Savulescu and colleagues.[44]

A related strategy that has been proposed for, among other reasons, avoiding publication bias[45] involves publishing protocols of studies at the time of inception. This might be accomplished more easily through the medium of electronic journals in which space is at less of a premium than in printed journals[46] and Richard Horton, editor of the *Lancet*, has recently invited investigators to submit trial protocols for peer review, with a view to publishing accepted protocols on the *Lancet*'s World Wide Web site.[47]

The empirical studies of publication bias, coupled with prior research, demonstrate that publication bias is a potentially serious problem when performing systematic reviews, or even when evaluating individual studies. Although there is some evidence that publication bias is not as severe for randomised trials as for non-randomised trials,[11,15] the potential for bias to exist should not be dismissed solely on the basis of the presence of randomisation. In any systematic review, funnel plots or related analytical approaches should be used to evaluate the potential for publication bias. If there is evidence suggestive of publication bias, the results of the analysis need to be interpreted cautiously.

Ethical issues

Publication bias and related sources of bias raise several ethical issues that are important to note. Perhaps the most important of these relates to the obligation to make study results publicly available. Ethics committees and funding agencies, in addition to requiring registration of studies, should also require a commitment from investigators to make their findings publicly accessible, arguing that not doing so constitutes an ethical violation. The importance of publishing is nicely summarised by Chalmers in a proposal to outlaw the term negative trial,[48] "All trials that have been well conceived and well conducted—whatever their results—represent positive contributions to knowledge".

Quality of reporting of randomised controlled trials

Even if all trials somehow came to our attention, we need to ascertain whether the information they contain is of reasonable quality. For this discussion to be informative, a meaningful definition of quality is required. The focus here is on one aspect of methodological quality—internal validity—and is defined as "the confidence that the trial design, conduct, analysis, and presentation have minimised or avoided biased comparisons of the intervention(s) under evaluation".[49] This definition is evidence based (concerned with those factors that can systematically influence the results of an intervention).

It is important to distinguish between the quality of an individual trial and the quality of its report. It is possible to have a study designed with many biases that is well reported. Conversely, a well designed and conducted study can be poorly reported. However, the evidence, to date, suggests that quality of reporting of randomised controlled trials and their design and conduct are often highly correlated. Liberati and colleagues evaluated the internal and external validity of 63 reports of randomised controlled trials using a scale with a maximum total score of 100 points.[50] The mean score for all trials was 50% (95% CI 46%–54%). To elaborate on various aspects of the trial reports the authors conducted telephone interviews with 62 (of 63) corresponding authors. This resulted in a 7% (mean) improvement in the quality scores.

Historical perspectives

Several guidelines have been published[51–54] to facilitate the reporting of randomised controlled trials, describing what needs to be included when reporting a trial. In addition, some journals[55] have published checklists of items for assessing randomised controlled trials to be used by authors, referees, and readers. Other journals[56] have published their policy on the statistical assessment of trials. With the possible exception of the *British Journal of Obstetrics and Gynaecology*,[57] these efforts have not had their intended impact of improving the quality of reporting of clinical research.[58] Perhaps one of the reasons for this disappointment is because these efforts were not evidence based.

In an early study, Mahon and Daniel[59] reviewed 203 reports of drug trials published between 1956 and 1960 in the *Canadian Medical Association Journal*. Only 11 (5.4%) reports fulfilled their criteria of a valid report. In a review of 45 trials published during 1985 in three leading general medical journals, Pocock and colleagues[60] reported that a statement about sample size was only mentioned in five (11.1%) of the reports, that only six (13.3%)

made use of confidence intervals and that the statistical analysis tended to exaggerate intervention efficacy. Altman and Doré reviewed 80 reports of trials published in 1987 and 1988 and found that information about the type of randomisation was only reported in 32 (40.0%) of the trials.[61] Schulz and colleagues reviewed 206 reports of trials published during 1990 and 1991 in two British and two American obstetrics and gynaecology journals.[57] Only 66 (32.0%) of the trials reported on how the randomisation sequence was generated and only 47 (22.8%) on how intervention assignment was concealed until the allocation of therapy, something possible in all trials. Gøtzsche[62] has suggested that the quality of randomised controlled trial reports in rheumatology may be so weak that it may be impossible to place any confidence in the statistical analysis or conclusions. Similar concerns have also been reported in the surgical literature. Solomon and McLeod reviewed 43 randomised controlled trials published in three leading surgical journals in 1990 and reported that in 21% of cases the results did not justify the conclusions.[63]

To the sceptic these surveys provide some evidence for the need to improve the reporting of randomised controlled trials. However, they do not answer the fundamental question as to whether inadequate reporting affects what is said about the effectiveness of interventions. Schulz and colleagues have recently produced evidence, in one area, to address this point.[64] They have shown empirically that trials in which the allocation sequence had been inadequately concealed yielded larger estimates of treatment effects (ORs lower, on average, by 30% to 40%) compared with trials in which authors reported adequate allocation concealment (keeping the intervention assignments hidden from all those participating in the trial until the point of allocation). One possible interpretation is that some trials with inadequate reporting of allocation concealment actually had faulty randomisation in their design and/or conduct, leading to the introduction of bias.

A few years ago, to improve the quality of reporting of clinical research, more informative abstracts were developed.[65] Such abstracts provide readers with a series of headings pertaining to the design, conduct, and analysis of a trial and standardised information within each heading. Evidence to date indicates that more informative abstracts have had a positive impact on how the results of those abstracts are communicated.[66] More informative abstracts also seem to be of better quality than more traditional ones. Taddio and colleagues[67] compared the quality of reporting of 150 non-structured abstracts (published in 1988 and 1989) and 150 structured abstracts (published in 1991 and 1992) published in the *British Medical Journal*, the *Canadian Medical Association Journal*, and the *Journal of the American Medical Association*. Quality was assessed using a 32 item checklist. The scoring range was between 0 and 100 with higher scores indicating superior quality. Assessors completed their quality assessment blind to journal, author and author affiliation, and references. These authors reported a significantly higher overall quality score for structured abstracts (74%) compared with non-structured ones (57%). This result was consistent across all three journals.

Proposed reporting standards

SORT

More recently, there has been a call to extend more informative abstracts to include structured reporting of the text of each randomised controlled trial.[68] The Standards of Reporting Trials (SORT) Group met on 7 and 8 October 1993. At the conclusion of this workshop the SORT Group issued a new proposal for the reporting of randomised controlled trials: structured reporting, defined as "providing sufficiently detailed information about the design, conduct, and analysis of a trial for the reader to have confidence that the report is an accurate reflection of what occurred during the various stages of the trial". Structured reporting set out 24 essential items that needed to be included in the report of a trial, and provided empirical evidence as to why the items should be included and a format as to how they could be included.

Asilomar

Independently, and about five months later (14 to 16 March 1994) another group, the Asilomar Working Group on Recommendations for Reporting of Clinical Trials in the Biomedical Literature, met to discuss similar challenges facing the reporting of clinical trials. Their proposal[69] consisted of a checklist of items that should be included when reporting a clinical trial, along with a suggestion that editors add it to the "Instructions to Authors".

A subsequent editorial urged both groups to meet and decide which recommendations from each group's proposal should be retained.[76] Besides being pragmatic, this suggestion had the potential for increasing consensus, which in turn may afford a greater chance of improving the quality of reporting of clinical trials among a wider audience. On 20 September 1995 a meeting was held in Chicago that included nine members (including editors, clinical epidemiologists, and statisticians) of both the SORT Group and Asilomar Working Group. Two other people participated in the meeting: a journal editor who expressed interest in helping to improve the reporting of clinical trials, and the senior author of a trial report that used the SORT approach.[71]

CONSORT

The day started with a review of both the SORT and Asilomar checklists to ascertain which items covered similar content areas and which ones were unique. Those items having similar content areas were then reviewed individually. It was decided, a priori, to keep only those items for which there was empirical evidence that omission resulted in biased estimates of the effects of interventions. Common sense was used for those items included for which there was no empirical evidence. The selection of items was achieved using a modified Delphi process. In developing a consensus, the group emphasised the need to keep the number of items to a minimum while maintaining adequate standards of reporting trials. A similar approach was used in deciding which of the unique items should remain in the resulting checklist. The day ended with a discussion on the use of the flow diagram proposed by the SORT Group and the format of a trial report. Shortly after the meeting a draft report was circulated to the entire group for further refinement. This process was continued until the report accurately represented what went on during the meeting.

This meeting resulted in the Consolidated Standards of Reporting Trials—CONSORT Statement[72]—a checklist (table 12.1) and flow diagram (fig 12.2). The checklist consists of 21 items that pertain mainly to the methods, results, and discussion of a randomised controlled trial report and identify key pieces of information necessary to evaluate the internal and external validity of the report. One reference for each item, where appropriate (table 12.1), has been included. The flow diagram provides information about the progress of patients throughout a two group parallel design randomised trial, perhaps the type of trial most commonly reported.[73] Appropriate adjustments will need to be made when reporting trials with a larger number of groups or those using a different design.

Although any optimally reported trial will address the items on the checklist and contain the flow diagram, the manner in which they are reported (their format) is also important. The format favoured by the CONSORT Group includes a combination of five new "subheadings" in the text of the trial report, and the use of the checklist during the journal submission process. Three of the subheadings fall within the "methods" section of a trial report: protocol, assignment, and masking (blinding). For example, under the subheading "assignment" authors would describe the "unit of randomisation" (for example, individual patient). The remaining two subheadings are included when reporting the results: participant flow and

---

FIG 12.2—*(opposite) Flow diagram of progress through the various stages of a trial, including flow of participants, withdrawals, and timing of primary and secondary outcome measures. From Begg* et al.[72]

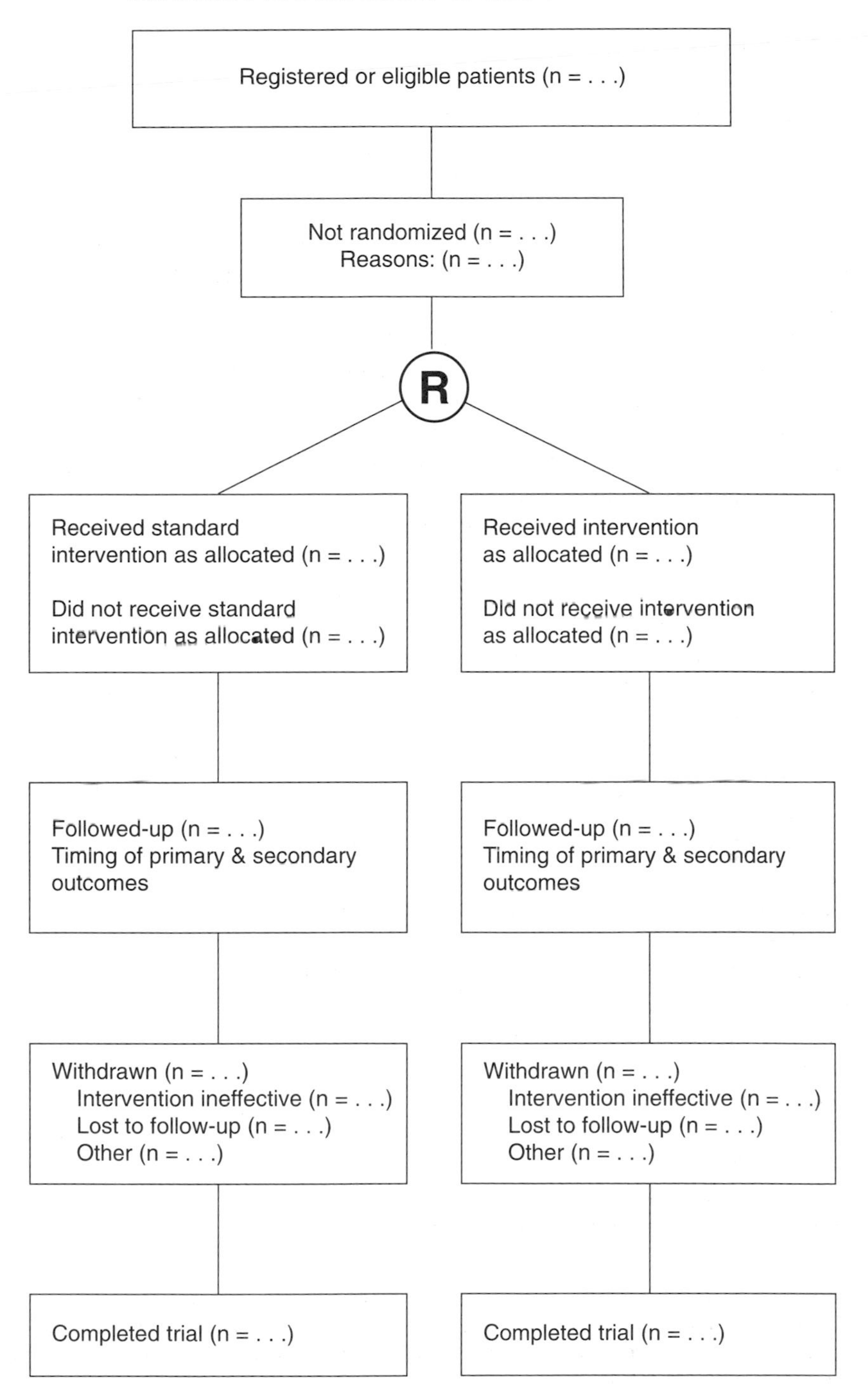
Registered or eligible patients (n = . . .)
Not randomized (n = . . .)
Reasons: (n = . . .)
R
Received standard intervention as allocated (n = . . .)
Did not receive standard intervention as allocated (n = . . .)
Received intervention as allocated (n = . . .)
Did not receive intervention as allocated (n = . . .)
Followed-up (n = . . .)
Timing of primary & secondary outcomes
Followed-up (n = . . .)
Timing of primary & secondary outcomes
Withdrawn (n = . . .)
Intervention ineffective (n = . . .)
Lost to follow-up (n = . . .)
Other (n = . . .)
Withdrawn (n = . . .)
Intervention ineffective (n = . . .)
Lost to follow-up (n = . . .)
Other (n = . . .)
Completed trial (n = . . .)
Completed trial (n = . . .)

FIG 12.2

TABLE 12.1—*Consolidation of standards of reporting trials: CONSORT checklist*

Heading	Subheading	Descriptor	Is the item reported?	Reported on Page No?
Title		Identify the study as a randomised trial.[7]		
Abstract		Use a structured format.[8,9]		
Introduction		State prospectively defined hypotheses, clinical objectives, and planned subgroup or covariate analyses.[10]		
		Describe:		
Methods	Protocol	Planned study population, together with inclusion/exclusion criteria.		
		Planned interventions and their timing.		
		Primary and secondary outcome measure(s) and minimum important difference(s), and indicate how the target sample size was projected.[2,11]		
		Rationale and methods for statistical analyses, detailing main comparative analyses and whether they are completed on an intention to treat basis.[12–13]		
		Prospectively defined stopping rules (if warranted).[14]		
		Describe:		
	Assignment	Unit of randomisation (for example, individual, cluster, geographic).[15]		
		Method used to generate the allocation schedule.[16]		
		Method of allocation concealment and timing of assignment.[17]		
		Method to separate the generator from the executor of assignments.[17,18]		
	Masking (blinding)	Describe mechanism (for example, capsules, tablets); similarity of treatment characteristics (for example, appearance, taste); allocation schedule control (location of code during trial and when broken); and evidence for successful blinding amongst participants, person doing intervention, outcome assessors, and data analysts.[19,20]		
Results	Participant flow and follow up	Provide a trial profile (figure), summarising participant flow, numbers, and timing of randomisation assignment, interventions, and measurements, for each randomised group.[3,21]		
		State estimated effect of intervention on primary and secondary outcome measures, including a point estimate and measure of precision (confidence interval).[22,23]		
	Analysis	State results in absolute numbers where feasible (for example, 10/20 not 50%).		
		Present summary data and appropriate descriptive and inferential statistics in sufficient detail to permit alternative analyses and replication.[24]		
		Prognostic variables by treatment group and any attempt to adjust for them.[25]		
		Describe protocol deviations from study as planned, together with the reasons.		
Discussion		State specific interpretation of study findings, including sources of bias and imprecision (internal validity) and discussion of external validity, including appropriate quantitative measures where possible.		
		State general interpretation of the data in light of the totality of available evidence.		

Adapted from Begg *et al.*[72] Superscripts refer to original references quoted in Begg *et al.*[72]

follow up, and analysis. The participant flow and follow up subheading is used in conjunction with describing details of the flow diagram. These subheadings provide readers with consistency from report to report as to where they can expect to find relevant information. The completed checklist, which includes all five subheadings, would be required for all journal submissions. For example, corresponding authors would need to specify whether or not their trial report described the unit of randomisation, and, if so, where in the report this is documented. Different trials, because of unusual or complex methodology, will require modifications to the reporting structure.

The advantages of the CONSORT format include minimal change to the length and readability of the manuscript, enhanced clarity, and organisation in the actual report of a trial, by the addition of five new subheadings, while at the same time maximising the information that is submitted to editors and reviewers—namely, the completed checklist. This strategy avoids some of the criticisms of previously suggested reporting formats.

Some authors, editors, and even reviewers may find the CONSORT recommendations for the reporting of clinical trials difficult and even restrictive. Similar concerns were also raised when more informative structured abstracts were first introduced. However, the previous separate group efforts and the combined one, CONSORT, came about because of the need to provide readers with enough valid and meaningful information concerning the design, conduct, and analysis of a randomised controlled trial, to be able to evaluate its internal and external validity.

The CONSORT statement was published in the *Journal of the American Medical Association* on 28 August 1996. In an accompanying editorial[74] the *Journal* indicated its support for CONSORT. As of 1 January 1997 authors wishing to submit reports of randomised controlled trials to the *Journal* will be required to use the CONSORT approach (content and format) along with a completed checklist. In conjunction with this move the *Journal* will change its "instructions to authors" to reflect their adoption of these guides. Other journals, including the *British Medical Journal*, the *Lancet*, and the *Canadian Medical Association Journal* will also be adopting CONSORT in a similar manner.[75,77] More journals are giving the CONSORT statement serious consideration and are likely to adopt it in due course.

It will also be important to evaluate whether the CONSORT approach actually has its intended impact. Ideally, such an evaluation should be conducted using a randomised controlled trial. In reality, a randomised design may prove difficult to implement given the initial positive response to CONSORT by many journals. Even if some journals were willing to participate in such a trial, it seems likely that there would be contamination of any control group because of the likely influence of CONSORT given the large number of journals which have adopted it. However, there are other approaches, such as variants of the pretest-post-test methodology, that might prove useful for addressing this question. Whatever design is ultimately used the assessments need to be of both process and outcome, such as the readability of the report and word length as well as more standard quality assessments. In the near future work will begin on designing and implementing such an evaluation.

Quality of reporting of systematic reviews

There are other reasons to concentrate energies on the reporting of randomised controlled trials. The variability in the quality of reports of randomised controlled trials included in systematic reviews sometimes influences the results of those reviews. Khan and colleagues[78] conducted a systematic review of anti-oestrogen therapy in subfertile men with oligospermia involving nine randomised controlled trials. The quality of each trial report was assessed using a validated scale. When all trials were included in the analysis, therapy did not prove to be statistically beneficial (OR 1.6; 95% CI 0.9–2.6). However, a sensitivity analysis according to the quality of reports of randomised controlled trials indicated the intervention to be statistically beneficial (OR: 2.8, 95% CI 1.2–5.2) for low quality trials. Results similar to these, but in the opposite direction, have also been reported.[79,80]

There are also issues surrounding the reporting of systematic reviews and meta-analyses. A 1987 survey[81] of 86 English language meta-analyses assessed each publication on 14 items from six content areas thought to be important in the conduct and reporting of meta-analysis of randomised controlled trials: study design, combinability, control of bias, statistical analysis, sensitivity analysis, and problems of applicability. The results showed that only 24 (28%) of the 86 meta-analyses addressed all six content areas. It is also likely that some readers do not know how to read and interpret systematic reviews, making it difficult to judge their validity. This survey was updated in 1992 with little change in the results.[82]

Silagy surveyed 28 review articles published in primary care journals during 1991 using eight methodological criteria thought to be important in the reporting of systematic reviews.[83] Each criterion had a maximum score of two for a total score of 16. Silagy reported that only 25% of the articles obtained a total score of more than 8. In a recent article Jadad and McQuay[84] reviewed 80 meta-analyses using a validated tool which included a question concerning the overall scientific quality of a meta-analysis. The scoring range for this question is 1 to 7 with higher scores indicating superior quality. The authors reported a median score of 4, bordering on "major" flaws. They also found that the lower the quality the more likely the meta-analyses were to have a positive result. Assendelft and colleagues[85] used a similar methodology to assess the methodological quality of 51 systematic reviews of spinal manipulation. They reported a median score of 23 (out of a maximum of 100). The authors also reported that reviews with "positive" conclusions tended to have higher quality scores. This result is in the opposite direction to that reported by Jadad and McQuay.[84] The differences in the results between both studies are likely due to, in part, differences in how the respective scales were developed. Similar results have been reported in the literature on randomised controlled trials.[49]

This evidence suggests that unless more attention is devoted to improving the reporting of systematic reviews we are likely to encounter similar problems to those experienced with the reporting of randomised controlled trials. There is a certain urgency to addressing this problem. Systematic reviews are "younger" (at least in medicine) than randomised controlled trials. If action is taken now, it may be possible to minimise some of the problems that have plagued the reporting of randomised controlled trials for so long. Systematic reviews are also being published at a rapidly increasing rate and are likely to grow rapidly on this trajectory with the development of the Cochrane Collaboration,[86] an international network of individuals who are preparing and maintaining up to date systematic reviews in many aspects of health care.

Some researchers have already started thinking about how to improve the reporting of systematic reviews,[87,88] and the Cochrane Collaboration has already adopted evidence-based guidelines which are being modified as empirical evidence accumulates about how to improve methods for research synthesis.[89]

The ultimate test of systematic reviews, as with randomised controlled trials, is whether the reader has the confidence that the report is an accurate reflection of what went on during its various stages. After innumerable efforts, we are making progress towards improving the quality of reporting of randomised controlled trials. Concern about the quality of reporting of systematic reviews has emerged earlier in their development than it did for randomised controlled trials, and augurs well for this younger science.

1 Sterling TD, Rosenbaum WL, Weinkam JJ. Publication decisions revisited: the effect of the outcome of statistical tests on the decision to publish and vice versa. *American Statistician* 1995;**49**:108–12.
2 Sterling TD. Publication decisions and their possible effects on inferences drawn from tests of significance or vice versa. *Journal of the American Statistical Association* 1959;**54**: 30–4.
3 Greenwald AG. Consequences of prejudice against the null hypothesis. *Psychol Bull* 1975; **82**:2–12.
4 White KR. The relation between socioeconomic status and academic achievement. *Psychol Bull* 1982;**91**:461–81.
5 Glass GV, McGraw B, Smith ML. *Meta-analysis in social research.* Beverly Hills, CA: Sage Publications, 1981.

6 Smith ML. Publication bias and meta-analysis. *Evaluation in Education* 1980;**4**:22–4.
7 Coursol A, Wagner EE. Effect of positive findings on submission and acceptance rates: a note on meta-analysis bias. *Professional Psychology* 1986;**17**:136–7.
8 Dickersin K, Chan S, Chalmers TC, Sacks HS, Smith H Jr. Publication bias and clinical trials. *Controlled Clin Trials* 1987;**8**:33–53.
9 Begg CB, Berlin JA. Publication bias: a problem in interpreting medical data. *Journal of the Royal Statistical Society A* 1988;**151**:419–63.
10 Begg CB, Berlin JA. Publication bias and dissemination of clinical research. *J Natl Cancer Inst* 1989;**81**:107–15.
11 Berlin JA, Begg CB, Louis TA. An assessment of publication bias using a sample of published clinical trials. *Journal of the American Statistical Association* 1989;**84**:381–92.
12 Simes RJ. Confronting publication bias: a cohort design for meta-analysis. *Stat Med* 1987; **6**:11–29.
13 Simes RJ. Publication bias: the case for an international registry of clinical trials. *J Clin Oncol* 1986;**4**:1529–41.
14 United States Department of Health and Human Services. *Compilation of experimental cancer therapy protocol summaries.* Washington, DC: NIH Publication No 83–1116, seventh edition, 1983.
15 Easterbrook PJ, Berlin JA, Gopalan R, Matthews DR. Publication bias in clinical research. *Lancet* 1991;**337**:867–72.
16 Dickersin K, Min YI, Meinert CL. Factors influencing publication of research results: follow-up of applications submitted to two institutional review boards. *JAMA* 1992;**267**: 374–8.
17 Dickersin K, Min YI. NIH clinical trials and publication bias. *Online Journal of Current Clinical Trials* [serial online] 28 April; 1993. (Doc No 50.)
18 National Institutes of Health. *NIH inventory of clinical trials: fiscal year 1979 (unpublished).* Datatapes obtained from the Division of Research Grants, Research and Evaluation Branch, Bethesda, MD, 1980.
19 Simes J, Stern J, Ghersi D. *The importance of prospectively registering trials: evidence of publication bias from a cohort of research protocols.* Paper presented at 3rd Annual Cochrane Colloquium, Oslo, 4–8 October 1995.
20 Scherer RW, Dickersin K, Langenberg P. Full publication of results initially presented in abstracts. *JAMA* 1994;**272**:158–62.
21 Gøtzsche PC. Reference bias in reports of drug trials. *BMJ* 1987;**295**:654–6.
22 Gregoire G, Derderian F, LeLorier J. Selecting the language of the publications included in a meta-analysis: is there a tower of babel bias? *J Clin Epidemiol* 1995;**48**:159–63.
23 Moher D, Fortin P, Jadad AR, *et al.* Completeness of reporting of trials published in languages other than English: implications for conduct and reporting of systematic reviews. *Lancet* 1996;**347**:363–6.
24 Egger M. *Language reporting bias among German-speaking authors of reports of controlled trials.* Paper presented to Clinical Trials and Epidemiology Seminars, Oxford, 5 November 1996.
25 Davidson RA. Source of funding and outcome of clinical trials. *J Gen Intern Med* 1986; **1**:155–8.
26 Cho MK, Bero LA. the quality of drug studies published in symposium proceedings. *Ann Intern Med* 1996;**124**:485–9.
27 Hemminki E. Study of information submitted by drug companies to licensing authorities. *BMJ* 1980;**280**:833–6.
28 Mahoney MJ. Publication prejudices: an experimental study of confirmatory bias in the peer review system. *Cognitive Therapy Research* 1977;**1**:161–75.
29 Light RJ, Pillemer DB. *Summing up: the science of reviewing research.* Cambridge, MA: Harvard University Press, 1984.
30 Rosenthal R. The file drawer problem and tolerance for null results. *Psychol Bull* 1979; **86**:638–41.
31 Begg CB, Mazumdar M. Operating characteristics of a rank correlation test for publication bias. *Biometrics* 1994;**50**:1088–101.

32 Dear KBG, Begg CB. An approach for assessing publication bias prior to performing a meta-analysis. *Statistical Science* 1992;**7**:237–45.
33 Iyengar S, Greenhouse JB. Selection models and the file-drawer problem. *Statistical Science* 1988;**3**:109–17.
34 Vevea JL, Hedges LV. A general linear model for estimating effect size in the presence of publication bias. *Psychometrika* 1995;**60**:419–35.
35 Early Breast Cancer Trialists' Collaborative Group. *Treatment of early breast cancer. Vol I. Worldwide evidence, 1985–1990.* New York: Oxford University Press, 1990.
36 Hetherington J, Dickersin K, Chalmers I, *et al.* Retrospective and prospective identification of unpublished controlled trials: lessons from a survey of obstetricians and pediatricians. *Pediatrics* 1989;**84**:374–80.
37 Chalmers TC, Berrier J, Sacks HS, Levin H, Reitman D, Nagalingam R. Meta-analysis of clinical trials as a scientific discipline. II: Replicate variability and comparison of studies that agree and disagree. *Stat Med* 1987;**6**:733–44.
38 Cook DJ, Guyatt GH, Ryan G, *et al.* Should unpublished data be included in meta-analyses? Current convictions and controversies. *JAMA* 1993;**269**:2749–53.
39 Meinert CL. Toward prospective registration of clinical trials. *Control Clin Trials* 1988;**9**: 1–5.
40 Dickersin K. Report from the panel on the case for registers of clinical trials at the eighth Annual Meeting of the Society for Clinical Trials. *Control Clin Trials* 1988;**9**:76–81.
41 Dickersin K. Why register clinical trials?-Revisited. *Control Clin Trials* 1992;**13**:170–7.
42 Making clinical trialists register. *Lancet* 1992;**338**:244–5.
43 Chalmers I, Dickersin K, Chalmers TC. Getting to grips with Archie Cochrane's agenda: all randomised controlled trials should be registered and reported. *BMJ* 1992;**305**:788–8.
44 Savulescu J, Chalmers I, Blunt J. Are research ethics committees behaving unethically? Some suggestions for improving performance and accountability. *BMJ* 1992;**305**:786–88.
45 Chalmers I. *Publication of protocols for new research: one way in which medical journal editors could help to promote well designed clinical research.* Conference on Promoting International Cooperation Among Medical Journal Editors, Bellagio, 7–13 March 1995.
46 Berlin JA. Will publication bias vanish in an age of online journals. Online *Journal of Current Clinical Trials* [serial online] July 8; 1992. (Doc No 12.)
47 Horton R. Luck, lotteries, and loopholes of grant review. *Lancet* 1996;**348**:1255–6.
48 Chalmers I. Proposal to outlaw the term "negative trial" [letter]. BMJ 1985;**290**:1002.
49 Moher D, Jadad AR, Tugwell P. Assessing the quality of randomized controlled trials: current issues and future directions. *Int J Technol Assess Health Care* 1996;**12**:195–208.
50 Liberati A, Himel HN, Chalmers TC. A quality assessment of randomized control trials of primary treatment of breast cancer. *J Clin Oncol* 1986;**4**:942–51.
51 Simon R, Wittes RE. Methodologic guidelines for reports of clinical trials. *Cancer Treatment Reports* 1985;**69**:1–3.
52 Grant A. Reporting controlled trials. *Br J Obstet Gynaecol* 1989;**96**:397–400.
53 Zelen M. Guidelines for publishing papers on cancer clinical trials: responsibilities of editors and authors. *J Clin Oncol* 1983;**1**:164–9.
54 Mosteller F, Gilbert JP, McPeek B. Reporting standards and research strategies for controlled trials. *Control Clin Trials* 1980;**1**:37–58.
55 Gardner MJ, Machin D, Campbell MJ. Use of checklists in assessing the statistical content of medical studies. *BMJ* 1986;**292**:810–12.
56 Gore SM, Jones G, Thompson SG. The Lancet's statistical review process: areas for improvement by authors. *Lancet* 1992;**340**:100–2.
57 Schulz KF, Chalmers I, Grimes DA, Altman DG. Assessing the quality of randomization from reports of controlled trials published in obstetrics and gynecology journals. *JAMA* 1994; **272**:125–8.
58 Altman DG. Statistics in medical journals: developments in the 1980s. *Stat Med* 1991; **10**:1897–913.
59 Mahon WA, Daniel EE. A method for the assessment of reports of drug trials. *Can Med Assoc J* 1964;**90**:565–9.
60 Pocock SJ, Hughes MD, Lee RJ. Statistical problems in the reporting of clinical trials. *N Engl J Med* 1987;**317**:426–32.

61 Altman DG, Doré CJ. Randomization and baseline comparisons in clinical trials. *Lancet* 1990;**335**:149–53.
62 Gøtzsche PC. Methodology and overt and hidden bias in reports of 196 double-blind trials of nonsteroidal antiinflammatory drugs in rheumatoid arthritis. *Control Clin Trials* 1989;**10**:31–56. (Erratum: p 356.)
63 Solomon MJ, McLeod RS. Clinical studies in surgical journals: have we improved? *Dis Colon Rectum* 1993;**36**:43–8.
64 Schulz KF, Chalmers I, Hayes RJ, Altman DG. Empirical evidence of bias: dimensions of methodological quality associated with estimates of treatment effects in controlled trials. *JAMA* 1995;**273**:408–12.
65 Ad Hoc Working Group for Critical Appraisal of the Medical Literature. A proposal for more informative abstracts of clinical articles. *Ann Intern Med* 1987;**106**:598–604.
66 Haynes RB, Mulrow CD, Huth EJ, Altman DG, Gardner MJ. More informative abstracts revisited. *Ann Intern Med* 1990;**113**:69–76.
67 Taddio A, Pain T, Fassos FF, Boon H, Ilersich AL, Einarson TR. Quality of nonstructured and structured abstracts of original research articles in the British Medical Journal, the Canadian Medical Association Journal and the Journal of the American Medical Association. *Can Med Assoc J* 1994;**150**:1611–15.
68 Standards of reporting trials group. A proposal for structured reporting of randomized controlled trials. *JAMA* 1994;**272**:1926–31.
69 Working Group on Recommendations for Reporting of Clinical Trials in the Biomedical Literature. Call for comments on a proposal to improve reporting of clinical trials in the biomedical literature: a position paper. *Ann Intern Med* 1994;**121**:894–5.
70 Rennie D. Reporting randomized controlled trials: an experiment and a call for responses from readers. *JAMA* 1995;**273**:1054–5.
71 Williams JW, Holleman DR, Samsa GP, Simel DL. Randomized controlled trial of 3 vs 10 days of trimethoprim/sulfamethoxazole for acute maxillary sinusitis. *JAMA* 1995;**273**: 1015–21.
72 Begg C, Cho M, Eastwood S, *et al.* Improving the quality of reporting of randomized controlled trials: the CONSORT statement. *JAMA* 1996;**276**:637–9.
73 Fletcher RH, Fletcher SW. Clinical research in general medical journals: a 30-year perspective. *N Engl J Med* 1979;**301**:180–3.
74 Rennie D. How to report randomized controlled trials: the CONSORT statement. *JAMA* 1996;**276**:649.
75 Altman DJ. Better reporting of randomised controlled trials: the CONSORT statement. *BMJ* 1996;**313**:570–1.
76 McNamee D, Horton R. Lies, damn lies, and reports of randomised controlled trials. *Lancet* 1996;**348**:562.
77 Huston P, Hoey J. CMAJ endorses the CONSORT statement. *Can Med Assoc J* 1996; **155**:1277–9.
78 Khan KS, Daya S, Jadad AR. The importance of quality of primary studies in producing unbiased systematic reviews. *Arch Intern Med* 1996;**156**:661–6.
79 Brown SA. Meta-analysis of diabetes patient education research: variations in intervention effects across studies. *Research in Nursing and Health* 1992;**15**:408–19.
80 Nurmohamed MT, Rosendaal PR, Buller HR, *et al.* Low molecular-weight heparin versus standard heparin in general and orthopedic surgery: a meta-analysis. *Lancet* 1992;**340**: 152–6.
81 Sacks HS, Berrier J, Reitman D, Ancona-Berk VA, Chalmers TC. Meta-analyses of randomized controlled trials. *N Engl J Med* 1987;**316**:450–5.
82 Sacks HS, Berrier J, Reitman D, Pagano D, Chalmers TC. Meta-analyses of randomized controlled trials: an update of the quality and methodology. In: Bailar JC, Mosteller F, eds. *Medical uses of statistics*. 2nd ed. Boston: NEJM Books, 1992.
83 Silagy CA. An analysis of review articles published in primary care journals. *Fam Pract* 1993;**10**:337–41.
84 Jadad AR, McQuay HJ. Meta-analyses to evaluate analgesic interventions: a systematic qualitative review of their methodology. *J Clin Epidemiol* 1996;**49**:235–43.

85 Assendelft WJJ, Koes BW, Knipschild PG, Bouter LM. The relationship between methodological quality and conclusions in reviews of spinal manipulation. *JAMA* 1995; **274**:1942–8.
86 Chalmers I. The Cochrane Collaboration: preparing, maintaining, and disseminating systematic reviews of the effects of health care. *Ann NY Acad Sci* 1993;**703**:156–65.
87 Rosenthal R. Writing meta-analytic reviews. *Psychol Bull* 1995;**118**:183–92.
88 Taylor-Halvorsen K. The reporting format. In: Cooper H, Hedges LV, eds. *The handbook of research synthesis*. New York: Russell Sage Foundation, 1994.
89 Mulrow CD, Oxman A. How to conduct a Cochrane systematic review. *Cochrane Collaboration Handbook. 3rd ed.* Oxford: The Cochrane Collaboration, October 1996.

13: Exploring lay perspectives on questions of effectiveness

SANDY OLIVER

Introduction

The science of asking and answering questions about effectiveness of health care has been developed to help health professionals decide whether or not, on balance, specific interventions do more good than harm, and therefore should be retained amongst a range of interventions available within health services. This information is necessary for informing decisions about service planning (such as caring for stroke patients in specialist units or general wards[1]) and practice guidelines (such as offering nicotine replacement therapy to heavy smokers,[2] or drug treatments for the parasitic disease giardiasis[3]). Information about the effectiveness of these treatments draws on randomised controlled trials and systematic reviews which embrace a wide variety of patients, with various characteristics and personal biases, attended by health professionals with varying skills and personal biases of their own, in various settings. The trials focus on the decision at a particular moment (what treatment is intended), such as provision of a specialist stroke unit, whatever second thoughts or mishaps may occur later (what treatment is ultimately received), such as admission to a general ward when beds or staff in the specialist unit are unavailable.

Health service users and those who offer them information and support within self help groups or consumer health information services, readily appreciate the value of randomised controlled trials and systematic reviews of evidence of effectiveness[4] and were quick to make use of such evidence[5] when it first became available in the form of the reference volumes *Effective care in pregnancy and childbirth*[6] and their pocket sized companion guide.[7] They also appreciate some of their shortcomings.[8,9] In this chapter I shall present what I have learnt from discussing questions of effectiveness with health service users and their informants, discuss how a lay perspective brings to mind different questions, and suggest steps for changing the focus of trials and systematic reviews of evidence of effectiveness to better inform decisions about health care. This is not a systematic review of the relevance of evidence of effectiveness to lay people but the result of a personal journey through the developing cultures of evidence-based health-care and consumer health information. The journey began by my search for information about my own care during pregnancy, later, as an antenatal teacher with the National Childbirth Trust offering information and support to expectant parents and, simultaneously, laying views to NHS research committees. This led me to systematically review health promotion evaluations for evidence of effectiveness and involvement of lay people in the research process, and to encourage lay involvement in the Cochrane Collaboration.

Lay responses to clinical trials and systematic reviews of effectiveness

To gather lay perspectives of questions of effectiveness I have listened to members of self help groups, who may be past or potential users of health services or lay providers of care for their own families or other people, and to staff of Consumer Health Information Services and health promotion units, who support people making personal decisions about health. I also bring my personal experience as a health service user and a mother.

In 1995 I had the opportunity to discuss research reports with staff from Consumer Health Information Services (drop in health shops and telephone help lines with a responsibility to provide the public with information on all aspects of health, illness, treatments, and health services, either directly or through health professionals), and members of self help groups. Critical Appraisal Skills Programme workshops, developed by the Oxford Institute of Health Sciences,[10] were adapted with funding from the King's Fund to enable those who respond to enquiries from the public about the effects of care to select and interpret reports of randomised controlled trials and systematic reviews.[4] These workshops were a useful forum for eliciting lay perspectives of trials and systematic reviews.[8] The topics for appraisal were chosen by workshop participants in advance to reflect typical questions from the public (about long term conditions, social support, and self care) and to allow participants to discuss questions of effectiveness in an area of health care familiar to them.

We discussed a trial of a walking fitness programme for people with arthritis of the knee,[11] which addressed a variety of outcome measures including how far patients could walk in six minutes up and down a smooth hospital corridor. Other outcome measures were scales—a physical activity scale, physical/ mental/ and social wellbeing scale, a pain scale, and a medication scale. The workshop participants readily understood the logic of applying randomised trials and quickly acquired the skills to recognise the quality of the methods used, but the published report of this trial was of limited use to them because the numerical values used to report the results could not be translated into meaningful lessons for them. Without examples illustrating how numbers might relate to functional ability, such as getting to the shops and back safely, this paper did not give readers enough information to explain to members of the public how this walking fitness programme might affect their lives.

Broader issues were raised by discussing a clinical trial of a drug treatment for Alzheimer's disease.[12] Again the descriptions of functional ability were reduced to numbers which could not be translated into terms of what the people were able to do in practice. The workshop participants were also disappointed to see that the trial did not investigate people's emotional wellbeing or the stress experienced by their family or carers. Without this information no one could judge whether the effect of the intervention was to relieve or to prolong the adverse effects of the illness.

The wellbeing of the family was also raised in discussion of a Cochrane review of professional support for families of people with schizophrenia.[13] The outcomes measured in the included trials were relapse, hospital readmission, drug compliance, and emotional involvement within the family. The workshop participants pointed out that hospital readmission might be a welcome break for other family members, and that the trials did not address the stress experienced by the family.

This was not an oversight of the review's authors. Indeed, although they could only report those outcomes which had been addressed in the primary studies, they did discuss the outcomes which were missing and remained to be addressed. Thus *The Cochrane Library* is able to disseminate widely information currently available about the effects of care and simultaneously highlight important information that is lacking. It offers an important opportunity to highlight questions that matter to lay people and to encourage a new emphasis to the research agenda. This review of family interventions was also highly valued by Consumer Health Information Service staff because it was easy to read. The reviewers had invited the father of a woman with schizophrenia to help with editing the review (C Adams, personal communication) and the result was much appreciated by readers, especially those without medical training.

Exploring questions of effectiveness of care

Exposing research of a high technical quality to a lay readership reveals how conventional approaches to assessing effectiveness of care may not satisfy the information needs of people making decisions about their own care. Exploring controlled trials in terms of the choice of outcomes measured, the populations recruited, and the interventions compared, suggest that multidisciplinary approaches are likely to be more successful in providing useful information on which to base personal decisions about care.

Choice of outcome measures

At first one might be tempted to think that health service users are being too demanding, and that their requests for a broad range of functional outcome measures would make trials impractical and frustrate attempts to answer more important questions. But examples of trials which assess health in broad terms can be found in *The Cochrane Library*, and it is interesting to compare these with similar trials employing a narrow range of outcomes.

For instance, the evidence underpinning efforts to help pregnant women stop smoking appears to isolate physical health from social and emotional wellbeing. This compares poorly with research into the effects of supporting disadvantaged mothers. Epidemiological data suggest that there is a large overlap between those women who are disadvantaged socially or economically and those who smoke.[14] However, different approaches to disadvantaged or smoking mothers are evaluated very differently (table 13.1).

TABLE 13.1—*Outcomes applied in randomised controlled trials included in systematic reviews to assess the effectiveness of social support for disadvantaged mothers and cessation strategies for smoking in pregnancy*

Support for disadvantaged mothers	*Strategies for women smoking in pregnancy*
• Feelings about first year	• Continued smoking
• Feeling tired	• Low birth weight
• Headaches	• Preterm birth
• Feeling miserable	• Perinatal mortality
• Negative feelings	
• Staying indoors	
• Returning to school	
• Broad range of outcome measures of baby's health	

Those trials which consider the effects of social support for disadvantaged mothers look at a broad range of outcome measures of the babies' health.[15] They also check how the women feel physically and emotionally and how they cope socially. But this broad range of outcomes is not addressed when strategies to help pregnant women give up smoking are evaluated.[16] But for many women smoking is how they cope with stress, taking "time out" from domestic pressures—we know this from listening to the women themselves.[17,18] So it seems irrational to try to take away a coping mechanism and not look for any social and emotional consequences such as strained family relationships or battered children.

A narrow range of outcome measures may satisfy some clinicians' questions about obstetric care, but they were seen as very inadequate by health promotion specialists when I used a review of smoking cessation interventions to introduce them to the *Cochrane Database of Systematic Reviews*. The logic and simplicity of randomised controlled trials may allow them an undue influence if, in the structured report of their review, they are divorced from their wider context, even when this wider context has been discussed by the review's author elsewhere.[19]

Another interesting comparison arises from looking at different approaches to helping women in labour. Both epidural anaesthesia and social support have been assessed in randomised controlled trials using outcome measures for pain, length of labour, complications and interventions during labour, fetal distress and neonatal wellbeing (table

TABLE 13.2—*Outcomes applied in randomised controlled trials included in systematic reviews to assess the effectiveness of epidural anaesthesia and social support for women in labour*

Epidurals for women in labour	*Social support for women in labour*
• Pain*	• All marked*
• Length of labour*	• Complications following labour
• Oxytocin to speed labour*	• Mothers' views of their experiences
• Medical interventions*	• Fathers' views of their experiences
• Complications in labour*	• Pain relief used
• Type of delivery*	• Amount of support received
• Fetal distress*	• Perceived control during labour and birth
• Apgar*	• Relationships within the labour room
• Neonatal blood pH	• Anxiety during labour
• Chemical indicators of stress	• Breastfeeding
• Neurobehavioural measures	• Mothers' interactions with their infants
• Neonatal jaundice	• Neonatal intensive care
	• Mothers' emotional wellbeing
	• Perceived difficulty in mothering

13.2).[20,21] Additional laboratory measures have been used to evaluate epidurals, whereas additional social, emotional, and mothering outcomes have been used to evaluate social support.

If the baby's blood pH, chemical measures of stress, neurobehavioural measures, and jaundice are important indicators of health to inform decisions about epidural anaesthesia, why are they not required for informing decisions about social support? And why are the mother's views of her labour and how she interacts with her baby (including breastfeeding) important for evaluating social support but not for evaluating epidural anaesthesia?

It seems that trials investigating the effects of epidural anaesthesia, a high-technology care, have answered the questions of the anaesthetist with the aid of some high technology measures, and trials investigating the effects of continuous support in labour, a social intervention, have answered the questions of the midwife with greater emphasis on subsequent social interactions. But we have very patchy answers for the woman who wanted to know what could help her in labour and leave her and her baby healthy and thriving. Is a woman better off choosing epidural anaesthesia or continuous social support in labour? If a woman has continuous social support, can additional benefit be gained from epidural anaesthesia? Is continuous social support unnecessary alongside epidural anaesthesia? Does epidural anaesthesia interfere with social support by diverting attention away from the labouring woman towards the continuous fetal heart monitor and thereby deprive the woman and her baby of all the positive effects of continuous social support in labour: reduced analgesia and anaesthesia in labour, reduced complications during or following labour, reduced operative delivery, reduced perceptions of mothering as difficult, prolonged exclusive breastfeeding, and reduced postnatal depression?

There seems to be an anomaly if epidural anaesthesia (which frees the attention of carers from supporting labouring women) and social support (which reduces the need for epidural anaesthesia[21]) are not evaluated by the same criteria.

Interventions compared

Archie Cochrane thought that effectiveness and efficiency were important for evaluating "therapy" within health services, but only relevant in a small way to "board and lodging and tender loving care".[22] But board and lodging and tender, loving care is often appreciated particularly highly by service users. If this care requires investment or a change of practice, evidence of its effectiveness (from studies of, for instance, home visiting for people with schizophrenia and their families,[13] familiar carers for childbearing women,[23] and extra support if they are socially disadvantaged,[15] a cosy place to give birth,[24] encouragement for mothers to cuddle or breastfeed their newborn babies,[25] and help for them to teach their babies socially acceptable sleeping patterns[26]) may be required to justify the costs or, indeed, provide evidence of cost effective alternatives[27] if low technology care has to compete in a culture of evidence-based health care.

Choosing which interventions should be compared, and successfully comparing them for their relative effectiveness (whether high or low technology care) has implications for answering patients' questions. One example of a trial failing to answer the questions of service users is illustrated by the controversy surrounding routine amniotomy in labour. Many women find that their waters are broken early in labour with no apparent reason and little, if any discussion. They are told this will help them along, make things quicker. What many of them find is that following amniotomy they can no longer cope with their labour because the contractions become much fiercer very quickly. Many women ask "Can't I get along better without having my waters broken?" Recently a multicentre trial was mounted to compare the effects of routine early amniotomy with leaving the membranes intact as long as possible.[28] The intention to leave the membranes intact led only to a relatively modest difference in dilatation at membrane rupture, possibly due to the "strong current beliefs of many United Kingdom delivery staff about the relative benefits or risks of amniotomy". Consequently it was not possible to demonstrate any effects following considerable delay and no significant effects were seen following the short delay in the timing of membrane rupture (but still in the middle of the first stage of labour, when women find a sharp increase in the intensity of contractions particularly challenging) and women's questions remain unanswered.

Another issue which is commonly the subject of discussion and decision-making between pregnant women and their carers is the question of how best to deliver a breech presenting baby. Is a planned caesarean section more likely to lead to better health outcomes for mother and baby? Unfortunately, reference to the Cochrane systematic review[29] does not leave readers well informed about the relative effects of care because important details about care of the control group are lacking (G Gyte, personal communication). Two trials included in this review have compared the policy of an elective caesarean section with the policy of a planned vaginal delivery. Details reported in the review about care for a planned vaginal delivery refer to the use of *x* ray pelvimetry, oxytocin, continuous monitoring of the fetal heart and uterine contractions, analgesia, and forceps, but ignore details about opportunities and support for adopting upright positions during labour. Without this information we do not know whether planned caesarean section was compared with supine labour or upright and mobile labour.

Populations recruited

It is not only the choice of which interventions to compare, and which outcomes to measure, which determines the usefulness of a study to personal decision making, but who was recruited into the study. Trials focusing on cardiovascular disease in men may have limited use in providing information on the care of women. Growth charts for bottle fed babies can be misleading when applied to breast fed babies. Down's syndrome screening developed with a largely white population may be less reliable when applied to Asian women.[30] Advice about alcohol consumption may not be equally applicable to all racial groups. When disabled women have been excluded from trials of care in pregnancy and labour, how can they know whether information on the outcomes of care is applicable to them too?

Thus whereas randomised controlled trials and systematic reviews of effectiveness have focused on testing narrowly defined interventions and broadly defined populations with the aim of informing policy decisions, personal decision making would benefit from trials testing a broad choice of interventions in a narrowly defined population.

The ultimate in personally relevant trials are "n of 1" trials which include only the individual seeking the best treatment for their particular chronic problem. Different treatments are employed at randomly allocated time intervals to determine the most effective care for the individual patient. In some areas of health—for instance skin care—lay people are sceptical of the value of large randomised controlled trials because they know that not everyone sharing a condition responds equally well to the same treatments, and they fear that treatments which are seen as effective for a minority of people may be withdrawn from the health service. Searching for studies which test the effectiveness of "n of 1" trials in identifying effective treatments for individuals may be a priority for reviewing evidence of effectiveness from a lay perspective.

Implications of lay perspectives for the Cochrane Collaboration

Lessons learnt from examining trials from a lay perspective have implications for the Cochrane Collaboration. It cannot be assumed that lay people share the same priorities about questions of effectiveness as those people currently embarking on systematically reviewing the evidence.

The scope of Collaborative Review Groups

According to the Cochrane *Handbook* "the description of the scope of [Cochrane Review Groups at exploratory meetings] . . . helps to delineate the way in which that group conceptualises the topic. . . . As systematic reviews are prepared, this description helps to highlight areas of care where no trials have been identified." *The Cochrane Library* reveals that most review groups have defined their scope by listing the conditions and interventions of interest. Two review groups which have described their scope in terms of outcomes as well as interventions do not share all the same interests as lay people discussing the same issues.

The Cochrane Review Group on Effective Professional Practice, which reviews methods for implementing evidence based care, has described its scope in terms of problems targeted (performance of healthcare professionals), types of interventions (including distributing educational materials, outreach visits, and local consensus processes) and outcomes (professional performance, patient outcomes, or cost). When the implementation of research findings was discussed by people bringing a lay perspective they expressed an interest in additional outcomes.[31] Bearing in mind how challenging change can be, they want to know how stressful was the implementation process for everyone involved, and did everyone involved consider the achievements worthwhile?

Differences in perspectives were also illustrated when the Cochrane Subfertility Group invited self help groups and other non-medical personnel to contribute to a workshop in March 1996. About 18 people attended, mainly doctors but also counsellors, infertility nurses, purchasers of health services, and representatives from self help groups. The scope of the group had originally been described as reviewing drug treatment or surgery for infertile couples with outcome measures of pregnancy or other secondary or surrogate measures. By the end of the meeting the population, interventions, and outcomes of interest had been reassessed and broadened through the involvement of people with a non-medical background, whether lay or professional (table 13.3).

TABLE 13.3—*Focus of the Cochrane Subfertility Group, March 1996 and its potential focus identified through multidisciplinary discussions including lay people*

	Current focus of Cochrane Subfertility Group	*Potential focus of Cochrane Subfertility Group*
Population	Infertile couples	Couples wanting a baby and seeking help
Interventions	Drug treatments Surgery	Information giving, listening, peer support, counselling, drug treatments, surgery, laboratory services
Outcomes	Pregnancy Secondary/surrogate measures	Baby, pregnancy, anxiety, stress, problem solved, relationships

Identifying a broad range of health problems, interventions, and outcomes of interest when describing the scope of the group can influence individual reviews. When reporting the outcomes of primary studies reviewers may also highlight the gaps when discussing implications for research. Gaps in the evidence may be obvious when they appear in a familiar field, but less readily identifiable in other disciplines. Without drawing on a broad range of experiences, reviewers risk perpetuating their own professional interests in the interventions and missing opportunities to draw on other disciplines or highlight the service users' interests in their health problems.

Reviewing health care as a multidimensional issue

Such a multidisciplinary approach to service development and evaluation is essential for the promotion of health in a holistic framework. For instance, as a mother, I look to my children's schools for support in helping them choose healthy lifestyles, becoming independent adults, able to build mutually supportive relationships accompanied by children of their own if and when they wish. But the research literature gives little guidance on how schools might best approach this aim. Some reports focus on the benefits of sexual health programmes focused on HIV/AIDS while others focus on pregnancy prevention interventions[32] but the most common reason for "unprotected sex" among young people is use of the pill for pregnancy prevention.[33] At the same time other programmes aim to build self esteem and help children prepare for employment. Addressing these health problems in isolation may lead to undue emphasis on pregnancy prevention, increased use of oral contraceptives, and decreased use of condoms, thereby placing people at greater risk of HIV transmission. Meanwhile the potential for pre-employment programmes to delay unwanted pregnancies may be overlooked. To know how best to support our children as they come to terms with adult life, we need reports of the effectiveness of all these programmes to be collated and reviewed together. This is a multidisciplinary task which needs to draw on health promotion and social work, in health care, education and community settings, and the experiences and views of the young people themselves. Thus in some instances, the primary common factor for attracting appropriate expertise for reviewing evidence of effectiveness is not a specific disease or health problem, but an approach to encouraging good health, and this may provide a more useful focus for some review groups.

This exploration of questions of effectiveness has not only revealed how priorities for particular questions may differ with perspective, it has also repeatedly touched on the themes of coping and support—support for growing up, support for coping in labour, support for mothers coping with social disadvantage, support for families coping with schizophrenia, coping with Alzheimer's disease, coping with subfertility, coping with changes within health services, and smoking to cope with the pressures of domestic life. If the aim of personal decisions is to maximise coping rather than maximise health, this bias needs to be reflected in the way health care is evaluated.

Addressing bias

Much of the methodology for controlled trials and systematic reviews has been developed to minimise the effects of personal bias. Blinding those involved in a trial prevents their personal views influencing which method of care is given to whom and how their health is subsequently assessed. Including unpublished as well as published studies in systematic reviews overrides judgements made at various stages in reporting and publishing the findings. Searching and selecting studies according to predefined methods and quality criteria limits opportunities for authors of reviews to impose their personal views. Explicit reporting of all the criteria and subsequent judgements, such as which studies were included in the final analysis and which were not, allows the readers to decide for themselves to what extent bias was minimised. However, exploring trials and reviews from a lay perspective reveals that the "first and most important step in preparing a review [of asking] a clear question" (*Cochrane Handbook*) remains open to bias.

Avoiding bias is one of the six original principles (along with collaboration, building on people's enthusiasm and existing interests, minimising unnecessary duplication of effort, keeping up to date and ensuring access) underlying the work of the Cochrane Collaboration. But when applying this principle to the fundamental process of composing questions about effects of care, we find that it is undermined by another principle of the Collaboration, namely, building on people's enthusiasm and existing interests (which are necessarily accompanied by their personal biases). The potential for biased questions is exposed by drawing on the experiences and insights of a broad range of people with a vested interest in Cochrane reviews. For instance, in preparing this chapter I was informed by discussions with midwives, obstetricians, health promotion practitioners, social scientists, Consumer Health Information Service staff and self help groups. If our experiences, and those of others, could be pooled, our individual biases could be important contributions to shaping questions which are more effective in informing decisions in health care. Thus, the principle of collaboration is not only essential for sharing the workload and avoiding alienating people who could make important contributions (*Cochrane Handbook*), it is also an opening for developing methods for formulating research questions which draw on many different biases and for ensuring that the appropriate range of skills is available for each individual review. The explicit reporting of teamwork is as essential for readers to judge the balance of bias in posing the questions as is explicit reporting of the search strategy, selection criteria, and reviewers' decisions for readers to judge the balance of bias in producing the answers.

To determine methods for formulating questions about effectiveness by drawing on a range of perspectives, and explicit reporting of this process, we can learn from qualitative research methods, which recognise the inherent bias of the researcher; from methods for reporting the degree of involvement of partners in "healthy alliances", partnerships which bring together different sectors in the quest for improved public health[34]; and from organisations which survive best in times of change by looking outwards, building on their innovative achievements and involving non-traditional groups.[35] Not only is it important to know that the Cochrane Collaboration includes individuals from the full range of professional disciplines and lay people, but also how many and in what roles they are involved, and whether their involvement has an impact on reviews. Similar to the challenge of managing equal opportunity policies,[36] the principle of collaboration and broad participation must be matched by a strategy for monitoring progress and results.

Bringing lay perspectives to the Cochrane Collaboration

After many years of epidemiological research in the mining and agricultural communities of Wales, Archie Cochrane was "convinced that British communities like helping medical research if they are treated properly and things are clearly explained."[37]

Increasing attention to lay involvement in research prompts several questions. Are Archie Cochrane's conclusions generalisable? To what extent is enthusiastic lay involvement an international phenomenon? How far has it spread across different research methodologies? How far has it penetrated the Cochrane Collaboration? In the words of Archie Cochrane, how are lay enthusiasts treated and are things clearly explained to them? What is the impact of efforts to bring researchers and lay people into working partnerships?

Since the Collaboration's inception, policies have recognised the need for lay involvement to ensure the relevance of reviews. The UK Cochrane Centre began by inviting Ruth Evans at the National Consumer Council to join its steering group. Hilda Bastian, a consumer advocate in Australia, was funded by the Nuffield Provincial Hospitals Trust to visit the United Kingdom and develop a proposal for consumer participation in the Collaboration internationally.[38] This enabled her to attend the first Cochrane Colloquium in 1993, when she joined the Collaboration's first steering group, and since then she has developed the Cochrane Consumer Network for lay people to offer each other mutual support, however they are contributing, or planning to contribute, to the work of preparing or disseminating Cochrane reviews. This development and facilitation of consumer participation around the world is supported by the Australasian Cochrane Centre. Pockets of enthusiasm are providing opportunities to try different ways of involving lay people, such as describing the scope of review groups, commenting on review protocols and draft reports, hand searching journals, planning individual reviews, and as members of advisory groups for Collaborative Review Groups or Fields.

In maintaining and raising the standards of Cochrane reviews, the *Cochrane Handbook* suggests that users may be involved in interpreting results, commenting on draft reviews, publishing substantive criticism or dissenting opinions, and amending reviews in the light of valid criticism or new evidence. Methods for involving lay people in preparing systematic reviews are in their infancy but lessons can be learnt from similar initiatives with controlled trials. For instance, the National Perinatal Epidemiology Unit, among others, has willingly shared the planning and conduct of clinical trials with organised self help groups,[39] and a current initiative at the University of Toronto involves Portuguese speaking women, a so-called hard to reach group in Canada, in developing and evaluating (with a broad range of outcome measures) a culturally appropriate intervention to encourage their peers to have Pap smears, thereby reducing the high rates of preventable death and cervical cancer in this group of "underscreened" women (E Hodnett, personal communication).

In addition we can learn from the relatively few people who are already bringing a lay perspective to the Cochrane Collaboration. The National Childbirth Trust was challenged by Iain Chalmers to use and influence research and has provided volunteers with lay perspectives for the Pregnancy and Childbirth Group, the Effective Professional Practice Group, and the Vaccines Network. A poster on a hospital notice board, asking for volunteers to hand search journals, attracted a committed lay member of the Eye and Vision Group (E Hawes, personal communication). The Incontinence Group proposes to seek out all relevant self help groups, convene meetings, and support lay contributions to continuously influence their work (A Grant, personal communication). The Australasian Cochrane Centre has already run two workshops for lay people called "Making sense out of health care research"; more are planned and these will form the basis of written materials for lay readers, including a research glossary. The Cochrane Skin Group has planned and budgeted for training in critical appraisal and information technology support to enable staff members of patient groups and patient volunteers to contribute to Cochrane reviews. The Cochrane Brain and Spinal Cord Injury Group shares an interest in this approach.

This is pioneering work and difficulties must be expected. In March 1996 United Kingdom members of the Cochrane Consumer Network met to share their experiences of working with researchers in a variety of settings, to discuss difficulties and possible ways of overcoming them, and much of what follows draws on a report of that meeting.[40]

Members of the Cochrane Consumer Network perceived that lay people and health professionals have different agendas and the concept of partnership may be alien to them both. Voluntary groups may be inhibited by fears about their independence and the risk of seeming to endorse a particular result.[41] Lay people may lack motivation, interest, and understanding of the research process, doubting it has value for them, whereas researchers may find lay involvement threatening and be reluctant to involve lay people in research design. Finding lay people to collaborate may be difficult. There is a high cost to patients (financial and emotional) in taking part in research. Health care may not be an issue for healthy people, such as those who are not users of treatments and services, whereas patients are often at their most vulnerable and may be reluctant to complain or get involved. In some areas (for instance, acute illnesses) there is a lack of lay groups and lay representation. In other areas lay people lack credibility in the absence of proper representative channels, or there may be pseudorepresentation by bodies or individuals.

There is institutional, cultural, and professional resistance to lay involvement, but where lay people are successful in working with researchers, there is a danger of them becoming "professionalised". In other ventures lay involvement has had difficulty in overcoming academic exclusiveness.[42] Lay people and professionals have different languages and cultures and the greatest confusion may arise when they mistakenly think that they understand each other. For instance, a shared terminology with different meanings can lead to misunderstandings. A problem arose in critical appraisal skills workshops when the word "clinically" was understood in different ways by different groups of people.[43] To the lay mind, the word "clinically" is associated with medical settings and doctors and is often used to mean clean, clearcut, and unfeeling. The *Collins Thesaurus*, for instance, lists as synonyms: analytic, antiseptic, cold, detached, disinterested, dispassionate, emotionless, impersonal, objective, scientific, and unemotional. The *Oxford Concise Medical Dictionary*, by contrast, gives a medical definition of "clinical" medicine as the branch of medicine dealing with the study of actual patients and the diagnosis and treatment of disease at the bedside, as opposed to the study of disease by pathology or other laboratory work. So here are two almost diametrically opposed meanings: to patients it is associated with doctors and lack of warmth; but to doctors it is associated with real, living people and bedside care. We need to be sensitive to other opportunities for misunderstanding, especially as the Cochrane Collaboration has appropriated common terms such as "field" and "entity" and given them specific definitions.

Clarification comes with perseverance. The National Childbirth Trust found that when entering the research arena "the most fruitful partnerships result when time is allowed for health service users to understand the history, organisation, and aims of the research and for researchers to understand the experiences, organisation, and aims of health service user groups. Working together we can look for better ways to share information, opinions, decision making, and responsibility."[44]

Overcoming some of these barriers is seen as important by the UK Cochrane Centre which includes in its targets the objective "to explore, in association with others, ways in which people using health services might become involved in planning and developing protocols for Cochrane reviews ...". The Centre observes however, that substantial scepticism exists in the minds of some of the professional researchers involved in the Collaboration that this (explicit) principle merits support.[45] The potential value of lay involvement may be more widely recognised with more articles in the medical press giving lay perspectives, paying more attention to validity of patients' experiences, and qualitative as well as quantitative research. There is a need to clarify the role, nature, and potential of lay involvement, exploring a range of methods (for instance, newsletters, questionnaires, and focus groups) to gather and communicate lay views and explore the use of patient advocates to ensure that vulnerable and marginalised groups are involved. In preparing this chapter I have gleaned valuable insights from people familiar with systematic reviewing and strongly committed to the Collaboration as well as from people responding to their first introduction to the science and the organisation. No doubt a plethora of methods can inform us. Some may be better than others. Some may be more appropriate for particular subjects, with particular groups, or in particular settings. Now is the time to explore options for encouraging lay input into reviews, to identify barriers, and to attempt to overcome them. Lay involvement needs commitment, funding, and training in effective communication for both lay people and professionals. Above all there is a need for research into involving lay people in research. How are lay people found and how do they become involved? What experience and skills do they bring, and what skills do they subsequently develop? What resources and support do they need? What roles do they fulfil? To what extent can they represent the views of others? And, what impact do they have?

To take this work forward within the Cochrane Collaboration, members of the Cochrane Consumer Network are calling for a two way communication between professional collaborators and lay people and a debate about accountability. This invokes practical questions about access to technology, which may not be available to lay people and about individual or group representation on Consumer Network and Cochrane entities. Developing formal structures may encourage lay involvement or it may diminish the dynamism.

There is a lack of knowledge amongst consumer organisations about the Cochrane Collaboration and confusion about its role, how it works, and how lay people can become involved. Greater guidance on attracting and involving lay people could be provided by the Cochrane Consumer Network, and included in *The Cochrane Library*, with potential lay participants being given summaries of the tasks that might involve them. Alternatively this may be seen as either restrictive or "spoon feeding" and participants should be free to develop their own contribution.

Staff at the UK Cochrane Centre have suggested that one or more pilot schemes be established to explore how people using health services can become involved in using specialised registers of randomised controlled trials to describe and comment on the pattern of past and current research. They have also suggested surveying the extent to which, and in which ways, people representing those using health services have become involved in developing protocols for and preparing Cochrane reviews.

Implications of lay perspectives for informed choice

I find the prospect of involving lay people in the preparation of reviews both exciting and daunting. It is something to be developed hand in hand with greater use of evidence in their decision making. Information about health and ill health, services availability, and voluntary support groups is more readily available than information on effectiveness. Although there are initiatives to disseminate the results of systematic reviews widely, such as "Informed Choice" leaflets for pregnant women in the United Kingdom[46] and, in Canada, an inexpensive audiotape for postmenopausal women considering hormone replacement therapy,[47] these are innovative approaches rather than examples of routine practice.

A member of the Cochrane Consumer Network seeking help to conceive a second child found that a range of help was available (medical, surgical, social, and complementary), but that this help and the information about it was arbitrarily divided between the different professional groups. Counselling was only offered to those patients who had decided to embark on high technology interventions, and a medical consultant was unable to offer any information or signposts for complementary medicine. Neither did the consultant know that some reviews of effectiveness of interventions for subfertility were already published on the *Cochrane Database of Systematic Reviews*. The efforts of this determined, enquiring service user went unaided by her carers and she was refused access to the *Cochrane Database of Systematic Reviews* by the local NHS library, which owned a copy. Eventually she accessed this database through the Cochrane Consumer Network, and thus informed made a special request for counselling without a commitment to high tech care, and subsequently found the counselling the most helpful intervention she had received.

Alternative routes for accessing information about the effects of care, through the Consumer Health Information Services and self help groups, also need developing. Better access to the evidence, better skills for appraising the literature,[48] and better skills for supporting lay people while they assimilate complex information relevant to their own health are essential for a satisfactory information service.[43] To meet this challenge the NHS Executive's Patient Partnership Strategy includes the commissioning of a national health information resource centre, from April 1997, to offer advice, support, and training to facilitate the production of high quality evidence-based patient information. Encouraging cooperation and partnership between lay and professional people, whether they are producing or using information, will be fundamental to this work.

Whereas evidence of effectiveness is necessary for making informed choices, it is not sufficient and people may choose to disregard it. This is acknowledged in the National Childbirth Trust's policy on the importance of evaluation, which highlights the value of research evidence of healthcare effectiveness for decision making but also accepts that "whilst individuals may be guided by research evidence, they will be influenced by their own beliefs, wishes and priorities"[44]. For instance, the decision to circumcise baby sons is frequently made for social, traditional, and religious reasons despite the risk of medical complications.[49] Some women with breast cancer prefer minimal surgery whereas others, with different priorities, prefer to minimise the risk of regret should the cancer recur and choose mastectomy.[50]

Similarly, lay people involved in discussions about the provision of services bring experience and values, but they also need to be informed about other relevant issues (such as the health needs of the population, effectiveness, cost effectiveness, and financial constraints)[51] to be fully involved in setting priorities for service planning.

When it is possible for lay people to ask questions about effectiveness and discuss these and their related issues among themselves and with people working in health services, as equal partners, we can address the value of *The Cochrane Library* for lay people by asking: are Cochrane reviews sufficiently highly valued to attract investment for wide dissemination of their messages; and, to what extent do Cochrane reviews either satisfy people's need for information on which to base decisions about health care, or stimulate new primary studies to generate evidence which could do so.

Acknowledgements

The ideas presented in this chapter have grown slowly from reading about and discussing health, health care, and evaluation with health professionals, researchers and lay people. Over the years Heda Borton, Phyll Buchanan, Iain Chalmers, Gill Gyte, Ruairidh Milne, Mary Newburn, Ann Oakley, and Ann Truesdale have been particularly thought provoking. I am also grateful to Hilda Bastian, Mike Clarke, Patricia Donnithorne, Vikki Entwistle, Ellen Hodnett, Charlotte Howell, Barbara Meredith, and Lesley Stewart for their comments and stimulating ideas for this chapter. Many original contributions were made by participants in critical appraisal skills workshops whose criticisms enabled me to see trials and reviews in a new light.

1 Stroke Unit Trialists' Collaboration. A systematic review of specialist multidisciplinary team (stroke unit) care for stroke inpatients. In: Warlow C, van Gijn J, Sandercock P,

eds. Stroke module of the Cochrane Database of Systematic Reviews, [updated 03 June 1996]. Available in The Cochrane Library [database on disk and CD-ROM]. The Cochrane Collaboration; Issue 2. Oxford: Update Software; 1996. Updated quarterly. Available from: BMJ Publishing Group, London.

2 Silagy C, Man D, Fowler G, Lancaster T. The effect of nicotine replacement therapy on smoking cessation. In: Lancaster T, Silagy C, Fullerton D, eds. Tobacco addiction module of the Cochrane Database of Systematic Reviews, [updated 03 June 1996]. Available in The Cochrane Library [database on disk and CD-ROM]. The Cochrane Collaboration; Issue 2. Oxford: Update Software; 1996. Updated quarterly. Available from: BMJ Publishing Group, London.

3 Zaat JOM, Mank ThG, Assendelft WJJ. Treatment of giardiasis. In: Garner P, Gelband H, Olliaro P, Salinas R, Wilkinson D, eds. Tropical diseases module of the Cochrane Database of Systematic Reviews, [updated 12 June 1996]. Available in The Cochrane Library [database on disk and CD-ROM]. The Cochrane Collaboration; Issue 2. Oxford: Update Software; 1996. Updated quarterly. Available from: BMJ Publishing Group, London.

4 Milne R, Oliver S. Evidence-based consumer health information: developing teaching in critical appraisal skills. *Int J Qual Health Care* 1996 (in press).

5 Stocking B. Implementing the findings of effective care in pregnancy and childbirth in the United Kingdom. *Milbank Q* 1993; **71**:497–521.

6 Chalmers I, Enkin M, Keirse M. *Effective care in pregnancy and childbirth.* Oxford: Oxford University Press, 1989.

7 Enkin M. Keirse M, Chalmers I. eds. *A guide to effective care in pregnancy and childbirth.* Oxford: Oxford University Press, 1989.

8 Oliver S. Do clinical trials answer questions that matter to consumers? In: Collier J, Barnett H, eds. *From trial outcomes to clinical practice, proceedings of the fourth drug and therapeutics bulletin symposium.* London: Which? 1996:30–5.

9 Gyte G. Evaluation of the meta-analyses on the effects, on both mother and baby, of the various components of 'active' management of the third stage of labour. *Midwifery* 1994. **10**;183–99.

10 Milne R, Donald A. Piloting short workshops on the critical appraisal of reviews. *Health Trends* 1995;**27**:120–3.

11 Kovar PA, Allegrandte JP, MacKenzie R, *et al.* Supervised fitness walking in patients with osteoarthritis of the knee. A randomised controlled trial. *Ann Intern Med* 1992; **116**: 529–34.

12 McLachlan DR, Dalton AJ, Kruck TP, *et al.* Intramuscular desferrioxamine in patients with Alzheimer's disease. *Lancet* 1991; **337**:1304–8.

13 Mari JJ, Streiner D. Family intervention for those with schizophrenia. In: Adams C, Anderson J, de Jesus Mari J, eds. Schizophrenia module of the Cochrane Database of Systematic Reviews, [updated 06 June 1996]. Available in the Cochrane Library [database on disk and CD ROM]. The Cochrane Collaboration; Issue 2. Oxford: Update Software; 1996. Updated quarterly. Available from: BMJ Publishing Group, London.

14 Graham H, Hunt S. Women's smoking and measures of women's socio-economic status in the United Kingdom. *Health Promotion International* 1994;**9**:81–8.

15 Hodnett ED. Support from caregivers for socially disadvantaged mothers. In: Enkin MW, Keirse MJNC, Renfrew MJ, Neilson JP, eds. Pregnancy and childbirth module of the Cochrane Database of Systematic Reviews, 1996 [updated 29 February 1996]. Available in The Cochrane Library from BMJ Publishing Group, London.

16 Lumley, J. Strategies for reducing smoking in pregnancy. In: Neilson JP, Crowther CA, Hodnett ED, Hofmeyr GJ, Keirse MJNC, Renfrew MJ, eds. Pregnancy and Childbirth Module of The Cochrane Database of Systematic Reviews [updated 27 September 1993]. Available in The Cochrane Pregnancy and Childbirth Database, 1995, Issue 1.

17 Graham H. Women's smoking and family health. *Soc Sci Med* 1987; **25**:47–56.

18 Oakley A. Smoking in pregnancy—smoke screen or risk factor? Towards a materialist analysis. *Sociology of Health and Illness* 1989;**11**:311–35.

19 Lumley J. Stopping smoking—again. *Br J Obstet Gynaecol* 1991;**98**:847–9.

Cochrane's Obituary*

A L COCHRANE CBE, FRCP, FFCM

Professor A L Cochrane, who had been director of the Medical Research Council's epidemiology unit in Cardiff and was the first president of the Faculty of Community Medicine, died on 18 June.

Archibald Leman—Archie—was born on 12 January 1909 in Galashiels. He won scholarships, first to Uppingham and then to King's College, Cambridge, where he obtained a first in both parts of the natural science tripos. He graduated MB, BCh late (in 1938) after studying at University College Hospital, London. At first, like many of his generation, he was bemused by Freud and Marx. Unlike most of them he spent a year as a medical student with the International Brigade during the Spanish civil war and started a training analysis in Vienna. Unconvinced by either experience he returned to medical research and then joined the Royal Army Medical Corps in 1940. He was captured in Crete in 1941 (an event that he usually blamed on Evelyn Waugh, the intelligence officer of D Battalion "Layforce") and spent four years as a prisoner of war in Crete, Greece, and Germany, treating chiefly Soviet, French, and Yugoslav prisoners with tuberculosis. In 1945 he was awarded the MBE for his services as a prisoner of war medical officer.

In 1946 he was given a Rockefeller fellowship, which enabled him to take the DPH at the London School of Hygiene and Tropical Medicine, and spent a year in the United States studying the epidemiology of tuberculosis. On his return he joined the MRC's pneumoconiosis research unit, which had just been set up, as epidemiologist and *x* ray film reader. There the next 10 years were probably the most productive of his life. With an almost obsessional interest in reproducibility, low rates of refusal, and validation he showed that measurements could be made on populations defined geographically with about the same known inaccuracy as measurements made in laboratories. This helped to make epidemiology a quantitative science but had many other results, notably in pneumoconiosis among coalminers and the epidemiology of bronchitis, anaemia, and

* Written by Archie Cochrane
Reproduced from *BMJ* 1988;**297**:63.

rheumatoid arthritis and, later, health service research. In 1957 he survived a professor of surgery's prognosis that he had only three months to live.

He was, possibly unnecessarily, upset by the MRC's decision to hand over research on pneumoconiosis among coalworkers to the National Coal Board with limited participation from the MRC and finally became David Davies professor of chest diseases at the Welsh National School of Medicine and honorary director of the MRC's epidemiology unit. He was not a real success as a professor, either as a teacher or on the senate, though his kindness to students was proverbial, but it gave him a sort of breathing space to switch the direction of his research from epidemiology to health services research. He managed to break through by his evaluation of screening procedures (for glaucoma and anaemia).

He retired as a professor in 1969 to become a full time MRC director, in this second productive period emphasising the importance of discovering, by means of randomised clinical trials, the optimum place of treatment and the optimum length of stay. In 1972 the Nuffield Provincial Hospitals Trust published his book *Effectiveness and efficiency: random reflections on health services*, which, although undoubtedly lucky in its timing, had a widespread international effect. At the same time he accepted the job of being the first president of the Faculty of Community Medicine. It was rather out of character: he did it in a crisis out of a sense of duty, but it upset his research plans. He managed a difficult important job with competence and achieved what was needed.

He retired to what looked like an Indian summer, living in a three generation household at Rhoose; he completed 20 year follow up studies of the communities he had studied in the 1950s, travelled widely, and studied the health services of developed countries. It did not work out as he hoped, but he continued his research work after some severe setbacks, completing a 30 year follow up study of men in Rhondda in 1983.

He had many other interests and abilities at different ages. He showed above average competence at rugby football, squash, tennis, and skiing and enjoyed collecting pictures and sculptures and gardening. A small volume of his verse exists, written while he was a prisoner of war. He entertained generously, particularly foreign visitors, and always admitted the value of a private income in helping his career.

Another aspect of his life was the support he gave his unfortunate family, chiefly by diagnosis and seeing that they got the best treatment and care. There were 11 in his immediate family: three had porphyria, three severe diabetes, and one juvenile rheumatoid arthritis.

He was a man with severe porphyria who smoked too much and was without the consolation of a wife, a religious belief, or a merit award—but he didn't do so badly.—ALC.

Index

abstracts, informative 260
abuse 137
age
  asthma onset and 79
  optimal alcohol intake and 64–5
air pollution 82
alcohol consumption 58–72
  mortality and 59–63
  optimal level 63–4
  patterns 68–9, 71–2
  public health policy 70–1
  sex/age variations in optimal 64–5
  specific beverages 65–70
  under-reporting 63–4
allergens 81–2, 83–4, 87–8
allocation
  concealment 97, 100–1, 260
  foreknowledge of 202
  random *see* random allocation
altruism 44–6
Alzheimer's disease 274
amaurosis fugax 113
amniotomy 277–8
angina, unstable 115, 116
antiarrhythmic drugs, new 188–9
antihypertensive therapy 223–8
anti-oestrogen therapy 266
antioxidants 69
Antiplatelet Trialists' (APT) Collaborative Group 212, 215
Archie Cochrane lecture 58
Armitage, Peter 108
arthritis, knee 273–4
Asilomar Working Group 261
aspirin 107–19
  cognitive decline and 118–19
  new uses 117–18
  post-myocardial infarction 107, 109–16, 213–16
    first randomised controlled trial 110–13
    further randomised controlled trials 113–14, 213–16
    subgroup analyses 204–5
    systematic overviews 114–16, 215
Aspirin and Myocardial Infarction Study (AIMS) 115
asthma 76, 77–88
  causation 82–4
  effects of treatment 86–7
  mortality 77–8
  natural history 84–6
  prevalence 79–82
    geographical variations 79–80
    time trends 80–2
  prevention 83, 87–8
  provoking factors 83–4
  risk factors 82–3
atopy 83
Australasian Cochrane Centre 283, 284

β_2 agonists 78, 86
Bastian, Hilda 283
Bates, Hugh 31, 36, 37
beer 66, 67–8
behavioural therapies 126–7
Benjamin, Tom 31, 36
bias
  confirmatory 256–7
  lay perspectives 281–3
  low response rates 75
  outcome assessment 203
  patient management 203
  publication 250–8, 281–2
  random *see* random errors
  regression dilution 224
  selection 190
  in social work research 141–2
  in study references 254
  systematic
    avoiding moderate 200–5
    control 198
binge drinking 68–9, 72
Black, Sir Douglas 23, 154
blinding 202–3, 281
blood donors 42
blood pressure
  alcohol consumption and 69
  stroke/coronary heart disease and 223–8

Bradford Hill, Austin 12, 108, 185–6, 188
breast cancer 202, 216–18, 288
breech delivery 278
British Journal of Obstetrics and Gynaecology 259
British Medical Journal 260, 265
British National Child Development Study 85–6
Brotherston, John 14
Buxton, Martin 155

Cabot, Richard 123–4
Caerphilly Cohort Study 119
Caerphilly Collaborative Prospective Study of Heart Disease and Stroke 113
Cambridge-Somerville youth study 123–4, 125, 131
Canadian Medical Association Journal 259, 260, 265
captivity, of trial participants 50
cardiac arrhythmias 188–9
carers, lay 273
carotid endarterectomy 208–10
Cartwright, Ann 50
cataracts 118
Central Council for Education and Training in Social Work (CCETSW) 127, 144
Central Oxford research ethics committee (COREC) 252
cerebrovascular disease
  alcohol consumption and 62, 63
  aspirin and 214–15, 216
cervical cancer 284
Chalmers, Iain 117, 258, 284
chaos, in social work 142
chest *x* rays 32, 35
child protection/abuse 130, 132, 136, 137
circumcision 288
clinical, meaning of word 285
clinical trials 197 *see also* randomised controlled trials
  lay perspectives 273–4
  publication bias 252
  registration of initiated 257–8
Cochrane, Archibald Leman
  education 7
  illnesses 8–10
  interests 8, 9
  obituary 292
  personal characteristics 11, 12–13, 25
  in United States 4–5
  wartime experiences 7–8, 58, 109, 184–5, 231
Cochrane Airways Group 76, 83
Cochrane Collaboration 25, 116–17, 211, 231–49, 267
  chronology 243–7
  evolution and consolidation 233–5
  lay perspectives 236, 279–87
  potential and limitations 235–40
  prelude/inauguration 231–3
  strategic alliances and future 240–2
  strategic plan 241, 247–9
Cochrane Consumer Network 283, 284–5, 286–7
The Cochrane Database of Systematic Reviews 233, 237, 240, 287–8
Cochrane Handbook 283–4
The Cochrane Library 235, 246, 274, 275, 279, 288
Cochrane Review Group of Effective Professional Practice 279–80
Cochrane Subfertility Group 280
Cochrane units 110
cognitive-behavioural approaches 126–7
cognitive decline 118–19
Cohen, Dick 11, 14, 154
collaborative review groups 233–4, 279–80
Collins, R 9
colon cancer 117–18
communication 102
comprehensibility 49–50
concealment, allocation 97, 100–1, 260
concern, for trial participants 50
confirmatory evidence 256–7
consent, informed 41, 102, 103
  selection by 190–2
  simplification 210–11
  in social work 139–41
CONSORT (consolidated standards of reporting trials) 262–6
  checklist 262, 264
  flow diagram 263, 264

Consumer Health Information
Services 273, 274, 287–8
continuity, of staffing 50
contracts, with trial participants 50
control groups 84
benefits to 44–6, 140–1
copper 60
coronary care units 8, 107
Coronary Drug Prevention Studies
(CDP) 113
coronary heart disease *see* ischaemic
heart disease
corticosteroids, inhaled 86–7
cost(s)
need for measurements 152
NHS 150
opportunity 153, 160
social services 150
social work research 132–3
cost benefit analyses 151–2
cost effectiveness analysis 157, 159,
206
counselling
psychodynamic 126–7
social work 126, 131
Craven, LL 109–10
Critical Appraisal Skills Programme
workshops 273–4, 285
cross-sectional studies 75, 81

Davies, Morley 31
delinquency 123–4, 125, 131, 137
dementia 118–19
Department of Health Policy and
Management 4
developing world 6
diet, asthma and 82, 83
disability adjusted life year (DALY)
173
distributive justice 176, 190
Dollery, Colin 23
Doll, Richard 7, 58, 114, 154
double blind design 76, 141–2

Early Breast Cancer Trialists'
Collaborative Group
(EBCTCG) 212, 216–18, 257
economic evaluations 156–9
checklist 156–7
role in health services research
160–2
economics
Cochrane's view 151–4
health 149–63
post-war changes 149–50
education, trial participants 41
*Effective care in pregnancy and
childbirth* (1989) 272
effectiveness (efficacy) 151, 169
lay perspectives 274–9
*Effectiveness and efficiency: random
reflections on health services*
(Cochrane 1972) 12, 15–17, 76,
149, 231–2
1989 edition 58
American response 4–5, 15–16
citations 24
on health economics 151–4
historical context 149–51
reactions to 21–6
on social work 122
translations 18–20, 24
effect size 206, 251
efficiency 149, 151–2, 169, 180
allocative 162
elderly
aspirin and cognitive decline
118–19
optimal alcohol intake 65
participation in community care
138
electronic publication 258
eligibility criteria, trial participants
207–11
empiricism, social science attitudes
124, 133–6
empowerment 135, 138, 140
English language 255
epidemiology 48–9
democratic nature 54–5
field 75–6
Epidemiology Unit, south Wales 3,
11–12, 31, 47, 54
epidural anaesthesia 276–7
equality/equity 169–81
allocative efficiency and 162
aversion to lack of 173–6
Cochrane on 170–1
health care distribution 150–1,
155, 170
of outcome 171–3
quantification 176–7

random *v* non-random sampling 189–90
risks/benefits of medical innovations 184–92
selection of trial participants 190–2
uncertainty and 186–7
weights to QALYs 177–81
ethics
evidence based 181
publication bias 258
of randomisation 139–41, 187
selection of trial participants 189–90
social work research 130–3
ethics committees 51, 257, 258
Central Oxford 252
European Carotid Surgery Trial (ECST) 208–10
European Community Respiratory Health Survey 80
EuroQol EQ-5D system 177, 178
Evans, Dai Dan 31
Evans, Ruth 283
evidence based ethics 181
evidence based medicine 76
evidence based patient information 287–8
evidence based purchasing 152
evidence based social work 143–4
exclusions, post-randomisation 203, 212

Faculty of Community Medicine 12, 22
"fair innings" concept 172–6
family therapy 127
feedback 50–1
feminist perspective 128
fenoterol 78, 86
fibrinolytic therapy 200, 208, 210–11, 218–22
Fibrinolytic Trialists' (FTT) Collaborative Group 212, 220–2
fibrosis, progressive massive (PMF) 33, 43
field
epidemiology 75–6
workers 36–7
financial incentives
in decision to publish 256
trial participants 42
flavonoids 69
Fletcher, Charles 3, 25
follow-up studies 76
food additives 82
Framingham study 32–3
France 19–20
Frankenberg, Ron 31

gender differences *see* sex differences
general practice
aspirin trial in 114
research within 51, 52–4
in south Wales 45–7
General Practice Research Framework (GPRF) 40–1, 53–4
genetic factors 174
Ginzberg, Eli 24
GISSI studies 206, 218–22
glaucoma screening 11
Glyncorrwg research studies 38–40, 44
Godber, George 11
Gough, Jethro 33
Graham, Jimmy 110
Green College, Oxford University 9
Gubéran, Etienne 18

Hart, Julian Tudor 4, 31, 38–40
Hart, Phillip D'Arcy 31, 43
Hawthorne effect 44, 141
health care
access, trial participants 44–6
demand for 160
equality in distribution 150–1, 155, 170
multidisciplinary approach 280–1
need for formal assessments 94
rationale for assessing 93–4, 151
supply 160
health economics 149–63
absorption into research process 156–9
Cochrane's view 151–4
contribution to health services research 160–2
early days 154–5
health promotion units 273
Health Services Research Committee 158
heart transplantation 158
high density lipoprotein (HDL) cholesterol 69

Himsworth, Sir Harold 9
hormone replacement therapy (HRT) 40–1
Horst, Gérard 19
hospital building programme 154
house dust mites 77, 81–2, 83–4
hygiene 82
hypertension, treatment benefits 223–8

ill health, measurement 76–7
Illich, Ivan 23, 151
incentives
  in decision to publish 256
  implementing research results 162
  trial participants 42
infections 82
information, patient 287–8
informative abstracts 260
"Informed Choice" leaflets 287
Inglis, Brian 24
Institute of Medicine (IOM) 4, 5
institutional review boards 257
"intention to treat" principle 140, 203, 212
International Clinical Epidemiology Network (INCLEN) 6
International Epidemiological Association (IEA) 4, 5–6, 15
International Study of Asthma and Allergy in Childhood (ISAAC) 80
interventions
  allocated, foreknowledge of 202
  assembly of comparison groups 94–5
  detecting moderate effects 199–200
  differences between comparison groups 95–9
  lay perspectives 277–8
  need for formal assessments 94
  novel, risks and benefits 184–92
  rationale for assessing 93–4
  social work, "active ingredient" of 139
in vivo exposure, graded 139
ischaemic heart disease
  alcohol consumption and 58–72
  blood pressure lowering and 223–8
ISIS-2 trial 204–5, 206, 210, 213–16, 218–22
ISIS-4 trial 222–3
isoprenaline 78
Italy 18–20

Jarman, Frank 31, 35
Jick, Herschel 111, 113
Johns Hopkins University 4–5, 15–16, 25–3
Jonathan, Gwilym 31, 36, 37
Jones, Trefor Stanley 31
Journal of the American Medical Association 260, 265
justice, distributive 176, 190

Kay, Sir Andrew Watt 23
Kennedy, Ian 23–4

labour
  amniotomy in 277–8
  care of women in 276–7
The Lancet 258, 265
language, of published articles 256
large-scale randomised evidence 197–29 *see also* randomised controlled trials, large; systematic overviews
  clinical relevance 228–9
  examples of important results 213–28
  value 199–211
lay perspectives 272–88
  clinical trials/systematic overviews 273–4
  Cochrane Collaboration 236, 279–87
  effectiveness of care 274–9
  informed choice 287–8
learning theories 126–7
life expectancy 172–3
  differences in 173–6
  quality adjusted 173, 177, 179
lifestyle 175
LIMIT-2 trial 222–3
L'inflation médicale (Cochrane 1977) 19–20
living standards, asthma and 80
low density lipoprotein (LDL) cholesterol 69

Maccacaro, G 18
McKeown, Tom 11, 14, 23
McLachlan, Gordon 4, 5, 11, 14

magnesium infusion, myocardial infarction 222–3
Mather, Gordon 8, 107
Medical Research Council (MRC) 11, 158
  Epidemiology Unit, south Wales 3, 11–12, 31, 47, 54, 77
  General Practice Research Framework (GPRF) 40–1, 53–4
  Health Services Research Committee 158
  Pneumoniosis Research Unit, Cardiff 3, 8
medical sociology 151
mega-trials *see* randomised controlled trials, large
mental illness 133
meta-analyses *see* systematic overviews
Moore, Fred 31, 36–7
Morris, Jerry N 3, 4
multidisciplinary approach 280–1
myocardial infarction
  alcohol consumption and 67
  aspirin after 107, 109–16, 204–5
  detecting reductions in mortality 199–200
  fibrinolytic therapy 200, 208, 210–11, 218–22
  magnesium infusion 222–3

National Cancer Institute (NCI) 251, 253
National Childbirth Trust 273, 284, 285, 288
National Health Service (NHS)
  expenditure 150
  internal market 160, 162
  mass research needs 52–3
  Patient Partnership Strategy 287–8
  reforms 24–5
  Research and Development Programme 25, 232–3
  resource allocation *see* resource allocation
National Institutes of Health 253
National Perinatal Epidemiology Unit 284
National Union of Mineworkers (NUM) 35–6, 43, 44
negligence, contributory 175
New York Academy of Sciences 233
New Zealand 5, 42, 78
NHS *see* National Health Service
non-respondents/participants
  characteristics 33–5, 190–2
  in social work research 140, 141
non-steroidal anti-inflammatory drugs 159, 255
Nuffield Provincial Hospitals Trust (NPHT) 4, 5, 11, 12, 14–17

O'Brien, John 109, 110, 113
obstetrics 232, 275–8
Office of Health Economics 25
oligospermia 266
One man's medicine (Cochrane 1989) 112, 118
opportunity cost 153, 160
oppression, social work research and 127–9
outcome measures
  in economic analysis 152–4
  lay perspectives 275–7
  in social work research 136–9
outcomes analysis 201
ovarian ablation 216–18
ovarian cancer 251
Oxford Institute of Health Sciences 273
oxygen therapy, premature infants 188

Palmer, John 108
participants, trial
  benefits to 44–6, 140–1
  entry procedures 207–11
  factors affecting recruitment 41–3, 190–2
  informed consent *see* consent, informed
  lay perspectives 278–9
  motivation 44–6
  payment 42
  post-randomisation exclusion 203, 212
  random *v* non-random selection 189–90
  response rates *see* response rates
  in social work research 140–1
participation, client 138–9

partnership, working in 138
Peto, Richard 9, 116
pharmaceutical industry 157, 159, 256
phobias 139
Pickering, George 14
platelets 69, 113
Platt Committee 8
pneumoconiosis 33, 43–4, 75–6
Pneumoconiosis Research Unit, Cardiff 3, 8
Pole, David 150
poliomyelitis vaccine 190–1
political ideology, social work and 133, 143
populations, studied 278–9
porphyria 13
pre-eclampsia 117
pregnancy
  prevention 281
  smoking in 85–6, 275–6
  social support in 128, 140, 275–6
prematurity, retinopathy of 188
primary care *see* general practice
prisoner of war (POW) camps 8, 109, 184–5, 231
probation 143–4
progressive massive fibrosis (PMF) 33, 43
psychodynamic counselling 126–7
psychological effects of care 102–3
publication bias 250–8, 281–2
  avoiding 257–8
  ethical issues 258
  evidence for 252–5
  related sources of bias 254–6

quality adjusted life years (QALY) 155, 157–8, 173
  cost per 158
  equity weighting 177–81
quality of life, health related 173
  measures 152, 153, 170, 206
  UK illustrative data 177–80
questionnaires, asthma 80

racism 128–9
random allocation
  advantages 95–9, 100–1, 200–2
  in British streptomycin trial 186
  ethics 131–2, 139–41, 187
  in limiting risk 188–9
  uncertainty and 186–7, 207–11
random errors
  avoiding moderate 200, 206–11
  control 198
randomised controlled trials 14, 76, 108–10
  avoiding moderate biases 200–5
  avoiding random errors 200, 206–11
  Cochrane Collaboration and 235
  cost and quality of life indices 207
  cultural differences in attitudes 18–20
  detecting moderate effects 199–200
  economic evaluations in 156–9
  effect size 206, 251
  entry procedures 207–11
  generalisability of results 101–3
  large (mega-trials) 198, 206–7
    clinical relevance 228–9
    examples of important 213–16, 218–23
  lay perspectives 272
  machinery of proper conduct 202–3
  participants *see* participants, trial
  registration 235, 257
  reporting *see* reporting, of randomised controlled trials
  response rates 40–3
  similarities to other designs 99–101
  in social work *see* social work, randomised controlled trials
  special features 95–9
  systematic overviews *see* systematic overviews
  viewpoints of 103–5
randomised evidence, large-scale *see* large-scale randomised evidence
random sampling 189–90
references, biased use 255
registers, study 235, 257
Reik, Theodor 7
Renan, Ernest 20
Renaud, Serge 113
Renton, Ross 110
reporting
  of randomised controlled trials 250–65
    historical perspectives 259–60

proposed standards 261–6
publication bias 250–8, 281–2
quality 259
structured 260–1
of systematic overviews 266–7
resource allocation
Cochrane's views 152–4
equitable 162
inequalities in 150–1, 155
influences of health economics 158
market forces and 160
resource allocation working party (RAWP) 155
respect 49
respiratory diseases, asthma and 84–5
response rates 31–55, 75–6
Cochrane units 110
in Glyncorrwg studies 38–40
methodological rigour and 32–3
methods of promoting high 35–7, 39
order effects 33–5
preconditions for high/sustained 49–51
in randomised controlled trials 40–3
in Rhondda Fach studies 32–7, 43–4
social influences 43–4
retinopathy of prematurity 188
review groups, collaborative 233–4, 279–80
Rhondda Fach studies 31–7, 42, 43–6
Rhoose Farm House 8, 9, 19
risk
limiting 188–9
maldistribution 190–2
Robson, Norrie 15
Rock Carling Fellowship 12, 14–15, 22
Rockefeller Foundation 5–6
Rosser, Rachel 154–5
Rougemont, André 18
Royal College of General Practitioners (RCGP) 53, 113–14
Russian prisoner of war 152, 231

Salk poliomyelitis vaccine 190–1
salt intake 82
sample size 206, 251
sampling, random *v* non-random 189–90
schizophrenia 274
scientific methodology, social science objections 124, 125–33
screening, mass 11, 14
Screening in medical care (Nuffield Provincial Hospitals Trust 1968) 14, 15–16
Seebohm, Frederick 122, 133
self help groups 273, 284, 287–8
sex differences
aspirin in myocardial infarction 115
asthma prevalence 79
life expectancy 174–5
optimal alcohol consumption 64–5
sexism 128–9
Seys-Prosser, Diana 31
shared experience 51
Sickness in Salonica: my first, worst and most successful clinical trial (Cochrane 1984) 109
side effects, treatment 205
limiting risk 188–9
publication and 256
smoking
"fair innings" approach 175
in pregnancy 85–6, 275–6
social change, post-war 149–50
social class
differences in health 170, 175–6
equity weighting of QALYs and 177–80
trial participants 41, 190–1
social factors, response rates 43–4
social medicine 47–9
social policy 133, 143
social support
in pregnancy 128, 140, 275–6
women in labour 276–7
social work 22, 122–44
costs 150
randomised controlled trials 122–3
early 123–5
ethical objections 125, 130–3
informed consent 139–41
philosophical objections 125–30
preferred alternatives 129–30
technical objections 125, 136–42

research
  cautionary note 142–4
  dealing with bias 141–2
  isolating the "active ingredient" 139
  need for better controlled 133–6
  need for formal 94
  outcome measures 136–9
  rationale 93–4
  working within chaos 142
solidarity 44–6
sortilege 187
SORT (Standards of Reporting Trials) group 261
south Wales 31–55
spirits, alcoholic 66, 67–8
statistical analysis
  "intention to treat" basis 203, 212
  subgroups 203–5, 212, 228–9
statistical significance
  confirmatory bias 256–7
  publication of results and 251, 252–5
streptokinase 219
streptomycin 185–6, 187, 188
stroke
  alcohol consumption and 62, 63
  aspirin and 214–15, 216
  blood pressure lowering and 223–8
subgroup analyses 203–5, 212, 228–9
Sweetnam, Peter 110, 116
systematic errors *see* bias, systematic
systematic overviews (meta-analyses) 47–8, 198, 200, 211–13, 232
  in Cochrane Collaboration 233–5
  examples of important 216–18, 220–2
  lay perspectives 272, 273–4
  potential and limitations 235–40
  publication bias and 250, 251, 253–5
  quality of reporting 266–7
  reliability 212–13
  role of aspirin 114–16
  unpublished data in 257

tamoxifen 216–18
Thomas, Hugh F 21, 60
Thomas, Mary 31, 38
Thomas, Merlin 31
Toronto University 284
training, in systematic overview methods 234
treatments *see* interventions
tuberculosis
  British streptomycin trials 185–6, 187, 188
  Rhondda Fach studies 32–5, 76

UK Cochrane Centre 233, 283, 285–7
uncertainty
  professional 102
  randomisation and 186–7, 207–11
United States 4–6, 15–16
unpublished studies, data on 257
urban areas, asthma prevalence 80

validity, internal and external 259
vascular disease
  alcohol consumption and 61–3
  aspirin and 214–16
  blood pressure lowering and 223–8
Vessey, Martin 111
vitamin B12 5
volunteers 190, 191

warfarin 39, 40
wheezing disorders 84–5
White, Kerr 3, 15–16
Williams, Alan 16, 150, 153, 154–5, 156–8, 160, 162
Williams, Bill 15
Wilson, Max 11, 14
wine consumption 58–61
  mortality and 59–61, 69–70, 71
  v other alcoholic beverages 65–9

x rays, mass screening 32, 35

young adults, optimal alcohol intake 64–5
young offenders, detention of 133

Zimbabwe 80

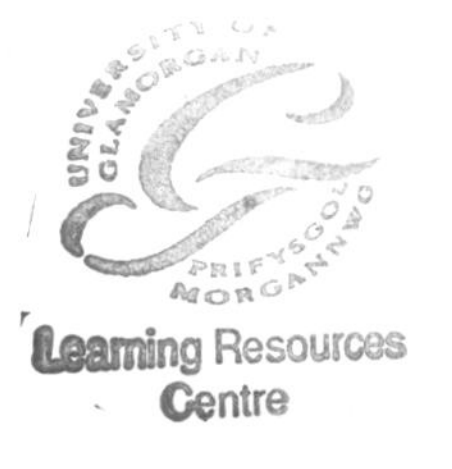